MISERY TO MIRTH

Misery to Mirth

*Recovery from Illness in
Early Modern England*

HANNAH NEWTON

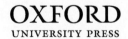
OXFORD
UNIVERSITY PRESS

OXFORD
UNIVERSITY PRESS

Great Clarendon Street, Oxford, OX2 6DP,
United Kingdom

Oxford University Press is a department of the University of Oxford.
It furthers the University's objective of excellence in research, scholarship,
and education by publishing worldwide. Oxford is a registered trade mark of
Oxford University Press in the UK and in certain other countries

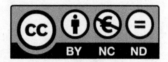
Published in the United States of America by Oxford University Press
198 Madison Avenue, New York, NY 10016, United States of America

British Library Cataloguing in Publication Data
Data available

Library of Congress Control Number: 2017959216

ISBN 978-0-19-877902-5

Printed and bound by
CPI Group (UK) Ltd, Croydon, CR0 4YY

Links to third party websites are provided by Oxford in good faith and
for information only. Oxford disclaims any responsibility for the materials
contained in any third party website referenced in this work.

For Dad

Acknowledgements

This book is based on research undertaken as a Wellcome Trust Medical Humanities Fellow at the University of Cambridge in 2011–14 (095760/Z/11/Z). My immense thanks to Wellcome, and to my sponsor at the History and Philosophy of Science Department in Cambridge, Dr Lauren Kassell, for making this possible. Throughout the Fellowship, I was very fortunate to benefit from the continued guidance of my wonderful PhD supervisor, Professor Alexandra Walsham, who happened to relocate from Exeter to Cambridge to take up a Professorship the preceding year—she couldn't escape me that easily! I would also like to express gratitude to other former PhD supervisors and examiners, Professors Sarah Toulalan and Jonathan Barry, and Dr Margaret Pelling, for their invaluable advice on chapters, articles, and funding applications throughout my time at Cambridge and beyond.

The road to recovery has been assisted enormously by Professor Peregrine Horden, who has read and commented on the whole book, and who helped me with my application for a Wellcome Trust University Award at the University of Reading: I cannot thank him enough. I would also like to show my appreciation to those academics who have been so kind to provide perceptive feedback on portions of my book, including Andrew Wear and John Henderson (Chapter 1), Sandra Cavallo and Tessa Storey (Chapter 2), Jan Frans van Dijkhuizen and Jonathan Reinarz (Chapter 3), Alec Ryrie and Alex Walsham (Chapter 4), Ralph Houlbrooke (Chapter 5), and Jeremy Burchardt (Chapter 6).

During the research, I consulted a number of experts on particular topics, to whom I owe further thanks—Sasha Handley, Alice Dolan, and Elizabeth Hunter (on sleep and bedclothes), Simon Schaffer, Andrew Cunningham, and Martin Edwards (Nature), Patrick Wallis (metaphors), Olivia Weisser, Elaine Leong, Jennifer Evans, Alun Withey, Leah Astbury, and Alanna Skuse (patients, gender, and recipes), Keith Thomas, Amy Erickson, Andy Burn, Charmian Mansell, and Brodie Waddell (work), Erin Sullivan, Colin Jones, and Thomas Dixon (emotions), Vivian Nutton (Galen), Jo Hedesan (Helmont), Simon Jackson (music), Mark Hailwood (alehouses), Fabiola van Dam (concoction), David Cressy (thanksgiving), Ken Albala and David Gentilcore (food), Maaike van der Lugt (neutrum), Mary Fissell (medical texts), Naomi Tadmor (family and friends), Paul Davies (paintings), Leona Archer (space and gender), and Stephen Pender and Joanna Bourke (pain and the senses). I apologize if I have missed anyone! Other friends and scholars to whom I am keen to express gratitude are Rohan Deb Roy, Dina Rezk, and Sian Pooley, whose fresh perspectives and listening ears have helped me to overcome numerous challenges. I would also like to thank all my fantastic new colleagues at the University of Reading, where I am now based, for supporting my Wellcome application, and for taking such interest in this project.

Most of the archival research for this book was carried out in the Cambridge libraries, British Library, and Wellcome Library, so I would like to thank the staff at these institutions for their assistance. My thanks go also to Dr Ollie Douglas at the Museum of English Rural Life, for alerting me to an extant seventeenth-century mattress in their collections, and to Dr Caroline Bowden, for conducting a fruitful search of the Cecil correspondence database on my behalf. Particular thanks are owed to Dr Anthony Buxton, who generously allowed me to reproduce drawings from his book, *Domestic Culture in Early Modern England* (Boydell and Brewer, 2015) of house layouts in Chapter 6, and to Dr Charles Shanahan, for creating a 'hierarchy of the senses' for Chapter 3. Part of Chapter 1 has been published as an article in *Social History of Medicine* (2015), and Chapter 2 is based on a contribution in Sandra Cavallo and Tessa Storey's edited volume, *Conserving Health in Early Modern Culture* (Manchester University Press, 2017). I am grateful to the referees who provided useful feedback on these pieces, and to the editors for permitting me to include the material in this book. I would also like to express my heartfelt thanks to the Readers commissioned by Oxford University Press for their constructive suggestions and comments on my book proposal and draft manuscript, and to Stephanie Ireland, Cathryn Steele, and Vijaya Manimaran for guiding me through the publication process so smoothly and pleasantly.

It seems apt that the writing up of this happy history has coincided with what has been perhaps the happiest year of my life: I have married the loveliest man, Dáire Shanahan. I would like to thank Dáire, and his family—Rose, Charlie, Hilary, Aoife, and De—for making me feel so at home in the Shan Clan! Finally, I send a huge thank you to my own dear family, Mum and Dad, Granny, Kathryn and John, Lydie and Alex, and little Penny, for being a constant source of love, encouragement, and fun. A special thanks is owed to Mum, who has read every word of this book, and has shared in all my highs and lows ever since (and indeed, long before!) the project began.

Contents

List of Figures

List of Abbreviations

BL	British Library, London
Bod	Bodleian Library, Oxford
Cowper, *Diary*	Sarah Cowper, 'Daily Diary', 7 vols., 1700–15 (MSS D/EP/F29-35, Hertfordshire Archives and Local Studies), scanned onto microfilm in Amanda Vickery (ed.), *Women's Languages and Experiences, 1500–1940: Women's Diaries and Related Sources: Part 1, Sources from the Bedfordshire and Hertfordshire Record Office* (Marlborough, 1996), reels 5–7
DBI	*Dictionary of Biblical Imagery*, ed. Leland Ryken, James Wilhoit, Tremper Longman III (Nottingham, 1998)
KJV	King James Version of the Bible
ODNB	Oxford Dictionary of National Biography (www.oxforddnb.com)
OED	Oxford English Dictionary Online (www.oed.com)
POB	Proceedings of the Old Bailey (www.oldbaileyonline.org)
RCP	Royal College of Physicians Library, London
SHC	Somerset Heritage Centre, Taunton
SHM	*Social History of Medicine*
WL	Wellcome Library, London

All the quotations from contemporary manuscript and printed works retain original punctuation, capitalization, italics, and spelling. The use of i, j, u, and v, however, have been modernized, and the archaic letter 'thorn' has been transcribed as 'th'. Standard abbreviations and contractions have been silently expanded, and long titles have been curtailed. In the bibliography and footnotes, the place of publication is London, unless otherwise stated.

Introduction

The history of early modern medicine often makes for depressing reading. It implies that people fell ill, took ineffective remedies, and died. A few snippets from Roy and Dorothy Porter's classic study, *In Sickness and in Health*, encapsulate this pessimism: they speak of the 'universal sickness, suffering, and woe' of the early modern past, a time in which 'people died like flies' from infections against which 'pre-modern medicine had few effective weapons'.[1] Even those who were lucky enough to survive illness could expect nothing more than a life 'repeatedly blighted' by chronic illness and disability.[2] Indeed, the recovery of full health is sometimes said to have been so rare, that it barely existed as a concept at this time, or at least not in any form that would be recognized today. Nancy Siraisi, for instance, has stated that 'cure was not necessarily conceived of as a ... recognizable return to total health': early modern people held 'a more vague and diffused concept of recovery'.[3] For these reasons, numerous histories have been written on disease and death, but none have been devoted to the subjects of recovery and survival. Such a focus may also reflect a more general penchant for sad topics, a tendency visible in many historiographical fields and chronologies, especially the history of emotion, an area largely dominated by the study of negative feelings.[4] Psychologists would not be surprised—they believe humankind suffers from a 'negativity bias', or 'positive-negative asymmetry

---

[1] Roy Porter and Dorothy Porter, *In Sickness and in Health: The British Experience 1650–1850* (1988), 1–3. See also Lucinda Beier, *Sufferers and Healers: The Experience of Illness in Seventeenth-Century England* (1987), 133. This impression has been accentuated by new work on accidental death, which implies that even in the absence of illness, one might succumb to innumerable other causes of death; for example, Craig Spence, *Accidents and Violent Death in Early Modern London, 1650–1750* (Woodbridge, 2016).

[2] Mary Lindemann, *Medicine and Society in Early Modern Europe* (Cambridge, 2010, first publ. 1999), 11. See also Keith Thomas, *Religion and the Decline of Magic: Studies in Popular Beliefs in Sixteenth- and Seventeenth-Century England* (1991, first publ. 1971), 6.

[3] Nancy Siraisi, *Medieval and Early Renaissance Medicine: An Introduction to Knowledge and Practice* (Chicago, 1990), 136–7. See also note 31 in this chapter.

[4] Here is a small selection of high quality studies: Jennifer Vaught (ed.), *Grief and Gender, 700–1700* (Basingstoke, 2003); Karl Enenkel and Anita Traninger (eds.), *Discourses of Anger in the Early Modern Period* (Leiden, 2015); Joanna Bourke, *Fear: A Cultural History* (2006); Erin Sullivan, *Beyond Melancholy: Sadness and Selfhood in Renaissance England* (Oxford, 2016). On guilt and despair, see Chapter 4, notes 11, 12. Even histories of love often take a negative angle—for instance, Aurelie Griffin, 'Love Melancholy and the Senses in Mary Wroth's Works', in Simon Smith, Jackie Watson, and Amy Kenny (eds.), *The Senses in Early Modern England, 1558–1660* (Manchester, 2015), 148–64. Notable exceptions to this focus on negative emotions include the intellectual histories by Ruth Caston and Robert Kaster (eds.), *Hope, Joy and Affection in the Classical World* (Oxford, 2016); Darrin McMahon, *In Pursuit of Happiness: A History from the Greeks to the Present* (2006). Michael Braddick and Joanna Innes' new edited collection, *Suffering and Happiness in England 1550–1850* (Oxford, 2017), was published when *Misery to Mirth* was already under publication, and therefore, unfortunately, it has not been possible to evaluate its contribution to the history of positive emotions.

effect'.[5] This trend was noticed in the early modern period too: ''Tis strange that we should be more ready to mourn than to rejoyce; and that our Sorrows should be more...fluent than our joys', mused the London clergyman Timothy Rogers in 1691.[6]

Such a gloomy picture of the past does not adequately capture the diversity of human experiences, however. While preparing my first book, *The Sick Child in Early Modern England*, I found, scattered amidst the heartrending stories of suffering and death, joyful recoveries. One in particular stood out. In 1652, eleven-year-old Martha Hatfield from Yorkshire fell gravely ill of 'Spleen-winde', a disease characterized by 'violent vomiting' and 'rigid convulsions'. For nine months, her parents and other relations were 'continually under sadnesse, and their sleep broken'; they longed for God to 'raise her up...to health', and 'ease...her pain, [so] that [their] eares...might not be filled with such dolefull cries, nor their hearts with those fears and amazements'. At nine o'clock one December evening, Martha suddenly felt strength returning to her limbs. She told her father, 'It trickled down, and came into [my] thighs, knees, and ancles, like warm water'. Seeing her mother by her bedside, she 'rejoyced...with laughing...and clasping her armes about her neck' in an embrace. The next morning, Martha 'took some food without spilling', and told her parents she'd had 'a very good night', not waking until 'seven a clock'. In the afternoon, she 'played with some...toys...which Neighbours had brought her in a...Basket', and towards the evening, her older sister Hannah, who had been 'very tender of her' during her illness, 'took her up, and set her upon her feet, and she stood by herself without holding, which she had not done for three quarters of a year'. Over the following weeks, Martha 'encreased in strength' beyond 'all expectation', and finally announced to her family, 'me is pretty well, I praise God...I am neither sick, nor have any pain'. A day of thanksgiving was arranged to praise the Lord for 'such a glorious end to this affliction': one of the guests recalled that the sight of Martha 'com[ing] forth into the Hall to...welcome us...was wonderfull in our eyes, so that our hearts did rejoyce with a kind of trembling'.[7]

Martha's story was penned and published by her uncle, the Sheffield minister James Fisher, to celebrate and commemorate his niece's restoration to health (Figure 1). Although it is partly didactic in nature, designed to 'teach...all that hear of it to depend upon the Lord', the author portrays recovery in a way that would have made sense to many people at this time.[8] Getting better is depicted as a 'happie motion' from anguish to elation, a trajectory marked and measured by a number of key milestones, such as sleeping through the night, eating solid foods,

[5] Paul Rozin and Edward Royzman, 'Negativity Bias, Negativity Dominance, and Contagion', *Personality and Social Psychology Review*, 5 (2001), 296–320; G. Peeters and J. Czapiniski, 'Positive-Negative Asymmetry in Evaluations: The Distinction between Affective and Informational Negativity Effects', in W. Stroebe and M. Hewstone (eds.), *European Review of Social Psychology* (New York, 1990), 33–60.

[6] Timothy Rogers, *Practical discourses on sickness & recovery* (1691), 265.

[7] James Fisher, *The wise virgin, or, a wonderful narration of the various dispensations towards a childe of eleven years of age* (1653), 138–50.

[8] Ibid., 144.

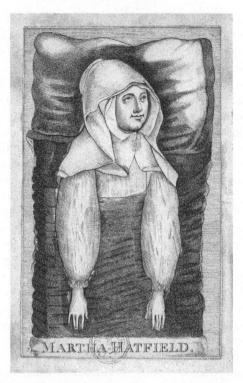

Figure 1. Martha Hatfield, from James Fisher, *The wise virgin* (1653); reproduced by kind permission of Cambridge University Library.

and standing unaided. The account inspired the subject of the present study not only by revealing that recovery *was* thought to be possible in early modern England, but by showing that descriptions of this outcome of illness have the potential to shine light into practically every corner of life in the past. In times of health, people were often too busy to remark on such things as breakfast routines, bodily sensation, and family relationships; in severe sickness, they were usually too unwell to be able to do so. But, the transformation from sickness to health propelled all the normally unnoticed facets of human existence to the forefront of people's minds and personal writings. As a result, this book is able to advance knowledge in a range of fields within cultural and social history, while acting as a bridge between medical history and other areas traditionally excluded from this arena. Lately, a number of scholarly centres for medical humanities have been restyled as centres for 'health humanities', a linguistic adjustment indicative of a growing desire to expand the remits of the research to encompass a much greater array of physical and mental states, including health itself.[9] It thus seems an opportune moment to produce a book that traces the patient's journey back to health. The ultimate goal

[9] A landmark article on this issue is Paul Crawford, Brian Brown, Victoria Tischler, and Charley Baker, 'Health Humanities: The Future of Medical Humanities?', *Mental Health Review Journal*, 15 (2010), 4–10.

of the study, however, is to rebalance and brighten our overall impression of early modern health, demonstrating that recovery did exist conceptually in this era, and that it was a widely documented experience.[10] In so doing, I seek to promote a 'positive turn' in the discipline of history at large.[11]

Misery to Mirth is about recovery from serious physical illness in England between the late sixteenth and early eighteenth centuries. It investigates medical perceptions and personal experiences of the return to health. How was recovery defined and explained? What physiological processes were involved? Was there a concept of convalescent care? How did patients and their families respond emotionally and spiritually to the escape from death, and to the abatement of physical suffering? What was it like returning to normal social and working life after a severe illness? Through these enquiries, a variety of specific historiographical contributions will be made. In medical history, the study fills a glaring gap in our knowledge of the patient's story, enabling us to complete the 'cycle of illness', which hitherto had ended mid-sickness or at the point of death.[12] Since recovery occupies a liminal space, 'floating betwixt' disease and health, and dying and living, an analysis of this concept necessarily sheds fresh light on perceptions and experiences of these other crucial states. The book also unearths a number of far less familiar medical concepts, such as the 'neutral body', 'analeptics', and the internal healing agent, 'Nature'. By exploring religious, as well as medical, interpretations of recovery, *Misery to Mirth* reveals the links between spiritual and bodily health in early modern culture, and adds to the growing literature on 'lived religion'.[13] A recurring theme is gender— medical theories and personal experiences of recovery were shaped by ideas about femininity and masculinity.[14] The study also yields insights into family bonds and friendships, and the connections between sensory stimuli and emotions, as it attempts to reconstruct loved ones' reactions to the sounds and sights of the patient's improving health.[15] Particular scrutiny is accorded to verbal and gestural manifestations of joy and praise, along with the relationships between individual passions; these discussions will demonstrate that emotions were conceptualized and classified rather differently in the early modern period to how they are understood today. Finally, the accounts of the return to normal spatial and working life illuminate such topics as house layout, attitudes to employment, and perceptions of the outdoors.

---

[10] For the historiographical exceptions—historians who *do* acknowledge recovery was possible— see notes 34–5 in this chapter.

[11] This term has been coined by Darrin McMahon in 'Finding Joy in the History of Emotions', in Susan Matt and Peter Stearns (eds.), *Doing Emotions History* (Urbana IL, 2014), 104–19.

[12] See the 'Historiography' section in this chapter for this.

[13] For a particularly rich study of the 'lived experience' of religion, see Alec Ryrie, *Being Protestant in Early Modern England* (Oxford, 2013). For the literature on medicine and religion, see Chapter 4, note 6.

[14] See note 17 in this chapter on the historiography of gender and medicine.

[15] For historiography of family and friendship, see pp. 18–19 in this chapter. For an introduction to the emotions–senses relationship, see Herman Roodenburg, 'The Senses', in Susan Broomhall (ed.), *Early Modern Emotions: An Introduction* (Abingdon, 2016), 42–5.

HISTORIOGRAPHY

A whistle-stop tour of the historiography of early modern medicine helps to situate this book within the landscape of existing literature. In the scholarship on disease and bodies, historians have examined contemporary understandings of illness causation, and the ways in which the sick body was conceptualized.[16] Particular attention has been paid to the category of gender, and the extent to which male and female bodies were distinguished in medical theory and practice.[17] In the last decade, scholars have become increasingly sensitive to other categories of bodily differentiation, such as age, disability, beauty, and weight.[18] There has also been an upsurge of work on 'the body in parts'—specific bodily organs, diseases, and fluids.[19] In these studies, however, neither theories of recovery, nor depictions of the convalescing body, feature.

Another area of historiography relevant to the present study concerns patients and their practitioners, a field spearheaded by Roy Porter in the 1980s.[20] Scholars

---

[16] The literature is vast, but key texts include Barbara Duden, *The Woman Beneath the Skin: A Doctor's Patients in Eighteenth-Century Germany*, trans. Thomas Dunlap (1991); Gail Kern Paster, *The Body Embarrassed: Drama and the Disciplines of Shame in Early Modern England* (Ithaca NY, 1993); Andrew Wear, *Knowledge and Practice in English Medicine, 1550–1680* (Cambridge, 2000); Lindemann, *Medicine and Society*; Olivia Weisser, 'Boils, Pushes and Wheals: Reading Bumps on the Body in Early Modern England', *SHM*, 22 (2009), 321–39; Michael Stolberg, *Experiencing Illness and the Sick Body in Early Modern Europe*, trans. Leonhard Unglaub and Logan Kennedy (Basingstoke, 2011, first publ. in German in 2003), Part II.

[17] For a summary of this literature, see Wendy Churchill, *Female Patients in Early Modern Britain: Gender, Diagnosis and Treatment* (Farnham, 2012), 2–4. The pioneering text on sex difference, now much criticized, is Thomas Laqueur, *Making Sex: Body and Gender from the Greeks to Freud* (1990).

[18] On elderly medicine, see Daniel Schäfer, *Old Age and Disease in Early Modern England*, trans. Patrick Baker (2011). For a survey of scholarship on children's medicine, see Hannah Newton, *The Sick Child in Early Modern England, 1580–1720* (Oxford, 2012), 10–13. On babies, see Leah Astbury, ' "Ordering the Infant": Caring for Newborns in Early Modern England', in Sandra Cavallo and Tessa Storey (eds.), *Conserving Health in Early Modern Culture* (Manchester, 2017), 80–103. On disability studies, see David Turner and Kevin Stagg (eds.), *Social Histories of Disability and Deformity* (2006); David Turner, *Disability in Eighteenth-Century England: Imagining Physiological Impairment* (Abingdon, 2012); Emily Cockayne, 'Experiences of the Deaf in Early Modern England', *Historical Journal*, 46 (2003), 493–510. On beauty/ugliness: Anu Korhonen, 'To See and To Be Seen: Beauty in the Early Modern London Street', *Journal of Early Modern History*, 12 (2008), 335–60; Naomi Baker, *Plain Ugly: The Unattractive Body in Early Modern Culture* (Manchester, 2010). On weight, see Lucia Dacome, 'Useless and Pernicious Matter: Corpulence in Eighteenth-Century England', in Christopher Forth and Anna Carden-Coyne (eds.), *Cultures of the Abdomen: Diet, Digestion, and Fat in the Modern World* (New York, 2006), 185–204. Thinness has mainly been addressed in the context of religious fasting.

[19] For the body parts approach, see David Hillman and Carla Mazzio (eds.), *The Body in Parts: Fantasies of Corporeality in Early Modern Europe* (1997). The following organs/parts and diseases have received most attention: feet, stomach, heart, skin, womb, and kidneys; venereal disease, mental illnesses, women's diseases, skin ailments, plague, fever, and cancer. For example, Alanna Skuse, *Constructions of Cancer in Early Modern England: Ravenous Natures* (Basingstoke, 2015); Jeremy Schmidt, *Melancholy and the Care of the Soul: Religion, Moral Philosophy and Madness in Early Modern England* (Aldershot, 2007); Philip Wilson, *Surgery, Skin and Syphilis: Daniel Turner's London* (Amsterdam, 1999). The most studied fluids are the humours, sweat, tears, blood, faeces, and breastmilk; for example, Helen King and Claus Zittel (eds.), *Blood, Sweat and Tears: The Changing Concepts of Physiology from Antiquity into Early Modern Europe* (Leiden, 2012).

[20] Roy Porter, 'The Patient's View: Doing Medical History from Below', *Theory and Society*, 14 (1985), 175–98; Roy Porter (ed.), *Patients and Practitioners: Lay Perceptions of Medicine in Pre-Industrial*

have examined the eclectic 'medical marketplace' of services accessed by the sick, the roles of women in healthcare, and the relationships between patients and doctors.[21] Important themes include the gradual commercialization and professionalization of medicine over time, the cultivation of networks of medical knowledge between laypeople, and the dissemination of 'medical secrets'.[22] Recently, scholars have paid greater attention to the work of nurses, together with the special treatment provided to different groups of patients, such as the elderly, disabled, children, surgical patients, pregnant women, and the healthy.[23] The care of convalescents as a cohort, however, has been overlooked.[24]

Over the last twenty years, the field of patient studies has been revitalized by the rise of the histories of pain and emotions. Scholars have uncovered unpleasant sensations that occurred 'beneath the skin', and analysed patients' physical and emotional experiences of pain, surgery, and disability.[25] This research has been complemented by studies of death and bereavement, a branch of literature that has

Society (1985). An earlier call for a history of patients is D. Guthrie, 'The Patient: A Neglected Factor in the History of Medicine', *Proceedings of the Royal Society of Medicine*, 37 (1945), 490–4.

[21] For a critique of the 'marketplace' concept, see Mark Jenner and Patrick Wallis (eds.), *Medicine and the Market in England and its Colonies, c.1450–c.1850* (Basingstoke, 2007). The doctor–patient relationship is a theme in much of the historiography in the 1980s–1990s; for example, Roy Porter and Dorothy Porter, *Patient's Progress: Doctors and Doctoring in Eighteenth-Century England* (1989). On women/lay healthcare, see Chapter 3, note 7.

[22] For example, Roy Porter (ed.), *The Popularization of Medicine, 1650–1850* (1992); Michael Stolberg, 'Medical Popularization and the Patient in the Eighteenth Century', in Willem De Blecourt and Cornelie Usborne (eds.), *Cultural Approaches to the History of Medicine: Mediating Medicine in Early Modern and Modern Europe* (Basingstoke, 2004), 89–107. On lay medical networks, see Elaine Leong and Sara Pennell, 'Recipe Collections and the Currency of Medical Knowledge', in Jenner and Wallis (eds.), *Medicine and the Market*, 133–52. On medical secrets, see Elaine Leong and Alisha Rankin (eds.), *Secrets and Knowledge in Medicine and Science 1500–1800* (Farnham, 2011).

[23] On nursing, see Margaret Pelling, *The Common Lot: Sickness, Medical Occupations, and the Urban Poor in Early Modern England* (Harlow, 1998), 179–202; Anne Stobart, *Household Medicine in Seventeenth-Century England* (2016), 20–2, 157–9. On surgical patients, see Seth Stein LeJacq, 'The Bounds of Domestic Healing: Medical Recipes, Storytelling and Surgery in Early Modern England', *SHM*, 26 (2013), 451–68; Katherine Walker, 'Pain and Surgery in England, *circa* 1620–1740', *Medical History*, 59 (2015), 255–74. On pregnant/lying-in women, see Linda Pollock, 'Embarking on a Rough Passage: The Experience of Pregnancy in Early Modern Society', in Valerie Fildes (ed.), *Women as Mothers in Pre-Industrial England* (1990), 39–67; Sharon Howard, 'Imagining the Pain and Peril of Seventeenth-Century Childbirth: Travail and Deliverance in the Making of an Early Modern World', *SHM*, 16 (2003), 367–82; Adrian Wilson, *Ritual and Conflict: The Social Relations of Childbirth in Early Modern England* (Farnham, 2013). For the care of the elderly, children, and disabled people, see note 18 in this chapter. On health preservation, see Sandra Cavallo and Tessa Storey, *Healthy Living in Late Renaissance Italy* (Oxford, 2013); Cavallo and Storey (eds.), *Conserving Health*.

[24] A few notable exceptions are given in Chapter 2, notes 9–11.

[25] Here is a little selection: Raymond Anselment, ' "The Wantt of Health": An Early Eighteenth-Century Self-Portrait of Sickness', *Literature of Medicine*, 15 (1996), 225–43; Lisa Silverman, *Tortured Subjects: Pain, Truth, and the Body in Early Modern France* (2001), ch. 5; Jan Frans van Dijkhuizen and Karl Enenkel (eds.), *The Sense of Suffering: Constructions of Physical Pain in Early Modern Culture*, Yearbook for Early Modern Studies, vol. 12 (Leiden, 2008), 19–38, 323–45, 469–95; Lisa Smith, ' "An Account of an Unaccountable Distemper": The Experience of Pain in Early Eighteenth-Century England and France', *Eighteenth-Century Studies*, 41 (2008), 459–80; Stolberg, *Experiencing Illness*; Newton, *The Sick Child*, ch. 6; Walker, 'Pain and Surgery in England'; Olivia Weisser, *Ill Composed: Sickness, Gender, and Belief in Early Modern England* (2015); on disability and chronic illness, see Turner, *Disability*, esp. ch. 5.

successfully debunked the older view that grief was rare in this period.[26] The outcome of such work is that we now know a considerable amount about what it was like to succumb to a painful or life-threatening disease or disability, or to suffer the loss of a loved one, in the early modern period. However, the question of how the sick and their families responded emotionally to relief from pain and illness, or to the escape from death, has received scant notice.

While recovery has rarely been addressed explicitly by historians, it has featured implicitly in several contexts. Firstly, when explaining the theory of disease and medical treatment, historians have alluded to the physiological processes through which recovery occurred. It is generally agreed that the cause of disease was the imbalance, obstruction, or corruption of the body's 'humours', the four special fluids from which living creatures were thought to be composed, and medicines 'worked' by removing this surplus or morbid matter.[27] By implication, recovery involved the rebalancing or unblocking of the humours, through the use of purging medicines. These insights are valuable, but they only convey part of the story—by focusing on the role of medical intervention, other crucial agents and mechanisms have been overlooked. This book slots in the missing pieces, drawing attention to the vital agency of 'Nature', and the forgotten processes of 'concoction' and 'retention'.[28]

Recovery has also been mentioned in discussions of patients' motives for seeking medical treatment, and their expectations surrounding the efficacy of remedies. Historians have often been pessimistic on these fronts, suggesting that 'people did not actually expect... medicines to cure them'.[29] Instead, the sick are said to have wished for an evacuation of humours, analgesia, or the partial restoration of bodily function.[30] David Gentilcore, for example, states that:

> The complete recovery of health, in the modern sense, [was] not necessarily the sick person's main desire or expectation. There is a gap between 'health' as defined by modern biomedicine and what people of other societies... are prepared to put up with, while considering themselves free from sickness.[31]

Misery to Mirth revises this view. It contends that while patients were certainly grateful for any improvement brought by medicines, they did not consider themselves *fully* recovered until their disease had been entirely removed, and strength

---

[26] See Chapter 5, note 4 for this historiography.

[27] Selected examples include Beier, *Sufferers and Healers*, 31; Wear, *Knowledge and Practice, passim*; Lindemann, *Medicine and Society*, 17–18; Michael Schoenfeldt, *Bodies and Selves in Early Modern England: Physiology and Inwardness in Spenser, Shakespeare, Herbert, and Milton* (Cambridge, 1999), 16; Alisha Rankin, 'Duchess, Heal Thyself: Elisabeth of Rochlitz and the Patient's Perspective in Early Modern Germany', *Bulletin of the History of Medicine*, 82 (2008), 109–44, at 130, 133; Siraisi, *Medieval and Early Renaissance Medicine*, 117, 145. Michael Stolberg revises this model of causation, arguing that in most cases, it was more often the morbid quality of the humours, than their imbalance, that was blamed: *Experiencing Illness*, 25, 72, 94, 99, 114, 133; Michael Stolberg, *Uroscopy in Early Modern Europe* (Farnham, 2015), 51.

[28] 'Concoction' also referred to the digestion of food: see Chapter 1, note 88.

[29] Beier, *Sufferers and Healers*, 5.

[30] For instance, Duden, *The Woman Beneath the Skin*, 88, 91–4; Rankin, 'Duchess, Heal Thyself', 112, 135, 142; Silverman, *Tortured Subjects*, 148.

[31] David Gentilcore, *Healers and Healing in Early Modern Italy* (Manchester, 1998), 186, 196–7.

restored. In more tangible terms, this meant feeling better, and being able to resume normal life, unimpeded by bodily weaknesses or blemishes.[32] Doctors also distinguished between medicines that brought a partial and a complete recovery, as can be evinced from the use of the word 'palliate', which was defined in a medical dictionary from 1657 as, 'when a disease is not eradicated, but only mitigated or covered, whereby... the pain, or trouble... is somewhat eased'.[33]

Several scholars have addressed recovery more directly. James Riley's book, *Sickness, Recovery and Death* (1989), deploys an interdisciplinary, quantitative approach to show that 'risks posed by illness and injury [have] changed'. Whereas in early modern Europe, 'most sicknesses were resolved quickly' by either death or recovery, 'during the nineteenth century, protracted ill health began to take over'.[34] Riley is thus one of the few historians who have acknowledged explicitly that illness did not always result in death in early modern times.[35] However, his principal aim is to use past patterns of health to influence current and future policy-makers, rather than to find out how early modern people understood or experienced recovery.[36]

Another scholar who has discussed recovery explicitly is Gianna Pomata, in her important monograph, *Contracting a Cure: Patients, Healers, and the Law in Early Modern Bologna* (1994). The book charts the evolution and decline of the 'cure contract', an economic arrangement between the practitioner and patient, whereby the latter paid for medical services only when the treatment had been successful. Drawing on the records of Bologna's medical tribunal, Pomata proposes that 'In sharp contrast to modern medicine, illness and recovery were defined not by the physician but by the sick.'[37] Pomata's interest lies chiefly with power relations, rather than with perceptions or experiences of getting better. She does, however, offer some insights into how recovery was conceptualized, stating that it meant 'be[ing] able to do things just as one had done them before falling sick—slicing bread and eating, walking and talking normally'.[38] Building on Pomata's findings, *Misery to Mirth* shows that it was not just function that mattered, but feeling—to be recovered meant feeling better, an elusive term that will be interrogated in one of the chapters in this book.

A more recent study that resonates with this investigation is Olivia Weisser's masterful monograph, *Ill Composed: Sickness, Gender, and Belief in Early Modern*

---

[32] See, for instance, Caryl Joseph, *An exposition... upon the thirty second, the thirty third, and the thirty fourth chapters of the booke of Job* (1661), 416.

[33] *A physical dictionary, or an interpretation of such crabbed words... used in physick* (1657), image 80. See also Thomas Blount, *Glossographia, or, a dictionary* (1661), 231.

[34] James Riley, *Sickness, Recovery and Death: A History and Forecast of Ill Health* (Basingstoke, 1989), xi.

[35] Others who agree recovery was possible are Stolberg, *Experiencing Illness*, 22; Stobart, *Household Medicine*, 22–3; Weisser, *Ill Composed*, 37, 51, 122.

[36] See Margaret Pelling's book review in *Economic History Review*, 44 (1991), 566–7.

[37] Gianna Pomata, *Contracting a Cure: Patients, Healers, and the Law in Early Modern Bologna* (1998, first publ. 1994), 28. The word 'cure' also appears in the title of Elaine Leong and Alisha Rankin's Special Issue, *Testing Drugs and Trying Cures, Bulletin of the History of Medicine*, 91 (2017). This excellent volume highlights the role of testing in the development of drugs in pre-modern Europe. Its aim is not, however, to consider the meaning of 'cure' or recovery.

[38] Pomata, *Contracting a Cure*, 28.

England (2015). Although mainly concerned with the gendering of sickness narratives, Weisser mentions recovery when examining the perceived effects of joyful emotions on the body, and the occasions which led doctors to record patients' voices in their notebooks. She reveals, for example, that the happy news of a loved one's restored health was thought to cure a sick relative, a phenomenon also observed in this book.[39] Weisser helpfully identifies various differences between women and men's experiences of illness, some of which we will see are equally applicable to recovery, such as the tendency for heads of households to express relief when they were able to resume their economic roles as providers.

Finally, recovery has been discussed in the context of childbirth. David Cressy's book, *Birth, Marriage, and Death* (1997), contains a section on the ritual of 'lying-in', the month-long period of convalescence recommended for women after labour, which ended with a thanksgiving service called 'churching'.[40] Taking a more medical perspective, Leah Astbury has explored the physical complaints of newly delivered mothers, and argued that these women only deemed themselves recovered when they were able to return to their normal tasks.[41] My book occasionally draws parallels between recovery from childbirth and sickness, and suggests that there may have been considerable overlap, especially in the care provided during convalescence. In short, recovery has rarely been examined in a sustained or direct manner, and when it has been mentioned, scholars have tended to imply that it did not mean the full return to health, an assumption this book repudiates.

SUMMARY OF ARGUMENTS

Misery to Mirth takes several perspectives. The first is medical or physiological, asking what recovery meant, and how it was thought to happen according to doctors and laypeople. As will be revealed below, recovery denoted the transition from disease to health, and it comprised two stages, the first of which was the removal of disease, the subject of Chapter 1.[42] This action was carried out by the combined efforts of three forces: God, Nature, and the medical practitioner. While scholars are familiar with the first and last of these agents, the vital role of Nature has been largely overlooked.[43] Like it does today, the word 'nature' held many meanings in the early modern period, but in the context of Galenic physiology, it denoted a divinely endowed power in the body that performed various essential tasks, including recovery. Personified as a hardworking housewife, Nature removed disease through

---

[39] Weisser, *Ill Composed*, 37, 99, 107–8. See also Olivia Weisser, 'Grieved and Disordered: Gender and Emotion in Early Modern Patient Narratives', *Journal of Medieval and Early Modern Studies*, 43 (2013), 247–73, at 260, 264.

[40] David Cressy, *Birth, Marriage, and Death: Ritual, Religion and the Life Cycle in Tudor and Stuart England* (Oxford, 1997), 82–6. See also Wilson, *Ritual and Conflict*, ch. 4.

[41] Leah Astbury, 'Being Well, Looking Ill: Childbirth and the Return to Health in Seventeenth-Century England', *SHM*, 30 (2017), 500–19.

[42] See p. 15 in this chapter for this definition of recovery.

[43] See the introduction to Chapter 1 for the historiography of nature.

processes that resembled cooking and cleaning—'concoction' and 'expulsion'. In theory, the three agents operated in a strict hierarchy: Nature was God's instrument, and the physician, Nature's servant; but in practice, the power balance was rather more complicated, with the doctor sometimes appearing more like Nature's partner, or even her commander. I suggest that these ambivalences reflect wider cultural attitudes to womankind: female Nature was kind and caring, but also weak and 'exorbitant', requiring rescue and restraint from the male physician. By placing Nature at the centre of early modern therapeutics, the book casts off the last vestiges of earlier generations of whiggish medical histories, which focused mainly on the achievements of doctors. The whole rationale behind medical treatment rested on the premise that 'Nature is the healer of the disease, the physician only the servant'—medicine was designed to promote what this agent was already attempting. This new understanding will help transform our attitudes to pre-modern medical practices, rendering more explicable those treatments which at first glance seem utterly ludicrous, such as giving a laxative to a patient who is weak from vomiting. Nature's role is also relevant to religious history, serving to clarify the relationship between natural and supernatural events: if we study what Nature *could* accomplish in the body, we will be in a better position to understand happenings that were classed as 'above' this agent, such as miracle cures.

Serious illness often left the body 'sicklish & shattered'; it was not until full strength and flesh had returned that the patient was pronounced back to health.[44] After the removal of disease, the second stage of recovery could take place: the restoration of strength, or 'convalescence', the subject of Chapter 2. What were the signs of growing strength, and how did this process occur? I argue that both the measures, and the mechanisms, for the restoration of strength were intimately connected to the 'six non-natural things', the various dietary and life-style factors that were believed to affect the body—excretion, sleep, food, passions, air, and exercise.[45] Patients' sleeping patterns, appetites for foods, and emotions, along with other inclinations and behaviours that related to the non-naturals, were used to track their progression on 'the road to health'. Doctors and the patient's family sought to regulate each non-natural to promote the body's restoration, and to guard against possible relapse. It is suggested that this regulation, together with the assiduous monitoring of the patient's growing strength, constituted a concept of convalescent care, or to use the contemporary term, 'analeptics'. Convalescence has rarely been addressed in the historiography of early modern medicine, perhaps because scholars have assumed that it was a later, Victorian invention.[46] As this study shows, however, the concept has much older origins: it was rooted in ancient Hippocratic–Galenic medical traditions.[47] Convalescents were placed in the 'neutral' category of human bodies, alongside other individuals who were deemed 'neither sick nor sound', such as

[44] Royal College of Physicians, London, ALS/F136 A-I, letter c (letter from John Freind to Henry Watkins concerning the illness of Mr Hill).
[45] See Chapter 2, note 3 for the historiography on the non-naturals.
[46] See Chapter 2, notes 9–11 for historiographical exceptions.
[47] See note 83 in this chapter on these traditions.

the elderly, newborn babies, and lying-in women. The interpretive value of this forgotten category is substantial: it brings us to a closer appreciation of how early modern people judged ambiguous states of health. The discussions also shed fresh light on the meaning of 'health', showing that it was not just the absence of disease, but the presence of strength.

As well as examining medical understandings of recovery, this book is concerned with the personal experiences of recovering patients. It investigates the physical, emotional, spiritual, and social dimensions of getting better. Four areas of experience have been identified for analysis, each of which forms the focus for a chapter: 'Feeling Better' (Chapter 3), about the abatement of bodily pain and suffering; 'Thanking God' (Chapter 4), on religious responses to the belief that it was God who had ordained recovery; 'Escaping Death' (Chapter 5), on reactions to the realization that the danger of death was over; and finally, 'Resuming Life' (Chapter 6), which examines attitudes to the return to normal life, society, and work. The main argument running through these chapters is that overwhelmingly, recovery was experienced as a transformation from misery to mirth.[48] 'Scarce any misery equal to *sicknesse*', declared the poet and Dean of St Paul's Cathedral, John Donne (1572–1631), when convalescing from 'purple fever' in 1623.[49] This misery included pain and sleeplessness, loneliness and confinement, boredom and monotony, anxiety about money, spiritual guilt, and the fear of death and damnation. The return of health reversed these feelings, bringing ease and rest, company and freedom, stimulation and variety, financial improvement, spiritual unburdening, and joy to be 'back in the land of the living'. Thus, at the heart of recovery was contrast, as the Oxfordshire clergyman Robert Harris (*c.*1581–1658) confirmed: 'this motion from sickenesse to health[,] from sadnesse to mirth, from paine to ease, from prison to libertie, from death to life, must needs be a happie motion, worthie [of] thankes [to God]'.[50] Ultimately, the clue to the experience of recovery lies in the word itself: the verb 'recover' derives from the Anglo-Norman and Middle French, *recuvrer*, which means to repossess.[51] Patients regained not just their physical faculties, but all the other things they loved about life of which they had been deprived during sickness, such as visiting friends, strolling in the garden, and undertaking engaging work. Recollecting his own recent illness, Harris mused:

Sicknesse put me out of possession of all, but with health all is come back againe; my stomach is come to mee, my sleepe, my flesh, my strength, my joy, my friends, my house, my wealth[:] all is returned.[52]

---

[48] The word 'misery' was one of the most common terms used in descriptions of illness, hence its appearance in the title of this volume. It incorporated both the emotional and physical dimensions of suffering, as confirmed by the physician James Hart, who stated, 'tormenting *griefe* with...paine, is called *aerumna*, or *miserie*': James Hart, *Klinike, or the diet of the diseased* (1633), 343. The word 'mirth' is used in the book's title because it captures multiple aspects of the experience of recovery, including bodily ease and pleasure, emotional and spiritual joy, and social jollity and celebration.

[49] John Donne, *Devotions upon emergent occasions: and severall steps in my sicknes* (1624), 177, 92.

[50] Robert Harris, *Hezekiahs recovery. Or, a sermon, shewing what use Hezekiah did, and all should make of their deliverance from sicknesse* (1626), 36–7.

[51] OED, 'recover' (verb), etymology.   [52] Harris, *Hezekiahs recovery*, 31.

Through this argument, the book revises current ideas about early modern 'sick roles', suggesting that withdrawal from normal life and work to the sickbed was more common than has often been supposed.[53] Since recovery from serious illness was usually experienced as the re-covery of daily activities and employments, disease necessarily involved an element of retirement.

A recurring theme in these four chapters is the way getting better is often described as a 'double delight' of patients' bodies and souls. Upon recovery, both parts of the human being were healed together, since the disappearance of bodily disease was a sign that God had forgiven spiritual sickness—sin. Depicted as 'loving playmates', the patient's body and soul rejoiced in one another's newfound ease and health, and felt relieved that they would no longer have to part in death. Such accounts enhance our understanding of how early modern people conceptualized their own beings—they saw themselves as two, intimately connected parts. This double healing commonly inspired the outpouring of delightful spiritual emotions called 'holy affections', cheerful responses to divine deliverance which help to counter the largely negative picture dominating the scholarship on the psychological culture of early modern Protestantism.[54] The expression of these holy feelings was part of the 'art of recovery', a set of religious duties incumbent on recovered patients explored in Chapter 4, akin to 'the art of death' with which historians are familiar; it included resisting sin, praising God, and joining together in collective thanksgiving. This forgotten art was the spiritual equivalent to analeptics, the branch of medicine discussed in Chapter 2: it was designed to strengthen the soul against sin, and prevent relapse into spiritual sickness. These findings confirm the close ties between the body and soul, bodily and spiritual health, and medicine and religion in early modern culture.

Besides investigating medical perceptions, and patients' experiences, of recovery, this book examines the reactions of relations and friends to their loved one's restored life and health. This is the third and final perspective adopted in the study. I argue that these individuals usually shared the experiences of patients, undergoing a transition from agony to ecstasy. 'My griefe[s] ... are vanquished and ... wholy swallowed up into joy', wrote Dr John Hildeyard when his dear friend Robert Paston escaped death in 1675.[55] This mirroring of experiences was known as 'fellow-feeling' in early modern England, a concept which has not attracted much attention from historians.[56] Contemporaries attributed this response to the passion of love, a 'true sign' of which was that 'friends rejoyce & grieve for the same things'.[57] Unlike the related terms of sympathy and compassion, fellow-feeling encompassed happy feelings as well as suffering, and it was physical as well as emotional. This meant that during illness, loved ones frequently claimed to *feel* something akin to the patient's bodily pains, and upon recovery they too experienced 'sweet ease'.

---

[53] See Chapter 6, notes 3–5 for this historiography.
[54] For this historiography, see Chapter 4, notes 11–13.
[55] Robert Paston, *The Whirlpool of Misadventures: Letters of Robert Paston, First Earl of Yarmouth 1663–1679*, ed. Jean Agnew, Norfolk Record Society, vol. 76 (2012), 167.
[56] For the exceptions, see Chapter 3, note 136.
[57] Nicholas Coeffeteau, *A table of humane passions*, trans. Edward Grimeston (1621), 103–5.

As well as revealing the depth of affection between loved ones, this argument challenges the established view, associated with Elaine Scarry, that pain is an 'unsharable experience'.[58] Taking a new, sensory approach, I argue that the main avenues to fellow-feeling were the ears and eyes: the patient's 'piercing cries' and 'deathly lookes' were replaced by the joyful sounds and sights of laughter and smiles. Such findings open up opportunities for engagement with debates in the burgeoning field of sensory history, such as the question of how the senses were ranked and linked in early modern culture.[59] Perhaps the most similar aspect of recovery for patients and their loved ones was the aforementioned spiritual 'art of recovery': family and friends regarded the deliverance as a mercy for themselves as well as the patient, and as a sign of God's forgiveness for their own sins. The structure of the book reflects these commonalities: rather than discussing patients and their relations in separate chapters, the two are integrated.

While this study presents the return to health in largely positive terms, it does acknowledge that there could be a distressing side. For some patients, getting better took a long time, with the body remaining frail and sore for weeks or months, and of course, not everyone made a full recovery. 'I am never quite at Ease', lamented the Hertfordshire gentlewoman Sarah Cowper (1644–1720) in 1712.[60] Nor did recovery always follow a linear motion: patients and their relatives fretted over the possibility of relapse, worrying that the slightest thing—even combing one's hair—could rekindle illness. This vulnerability extended to the soul: patients might return 'like pigs to mud' to former sins, with the double disaster of spiritual *and* bodily relapse. For those who disliked their work, or enjoyed solitude, sickness could be a welcome break, and the return to former employments and interactions, a source of vexation. The most explicitly negative reactions, however, came from those individuals who had, during their illness, longed for heaven. Survival for these people could be the source of disappointment rather than joy, especially if their lives were unhappy. These experiences reveal the power of religious doctrine, and the extent to which ideas about salvation shaped attitudes to both death and life. Occasionally, relatives and friends also expressed disgruntlement at the patient's recovery, though such reactions tended to be sparked by more secular concerns about delayed inheritance.

The timeframe of this study—the late 1500s to the early 1700s—has been depicted as one of dramatic upheaval. Developments were occurring in the economy; the period saw an extension of governments' powers, and religious and civil strife. Leisure activities and material culture diversified, and the middling groups of society expanded.[61] In a medical context, new theories of disease were springing

---

[58] See Chapter 3, note 10.   [59] See Chapter 3, notes 17–19 on this historiography.

[60] Cowper, *Diary*, vol. 2, 216. This woman was suffering from chronic pains in her feet. On Cowper, see Anne Kugler, *Errant Plagiary: The Life and Writing of Lady Sarah Cowper, 1644–1720* (Stanford CA, 2002).

[61] On material culture, see Mark Overton, Jane Whittle, Darron Dean, and Andrew Hann, *Production and Consumption in English Households, 1600–1750* (2004); on leisure/social spaces, see Sasha Handley, *Sleep in Early Modern England* (2016), ch. 5; Amanda Flather, *Gender and Space in Early Modern England* (Woodbridge, 2006), ch. 4.

up in opposition to the ancient traditions of Galenism,[62] the volume of imported drugs was expanding,[63] and ready-made, 'proprietary medicines' and 'specifics' were being introduced.[64] Some scholars purport that changes were also occurring in the realms of religion and philosophy: by the close of the seventeenth century, fervent spiritual emotion—'enthusiasm'—was apparently being discouraged,[65] belief in providence and Hell may have been fading,[66] and the body and soul were no longer seen as so closely connected.[67]

Choosing this time-period therefore provides opportunities for the reassessment of some of these changes. It is argued that, despite the wider developments, the fundamental ways in which recovery was perceived and experienced remained relatively static. In Chapter 1, we will see that while there was some disagreement over the precise physiological mechanisms through which disease was removed, doctors of diverse theoretical perspectives concurred on the tripartite agents of recovery. Likewise, in Chapter 2, it is argued that the convalescent's growing strength was measured and promoted in similar ways throughout the period, even down to the staple ingredients in convalescents' broths. The experience of recovery was also characterized by continuity: relief from physical suffering, the escape from death, and the resumption of normal life, provoked similar emotional and spiritual responses in patients and their loved ones across the period, though there may have been subtle changes in the activities and venues to which patients returned after illness. This was partly because the philosophical and religious concepts that held most significance during sickness and recovery—the perceived sympathy between body and soul, and the providential origin of health states—actually remained prominent throughout the years.[68] While 'enthusiasm' may have been disparaged in some contexts, it seems that recovery was regarded as a legitimate cause for hyperbolic religious rapture, even amongst Anglicans.

---

[62] For discussions of these various theories and transformations, see Roger French and Andrew Wear (eds.), *The Medical Revolution of the Seventeenth Century* (Cambridge, 1989); Charles Webster, *The Great Instauration: Science, Medicine and Reform 1626–1660* (Oxford, 2002, first publ. 1975).

[63] Patrick Wallis, 'Exotic Drugs and English Medicine: England's Drug Trade, c.1550–c.1800', *SHM*, 25 (2012), 1–27; Patrick Wallis and T. Pirohakul, 'Medical Revolutions? The Growth of Medicine in England, 1660–1800', *Journal of Social History*, 49 (2016), 510–31.

[64] Harold Cook, 'Markets and Cultures: Medical Specifics and the Reconfiguration of the Body in Early Modern Europe', *Transactions of the Royal Historical Society*, 21 (2011), 123–45; Louise Hill Curth, 'Medical Advertising in the Popular Press: Almanacs and the Growth of Proprietary Medicines', in Curth (ed.), *From Physick to Pharmacology: Five Hundred Years of British Drug Retailing* (Basingstoke, 2006), 29–48.

[65] See Chapter 4, note 17.

[66] On the apparent decline of belief in providence, see Chapter 4, note 16; on Hell, see Chapter 5, note 3.

[67] The French philosopher René Descartes (1596–1650) is usually pronounced the pioneer of the new 'dualist' view of the body and soul. For recent critiques of this notion, see Charis Charalampous, *Rethinking the Mind–Body Relationship in Early Modern Literature, Philosophy and Medicine* (Abingdon, 2016); Laurie Johnson, John Sutton, and Evelyn Tribble (eds.), *Embodied Cognition and Shakespeare's Theatre: The Early Modern Body-Mind* (Abingdon, 2014).

[68] On the continuities in Protestant beliefs into the early 1700s, see Andrew Cambers, *Godly Reading: Print, Manuscript and Puritanism in England, 1580–1720* (Cambridge, 2011); W. M. Jacob, *Lay People and Religion in the Early Eighteenth Century* (Cambridge, 1996); Jane Shaw, *Miracles in Enlightenment England* (Oxford, 2006).

DEFINITIONS AND PARAMETERS

Recovery was rarely defined explicitly in early modern England, for the simple reason that the meaning was assumed to be too obvious to need stating. Occasional definitions can be cited, however. An English compilation of works attributed to Galen declares that it is 'nothing else, but the translation of the *disease* into *health*'.[69] The sixteenth-century medical writer from Suffolk, Philip Barrough, stated in his best-selling medical text, *The methode of phisicke* (1583), that recovery means 'to bring the sicke member unto health'.[70] About a century later, the famous royal physician, Walter Harris (1647–1732), referred to the '*change* from *Sickness* to *Health*', a description which the aforementioned clergyman, Robert Harris, would have endorsed—he called it a 'motion from sicknesse to health'.[71] All these statements indicate that recovery denoted the transition from a state of illness to health.[72] As will be shown in Chapters 1 and 2, this transition comprised two stages, the removal of disease, followed by the restoration of strength, or convalescence. Although not always explicit in the primary sources, this two-stage understanding is obvious from the frequent references to the need to remove or 'carry off' disease, before building up the weak and lean body.[73]

The word 'recover' was one of numerous terms used to denote the transition from disease to health in early modern England, of which the most common were 'cure', 'heal', 'deliver', and 'mend'. In dictionaries as well as personal documents and medical treatises, these words were used interchangeably, which suggests that they were synonyms. A French–English dictionary from 1677, for instance, states that the word *guerir* means 'to cure, to heal, or recover to health', or 'to mend, or recover his health'.[74] The Essex clergyman Ralph Josselin (1617–83) asked God to 'give a perfect cure and healing', and 'recover me perfectly', of a sore navel in 1648; a few decades later, the merchant and astrologer Samuel Jeake (1652–99) longed for '*the healing of my eyesight*' and '*the recovery of my sight*'.[75] Doctors also deployed

[69] Galen, *Galen's method of physic*, trans. Peter English (1656), 195.

[70] Philip Barrough, *The methode of phisicke* (1583), 274; this text went through seven editions by 1652. The extract appears in a discussion of treating cancer.

[71] Walter Harris, *Pharmacologia anti-empirica, or, A rational discourse of remedies both chymical and Galenical* (1683), 275; Harris, *Hezekiahs recovery*, 32.

[72] These definitions invite further definitions—of 'illness' and 'health', which are given in Chapter 1.

[73] References to the removal of disease include Nicholas Abraham de La Framboisière, *The art of physick made plain & easie*, trans. John Phillips (1684; originally publ. in Latin, 1628), 91, 103; Brice Bauderon, *The expert physician: learnedly treating of all agues and feavers* (1657), 47; John Macollo, *XCIX canons, or rules learnedly describing an excellent method for practitioners in physic* (1659), 80–1; John Pechey, *A plain introduction to the art of physic* (1697), 106. On weakness after illness, and the need for strengthening, see Chapter 2, esp. pp. 68–74.

[74] Guy Miege, *A new dictionary French and English* (1677), image 160. This dictionary went through at least seven editions between 1677 and 1699, and the wording remained similar—the 1691 edition states, '*to be cured, or healed; to mend, or recover his health*' (image 342).

[75] Ralph Josselin, *The Diary of Ralph Josselin 1616–1683*, ed. Alan Macfarlane (Oxford, 1991), 142, 145; Samuel Jeake, *An Astrological Diary of the Seventeenth Century: Samuel Jeake of Rye*, ed. Michael Hunter (Oxford, 1988), 124, 116.

these words in this manner.[76] Such indiscriminate use of language may seem strange from today's viewpoint, since we now tend to invoke these words in slightly different contexts. For example, in modern English-speaking regions, the word 'heal' is associated predominantly with the re-joining of flesh or bones after a wound or break, or with emotional or spiritual therapy; it would rarely be used in the context of a bodily disease or disability.[77] Likewise, 'deliver' now carries connotations of direct divine intervention, but in the early modern period it was also used to denote recovery brought about by 'second causes', like medicines.[78] In modern parlance, 'cure' is generally used in reference to the successful treatment of dangerous conditions, unlike in the early modern period, where the word could be applied to recovery from any disease, however trivial, and included those cases where the patient got better without the use of medicine.[79] In this study, 'recover' has been privileged over the other terms, on the grounds that it is the most neutral, lacking the strong medical or religious connotations of the other words.

Misery to Mirth focuses on recovery from serious physical illness. It is hoped that this initial research will lead to comparative studies of healing from other conditions, such as childbirth, surgery, wounds, and mental illness.[80] By 'serious', I mean diseases that caused considerable bodily suffering, loss of function, or posed a threat to life. This category may seem somewhat amorphous, but in the early modern period the common features of illnesses were emphasized much more than they are today. This was partly due to the way disease was defined in Galenic medical theory: it denoted impairment in the performance of faculties, caused by the 'distemperature' or corruption of the body's humours, a definition applicable to all ailments.[81] The Church reinforced this unifying approach to disease: Christian consolation literature, texts designed to comfort the afflicted, usually deal with sickness in a single chapter, teaching that all illnesses are the fruit of sin, and have in common such things as being 'confin'd to thy Bed' and 'wholly entertain'd with the Extremity of thy pains'.[82] The reason that life-threatening diseases feature heavily in this study is that recovery

---

[76] For the interchangeable use of 'healed' and 'delivered', see Robert Bayfield, *Tes iatrikes kartos... adorned with above three hundred choice and rare observations* (1663), 172. For the interchangeable use of 'recovered' and 'cured', see John Symcotts, *A Seventeenth Century Doctor and his Patients: John Symcotts, 1592?–1662*, ed. F. N. L. Poynter and W. J. Bishop, Bedfordshire Historical Record Society, vol. 31 (Streatley, 1951), 53.

[77] A search for 'healing' on PubMed generates thousands of articles; the first fifty deal mainly with wounds, fractures, and surgery: <https://www.ncbi.nlm.nih.gov/pubmed/>. On Amazon books, 'healing' brings up 140,000+ items; the first two pages deal mostly with spiritual/emotional healing: <https://www.amazon.co.uk>. Both websites accessed 26/01/17.

[78] For instance, see Barrough, *The methode*, 38; Ysbrand van Diemerbroeck, *The anatomy of human bodies... To which is added... several practical observations*, trans. William Salmon (1694, first publ. in Utrecht in 1664), 51, 70; John Hall, *Select observations on English bodies*, trans. James Cooke (1679), 86, 88, 160.

[79] For example, Oliver Heywood records that his cold was 'cured': *The Rev. Oliver Heywood, B.A: His Autobiography, Diaries, Anecdote and Event Books*, ed. Horsfall Turner, 4 vols. (1883), vol. 3, 275. The word 'cure' also referred to any course of treatment in the early modern period.

[80] This has already started: see Astbury, 'Being Well' (childbirth); Wilson, *Surgery, Skin and Syphilis*, ch. 7 (surgery).

[81] See Chapter 1, p. 44, for a definition of disease.

[82] For example, Richard Allestree, *The art of patience and balm of Gilead* (1694, first publ. 1684), Section 2, 'In Time of Sickness'.

was very often experienced as a close shave with death. For this reason, a chapter is devoted to reactions to survival.

Most of the doctors and laypeople encountered in this book draw on the 'Hippocratic–Galenic' tradition, the medical theory developed by the ancient physicians Hippocrates (*c*.460–370 BC) and Galen (AD 129–199/217). According to this theory, the body was composed of the aforementioned 'four humours', and disease resulted when these substances became imbalanced.[83] Of course, such a reading is somewhat reductive, since there existed no single version of 'humoral' or 'Galenic' medicine; rather, there were many different 'humoral medicines'.[84] Even within the Hippocratic corpus itself, the meaning and number of humours are not consistent, nor are Hippocrates' humours the same as those described by Galen.[85] Nonetheless, the basic belief in humours persisted throughout the period, hence the decision to retain the use of these terms in this study.[86] In recognition of the fact that Galenism *did* face a degree of opposition, however, we shall also consider the views of some of its rivals, followers of the Flemish physician and chemist Jan Baptista van Helmont (1579–1644), who dismissed the humours as 'frivolous…fictions'.[87]

With the title, *Misery to Mirth*, it will come as no surprise that emotions feature heavily in this book. In Aristotelian thinking, the dominant philosophical tradition in early modern England, the emotions were known as the 'passions' and 'affections' of the soul.[88] Passions were defined as 'motions' (physical movements) of the middle part of the triangular soul, the 'animal' or 'sensitive soul', instigated for the preservation of the human.[89] 'Affections' were emotions of a higher moral status, emanating from the top part of the soul, the 'rational soul'; they were understood to be spiritual feelings, kindled by the presence of the Holy Spirit.[90] Of crucial importance in discussions of the passions and affections were the heart and the 'spirits', the 'subtle airy' substances through which the functions of the body and mind were performed.[91] Upon experiencing a passion or an affection, the heart drove the spirits either outwards or inwards, depending on the nature of the

[83] For definitions of 'doctor' and 'laypeople', see Newton, *The Sick Child*, 8–9. On the Hippocratic–Galenic medical tradition, see Owsei Temkin, *Galenism: Rise and Decline of a Medical Philosopher* (Ithaca NY, 1973); Luis Garcia-Ballester, *Galen and Galenism: Theory and Medical Practice from Antiquity to the European Renaissance* (Burlington VT, 2002).
[84] On this issue, see Peregrine Horden and Elisabeth Hsu (eds.), *The Body in Balance: Humoral Medicines in Practice* (New York, 2013).
[85] Helen King, 'Female Fluids in the Hippocratic Corpus', in ibid., 25–52, at 25–35.
[86] On the persistence of humoral ideas in the 1700s, and their co-existence with other theories, see Séverine Pilloud and Micheline Louis-Courvoisier, 'The Intimate Experience of the Body in the Eighteenth Century: Between Interiority and Exteriority', *Medical History*, 47 (2003), 451–72; Weisser, *Ill Composed*, 19–20.
[87] Jean Baptiste van Helmont, *Van Helmont's works containing his most excellent philosophy, physick, chirurgery, anatomy* (1664), 1. See Chapter 1, note 13 for historiography on Helmontianism.
[88] On the structure of the soul, see Thomas Dixon, *From Passions to Emotions: The Creation of a Secular Psychological Category* (Cambridge, 2003). Erin Sullivan has pointed out that the Aristotelian tripartite soul, though highly influential, did not go unchallenged: *Beyond Melancholy*, 71.
[89] Coeffeteau, *A table*, 2.
[90] See Hannah Newton, 'The Holy Affections', in Susan Broomhall (ed.), *Early Modern Emotions* (2016), 67–70.
[91] On the spirits, see Chapter 1, p. 38.

particular feeling; it was these sudden movements that explained emotional gestures like smiling, jumping for joy, or trembling with fear.[92] These ideas will help us to make sense of the emotional experiences of recovering patients and their loved ones.

The final set of definitions concern the vocabulary pertaining to family and friends. In early modern England, the word 'friend' encompassed family members as well as non-related individuals; likewise, 'cousin' referred to many different relatives besides the children of aunts and uncles.[93] 'Family' denoted all the members of a household, including non-related individuals, such as servants and lodgers. For the sake of clarity, these words are used here in the modern sense, unless they appear within a contemporary quotation. In this study, members of the 'nuclear family' predominate, but an attempt has also been made to include non-related individuals, like friends and work colleagues, servants, and wider kin such as aunts, uncles, and cousins. This decision has been informed by Amy Froide's reminder that at least a fifth of men and women never married, and the same proportion of married couples did not bear children, a warning she has issued in response to the tendency for social historians to privilege the nuclear family.[94]

The discussions of the reactions of family and friends to the patient's recovery contribute to the historiography of social and family networks. A pioneer in this field, Lawrence Stone, believed that the early modern period saw the erosion of ties between members of the extended family, and the gradual rise of the modern 'companionate nuclear family'.[95] This view was rejected in the 1980s on the basis that links between wider kin had long been weak in comparison to the much warmer bonds within the nuclear family.[96] Nowadays, 'neo-revisionists' contest both positions, arguing that all forms of social network—nuclear, extended, and non-related—were important throughout the era, though varying according to individual circumstances.[97] By showcasing the diversity and depth of relationships enjoyed by many people at this time, *Misery to Mirth* supports this latest

---

[92] This conception of the emotions has been labelled by Gail Kern Paster the 'hydraulic model', since the passions seem to surge around the body like liquids: *Humoring the Body: Emotions and the Shakespearean Stage* (Chicago, 2004), 17; Ulinka Rublack, 'Fluxes: The Early Modern Body and the Emotions', *History Workshop Journal*, 53 (2002), 1–16.

[93] On the language of family/friendship, see Naomi Tadmor, *Family and Friends in Eighteenth-Century England: Household, Kinship, and Patronage* (Cambridge, 2001).

[94] Amy Froide, *Never Married: Singlewomen in Early Modern England* (Oxford, 2005), 2. See also Helen Berry and Elizabeth Foyster, 'Childless Men in Early Modern England', in Berry and Foyster (eds.), *The Family in Early Modern England* (Cambridge, 2007), 158–83. These figures are from Edward Wrigley and Roger Schofield, *The Population History of England, 1541–1871: A Reconstruction* (Cambridge, 1981), 255–65.

[95] Lawrence Stone, *The Family, Sex and Marriage in England 1500–1800* (1977); for the antecedents to Stone's thesis, see Naomi Tadmor, 'Early Modern English Kinship in the Long Run: Reflections on Continuity and Change', *Continuity and Change*, 25 (2010), 15–48.

[96] Many could be cited; here is a selection: Keith Wrightson, *English Society, 1580–1680* (1982); Linda Pollock, *Forgotten Children: Parent–Child Relations from 1500 to 1900* (Cambridge, 1983); Ralph Houlbrooke, *The English Family 1450–1700* (1984).

[97] The term 'neo-revisionist' was coined by Tadmor in 'Early Modern English Kinship'. She provides a summary of the multiple contexts within which scholars have examined relationships between wider kin and friends on pp. 16–20. Further examples are given in Berry and Foyster (eds.), *The Family*, 1–17.

interpretation, though adding the important caveat that there seems to have been a hierarchy of affection, with the most acute emotions being professed by spouses, parents, and children.

SOURCES

This study draws on a diverse array of sources, since it seeks to uncover a range of perspectives. To access physiological understandings of recovery, vernacular medical texts have been analysed, a heterogeneous body of literature that enjoyed an 'extraordinary flowering' in the 1600s.[98] Various genres are deployed, including 'methods of physic', treatises that outline the fundamental principles of medicine, together with texts on the diseases 'from the head to the foot', multivolume tomes which often contain a chapter on how to deal with 'great weakness after sickness'.[99] Medical books devoted to specific illnesses or treatments provide more detailed information about physiological processes, from which it has been possible to piece together what was thought to be happening inside the body during recovery. Other types of medical book used here are dictionaries and collections of aphorisms, lists of definitions and pithy sayings, some of which relate specifically to the agents and processes of recovery.[100] Rather more discursive in style are texts about Nature, a miscellaneous array of philosophical and medical writings that describe explicitly the role of this agent in recovery. Examples include *The secret miracles of nature*, by the Dutch physician Levinus Lemnius (1505–68), and a critical exposition of mainstream views of Nature by the natural philosopher and chemist Robert Boyle (1627–91).[101] Finally, I have drawn on 'medical regimens', guides for healthy living that originate in the 'dietetic doctrine' of the Hippocratic corpus; these texts are usually structured loosely around the six non-naturals, and contain tips on how to manage the patient's life-style after illness.[102]

The authors of the above texts were as varied as the genres themselves. Some were English physicians, alive in the timeframe of the investigation, but others were doctors from Europe or the Middle East, whose works had been translated or edited many years after their deaths. For example, the aforementioned text by Lemnius was first published in Latin in Antwerp in 1559; the English edition used

---

[98] Mary Fissell, 'The Marketplace of Print', in Jenner and Wallis (eds.), *Medicine and the Market*, 108–52, at 113. See also Irma Taavitsainen and Päivi Pahta (eds.), *Medical Writing in Early Modern English* (Cambridge, 2011), 9–25.

[99] For example, John Pechey's text, *The store-house of physical practice* (1695), describes treatments for 'Weakness' caused by 'great Diseases': 187.

[100] The genre of aphorisms owes much to the Hippocratic aphorisms; I will be using the following edition: *The aphorismes of Hippocrates*, trans. S.H. [possibly Stephen Hobbes] (1655).

[101] Levinus Lemnius, *The secret miracles of nature* (1658, first publ. 1559); Robert Boyle, *A free enquiry into the vulgarly receiv'd notion of nature* (1686).

[102] On regimens, see Pedro Gil Sotres, 'The Regimens of Health', in Mirko Grmek (ed.), *Western Medical Thought from Antiquity to the Middle Ages* (Cambridge MA, 1998), 291–318; for a summary of the scholarship of regimens, and a detailed discussion of the nature of these texts, see Cavallo and Storey, *Healthy Living*, ch. 1.

in this study came out almost a century later.[103] In some cases, it is not clear whether the authors and translators were actually physicians: Mary Fissell has warned that professional titles were adopted regardless of official conferment of medical degree or licence.[104] At this time knowledge of physic was not monopolized by university-educated doctors; literate laypeople could acquire expertise from reading medical texts, and some gentlemen went on to publish medical books themselves.[105] The question of authorship is further complicated by the tendency of writers to plagiarize one another, 'circulating not only ideas but also...whole paragraphs' from past and contemporary works.[106] In the light of these matters, medical texts should be regarded as 'patchworks of viewpoints', rather than as the creations of particular individuals.[107] The intended readership of these books is similarly varied. *Praxis medicinae, or, the physicians practice* (1632), by the German medic Walter Bruele, was 'published for the good, not onely of Physicians, Chirurgions, and Apothecaries, but very meete and profitable for all such which are solicitious of their health'.[108] The physical features of regimens are indicative of a broad readership, as Jennifer Richards has highlighted—they have a 'reader friendly' format, including chapter headings and alphabetical indexes, and there is evidence that readers actively engaged with these books.[109] Some of the texts, however, are more academic in style, and so cumbersome that it seems unlikely they would have been lugged beyond the libraries of universities and learned gentlemen.

The above medical texts have been supplemented by a number of doctors' casebooks and observations, documents which purport to describe the histories of 'real' patients.[110] The notebook of the eminent Stratford physician John Hall (1575–1635), for example, contains biographical information about 125 of his 178 clients.[111] These documents were either published as stand-alone pieces, or appended or incorporated into medical texts to illustrate particular treatments. For instance, the Norwich physician Robert Bayfield (b. 1629), '*adorned*' his treatise on the diseases of the head '*with above three hundred... observations*' for the benefit

---

[103] The title of the original edition is *Occulta naturae miracula* (hidden wonders of nature).

[104] Fissell, 'The Marketplace of Print', 120.

[105] For instance, the lawyer and humanist Sir Thomas Elyot (*c.*1490–1546) wrote *The castle of health* (1610, first publ. 1534). One of the first studies of the blurred boundary between lay and learned medicine is Doreen Nagy, *Popular Medicine in Seventeenth-Century England* (Bowling Green OH, 1988).

[106] Sarah Toulalan, ' "Age to Great, or to Little, Doeth Let Conception": Bodies, Sex and the Life Cycle, 1500–1750', in Sarah Toulalan and Kate Fisher (eds.), *The Routledge History of Sex and the Body 1500 to the Present* (Abingdon, 2013), 279–95, at 282.

[107] Jennifer Richards, 'Useful Books: Reading Vernacular Regimens in Early Modern England', *Journal of the History of Ideas*, 73 (2012), 247–71, at 258.

[108] Walter Bruele, *Praxis medicinae, or, the physicians practice* (1632).

[109] Richards, 'Useful Books', *passim*.

[110] On casebooks, see Lauren Kassell, 'Casebooks in Early Modern England', *Bulletin of the History of Medicine*, 88 (2014), 595–625. See her digital casebooks project: <http://www.magicandmedicine. hps.cam.ac.uk> (accessed 20/10/17).

[111] Joan Lane, *John Hall and his Patients: The Medical Practice of Shakespeare's Son-in-Law* (Stratford-upon-Avon, 1996), xxxi.

of 'young Students in Physick'.[112] Other casebooks were never published, and probably functioned as aide-mémoires, records of fees, or places for reflection.[113] For most historians, the resounding disadvantage of casebooks is the 'prevalence of happy endings': in an effort to enhance their professional reputations, physicians may have exaggerated successful treatments.[114] Fortunately, this is actually an advantage here, since the cases provide windows into how contemporaries explained the return to health, even if there was a degree of selection going on.[115]

The above sources reveal how doctors and medical authors understood recovery. To gain insights into the personal experiences of patients and their loved ones, a variety of 'egodocuments' have been examined, including diaries, autobiographies, meditations, and poems. These genres encompass a diverse array of literary forms, from travel accounts to conversion narratives, but what they have in common is a concern for health.[116] Sickness disrupted travel, for instance, as the surveyor Richard Norwood (1590–1675) found in the early 1600s, while journeying around Bermuda; he noted when he was able to resume his expedition during his convalescence.[117] Recovery was also spiritually important: it was believed to be ordained by God, and was often found to kick-start an individual's religious awakening.[118] The return to health was economically significant too—records of resuming work, and paying off apothecaries' bills, thus appear in diaries of a financial kind. Indeed, these last two purposes were linked, since wealth, as well as health, was interpreted providentially.[119] Poetry and meditations—underused sources in medical history—provide especially rich insights into the dual experiences of patients' bodies and souls, since a literary convention at this time was to structure verse as a 'dialogue betwixt the body and soul'.[120] Perhaps the most valuable of all these sources are those meditations dedicated entirely to the subjects of illness and recovery, such as John Donne's *Devotions upon emergent occasions: and*

[112] Robert Bayfield, *Tes iatrikes kartos…adorned with above three hundred choice and rare observations* (1663), to the reader.

[113] For example, BL, Sloane MS 153 (Casebook of Joseph Binns, 1633–63).

[114] Gianna Pomata, 'Sharing Cases: The Observations in Early Modern Medicine', *Early Science and Medicine*, 15 (2010), 193–236, at 210.

[115] Churchill, *Female Patients*, 7, 11–15, 22–4. For the evolution of casebooks, see Giana Pomata, '*Praxis Historialis*: The Uses of *Historia* in Early Modern Medicine', in Giana Pomata and Nancy Siraisi (eds.), *Historia: Empiricism and Erudition in Early Modern Europe* (Cambridge, 2005), 105–56.

[116] On the diverse genres, see Adam Smyth, *Autobiography in Early Modern England* (Cambridge, 2010), *passim*.

[117] Richard Norwood, *The Journal of Richard Norwood, Surveyor of Bermuda*, ed. Wesley Frank Craven and Walter Hayward (New York, 1945), 16, 18–19.

[118] On conversion narratives/spiritual autobiographies, see Bruce Hindmarsh, *The Evangelical Conversion Narrative: Spiritual Autobiography in Early Modern England* (Oxford, 2005); Kathleen Lynch, *Protestant Autobiography in the Seventeenth-Century Anglophone World* (Oxford, 2012).

[119] See Effie Botonaki, 'Seventeenth-Century Englishwomen's Spiritual Diaries: Self-Examination, Covenanting, and Account Keeping', *Sixteenth-Century Journal*, 30 (1999), 3–21.

[120] The value of poetry for this research has been highlighted by Raymond Anselment, *Realms of Apollo: Literature and Healing in Seventeenth-Century England* (1995); David Thorley, *Writing Illness and Identity in Seventeenth-Century Britain* (Basingstoke, 2016), 113–58.

severall steps in my sicknes (1624). Seldom written at the height of illness, these texts came into being during recovery, when the patient was able to put pen to paper.[121]

Other types of personal document deployed in this book are domestic letters, a literary genre on the rise in early modern England.[122] Two varieties of correspondence prove especially useful: firstly, patients' handwritten announcements of their recoveries. The clergyman Philip Henry (1631–96) wrote to a friend, 'two or three dayes [I have been] a Prisoner to my Bed under Distempers, & this is the First-fruit of my Recovery, the first time I sett Pen to Paper to write a letter' (Figure 2).[123] The act of writing a letter was a milestone on the road to health, since it signified the patient was well enough to sit up and hold a pen. The second epistolary form used in this study are letters of congratulations and advice, sent by relations, friends, and colleagues to the convalescent. The landowner and politician William Fitzwilliam (1643–1719) wrote to his steward Francis Guybon in 1703 to say, 'I…am glad to find you daily abroad…[but] You must take some gentle purgeing… to carry of[f] the [remnant] humour'.[124]

Sources that provide more detailed information about the family's involvement in convalescent care are domestic recipe books, manuscript compilations of instructions for the making of a multifarious array of household items, including medicines and foods for patients after illness.[125] For example, the Corylon family's 'Booke of divers medecines', dated 1606, describes a 'China Brothe' to 'restore your Losse of Substance and Strengthe'.[126] While these texts do not, as Wendy Wall has cautioned, constitute 'snapshots of what people daily concocted in their homes', the fact that the pages were annotated and marked with 'greasy stains' indicates that they were 'actively used in kitchens'.[127] These manuscript sources have been supplemented by a small selection of material objects, such as a posset pot and armchair, which afford more tangible clues into the embodied experiences of convalescents.[128] These items may not, as historians have warned, have been as 'everyday' as they appear, since their very survival may 'be virtue of their aesthetic or financial value', but we can suppose that certain pieces made it to the present

---

[121] Conventional wisdom taught that 'A Poet in adversity can hardly make Verses': N.R., *Proverbs English, French, Dutch, Italian, and Spanish* (1659), 1.

[122] James Daybell, *The Material Letter in Early Modern England: Manuscript Letters and the Culture and Practices of Letter-Writing, 1512–1635* (Basingstoke, 2012), 10.

[123] BL, Additional MS 42849, fol. 6r (Letters of the Henry family).

[124] William Fitzwilliam, *The Correspondence of Lord Fitzwilliam of Milton and Francis Guybon, His Steward 1697–1709*, ed. D. R. Hainsworth and Cherry Walker, Northampton Record Society, vol. 36 (1990), 126.

[125] For an overview of scholarship on recipes, see the introduction to Michelle DiMeo and Sara Pennell (eds.), *Reading and Writing Recipe Books, 1550–1800* (Manchester, 2013).

[126] WL, MS 213, fol. 108r (Mrs Corylon, 'A Booke of divers medecines', 1606).

[127] Wendy Wall, *Recipes for Thought: Knowledge and Taste in the Early Modern English Kitchen* (Philadelphia PA, 2016), 5. For up-to-date bibliographies and blogs on recipe use, see <http://recipes.hypotheses.org> (accessed 20/10/17).

[128] This approach was inspired by Handley's book, *Sleep*, 14–16. For an introduction to material objects as sources, see Karen Harvey (ed.), *History and Material Culture: A Student's Guide to Approaching Alternative Sources* (2009).

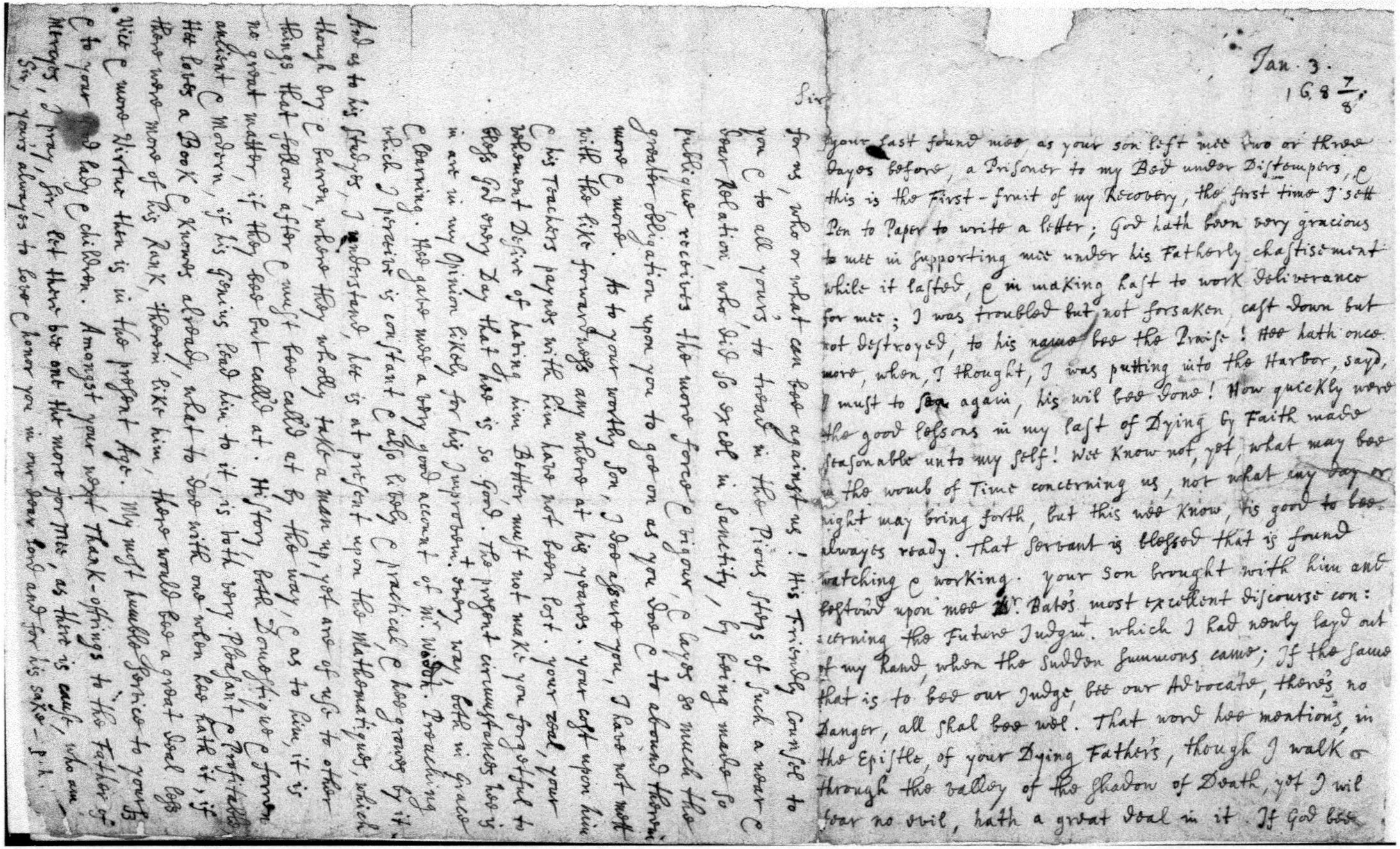

Sir,

your last Letter mett as your son left mee two or three dayes before, a Prisoner to my Bed under Distempers, ę this is the First-fruit of my Recovery, the first time I sett Pen to Paper to write a Letter; God hath been very gracious to mee in supporting mee under his Fatherly chastisemt while it lasted, ę in making hast to work Deliverance for mee; I was troubled but not forsaken, cast down but not Destroyed, to his name bee the prayse! Hee hath once more, when I thought I was putting into the Harbor, sayd, I must to Sea again, his will bee done! How quickly were the good Lessons in my Last of Dying by Faith made seasonable unto my self! wee know not, yet what may bee the womb of Time concerning us, not what any Day or night may bring forth, but this wee know, tis good to bee always ready, That Servant is blessed that is found watching ę working. Your son brought with him out bepping upon mee Dr. Baba's most excellent Discourse concerning the Future Judgm. which I Read newly layd out of my hand, when the Sudden summons came; If the same that is to bee our Judge bee our Advocate, theres no Danger, all shall bee well. That word his mentions in the Epistle of your Dying Fathers, though I walk through the valley of the Shadow of Death, yet I will fear no evil, hath a great seal in it. If God bless

for us, who or what can bee against us! His Friendly Counsel to you ę to all yours, to tread in the Pious steps of such a near ę dear Relation, who did so excel in Sanctity, by being made so publique receives the more force ę vigour, ę layes so much the greater obligation upon you to goe on as you doe ę to abound therein more ę more. As to your worthy Son, I doe assure you, I have not mett with the like forwardness any where at his yeares. your cost upon him ę his Teachers paynes with him have not been lost. your zeal, your vehement Desire of having him Better must not make you forgetful to bless God every Day that hee is so Good. The present circumstances hee is in are in my Opinion likely for his Improvemt. every way, both in Grace ę Learning. Hee gave mee a very good account of Mr. Woods. Preaching which I perceive is constant ę also lively ę practical, ę hee growes by it. And as to his studyes, I understand, hee is at present upon the Mathematiques, which though dry ę barren, where they wholly take a man up, yet are of use to other things that follow after ę must bee calld at by the way, ę as to him, it is no great matter, if they bee but calld at. History, both Domestique ę foreign antient ę modern, if his Genius lead him to it, is both very Pleasant ę Profitable. Hee loves a Book ę knowes already, what to doe with one when hee hath it, if there were more of his Rank, therein like him, there would bee a great deal less vice ę more virtue then is in the present Age. My most humble Service to yourself ę to your good lady ę children. Amongst your next Thank-offrings to the Father of Mercyes, I pray, Sir, let there bee one the more for Mee, as there is cause, who am Sir, yours always to love ę honor you in our dear Lord and for his sake — p. h.

Figure 2. Philip Henry's first letter after illness, 3 January 1688; © The British Library Board (Additional MS 42849, fol. 6r).

day by accident rather than design.[129] An example of such an item is a disposable mattress for the sick, found boarded up in a loft in Hampshire, which was apparently used for insulation purposes (see Figure 6 in Chapter 3).[130]

To glean more systematic insights into the spiritual side of recovery, published sermons and conduct books have been analysed, works that outstripped all other published forms in the seventeenth century.[131] A sub-genre of these texts was devoted specifically to recovery, termed here the 'art of recovery literature'. Numbering at least a dozen treatises, these texts set out the spiritual duties incumbent on patients and their relations upon deliverance from sickness. Classic examples include, *Hezekiahs recovery* (1626) by Robert Harris, and *Practical discourses on sickness & recovery* (1691) by the Presbyterian minister Timothy Rogers (1658–1728). Usually, these sermons would have been delivered at the thanksgiving service of a particular patient before being published, though Arnold Hunt has warned that printed versions were not necessarily identical to those preached.[132] It was also common for ministers to publish thanksgiving sermons after their own recoveries; this was the case for the Presbyterian Suffolk minister Thomas Steward (1668/9–1753), whose sermon *Sacrificium laudis* (1699) is 'a Testimony of *my* Thankfulness' to God, 'the *blessed Author*' of his recovery.[133] As didactic texts, we might expect these sources to tell us more about prescription than practice, but in fact, some provide rich insights into what it was like to get better. Rogers told his parishioners that, 'In these Discourses you will find a Relation of some part of my Affliction', which he hoped would enable them to experience vicariously the 'motion' from suffering to ease, so that they could share his new appreciation of the blessing of health.[134]

Finally, to gain a deeper understanding of the emotional responses of patients and their loved ones to recovery, a selection of philosophical treatises on the 'passions and affections' have been deployed.[135] These texts give definitions of particular emotions, and describe their 'signs and effects', crucial information when it comes to deciphering the meanings of contemporary emotion terminology. Two English translations that crop up frequently in this study are *A table of humane passions*, by the French philosopher and poet Nicholas Coeffeteau (1574–1623), and *The use of passions*, by another French thinker, Jean-François Senault (*c.*1601–72).[136] Despite

---

[129] Cavallo and Storey, *Healthy Living*, 62. This book discusses the problems of using these sources, at 61–3.

[130] My thanks to the curator at the Museum of English Rural Life in Reading, Dr Ollie Douglas, for this information.

[131] Ian Green, *Print and Protestantism in Early Modern England* (Oxford, 2000), 14–15.

[132] Arnold Hunt, *The Art of Hearing: English Preachers and their Audiences, 1590–1640* (Cambridge, 2010), ch. 3.

[133] Thomas Steward, *Sacrificium laudis, or a thank-offering* (1699), epistle dedicatory. Other examples include Nathaniel Hardy, *Two mites, or, a gratefull acknowledgement of God's singular goodnesse... occasioned by his... recovery of a desperate sickness* (1653), and Rogers, *Practical discourses*, which was '*lately preached in a congregation in London... after [Rogers'] recovery from a sickness*'.

[134] Rogers, *Practical discourses*, preface.

[135] See pp. 17–18 in this Introduction for definitions of these terms.

[136] Coeffeteau's treatise was published in French in 1620 under the title *Tableau des passions humaines*; the English translation appeared a year later; Senault's text was published in French as *De l'usage des passions* (1641), and was first put into English in 1649 by Henry Earl of Monmouth; the edition used here was published in 1671.

their French Catholic authorship, the ideas in these texts are consistent with those expressed by English Protestant writers, such as the Northampton puritan physician James Hart (d. 1639), whose medical regimen contains a section on the passions.[137]

It is important to ask how far the above sources reflect the perceptions and experiences of most people in society. Undoubtedly, the socio-economic elites are over-represented: to read, write, or own any of these texts required literacy and money.[138] Over 60 per cent of the letter-writers featured in this study, and more than a fifth of the diarists, were titled.[139] The majority of the male authors were university-educated, and roughly half were engaged in parliamentary or legal careers.[140] Of the female diarists and correspondents, just over 80 per cent were the wives or daughters of public officials.[141] Finance must have affected many aspects of recovery, such as the types of medicines and foods that could be afforded, and the physical environment and duration of convalescence. The experience of returning to employments like agricultural labour must have been very different to resuming the sort of work that could be done indoors. Nonetheless, if this study over-represents the middling and upper classes, it does manage to embrace a wide range of occupations within these groups.[142] Furthermore, some individuals *did* come from fairly humble backgrounds. Richard Norwood was apprenticed to a London fishmonger at the age of fifteen, and Roger Lowe (d. 1679) worked as a general shopkeeper, selling candles and scythes.[143] We also encounter a wigmaker, a woodturner, a ploughboy, and several servants.[144] In any case, even those from the upper echelons were vulnerable to financial trouble on occasions—this was a time of limited state welfare and considerable religious persecution.[145]

Nevertheless, there is still an undeniable skew towards the wealthier sectors, which must be corrected as far as possible. To this end, a selection of additional types of evidence has been analysed: firstly, records from the Proceedings of the Old Bailey, documents which refer incidentally to sickness and survival in the

[137] Hart, *Klinike*, 220–56. See also Humphrey Brooke, *Ugieine or A conservatory of health* (1650), 220–56.
[138] On the representativeness of diaries, see Elaine McKay, 'English Diarists: Gender, Geography and Occupation, 1500–1700', *History*, 90 (2005), 191–212. Literacy rates in males rose from 20% in 1558, to 45% in 1714, and 5% to 25% in females: David Cressy, *Literacy and the Social Order: Reading and Writing in Tudor and Stuart England* (Cambridge, 1980), 151–83.
[139] 'Diarists' includes autobiographers too; 'letter-writers' refers to the chief correspondent/recipient of each of the collections of correspondence.
[140] This figure combines male diarists and letter-writers, where the chief correspondent/recipient was male.
[141] Same as note 140, but in relation to women.
[142] This is shown in the discussions of resuming work in Chapter 6.
[143] Norwood, *The Journal*; Roger Lowe, *The Diary of Roger Lowe of Ashton-in-Makerfield, Lancashire, 1663–1674*, ed. William Sachse (1938).
[144] Edmund Harrold (wigmaker), Nehemiah Wallington (woodturner), Joseph Lister and Thomas Whythorne (servants), and John Cannon (ploughboy, who became a teacher)—see Primary Bibliography for references.
[145] On religious persecution see Alexandra Walsham, *Charitable Hatred: Tolerance and Intolerance in England, 1500–1700* (Manchester, 2009, first publ. 2006).

period after 1674.[146] Scholars have shown that although these documents convey 'the words of scribes, not the voices of the past', they do offer glimpses into the lives of people below the level of middling status.[147] Secondly, newspaper advertisements for remedies have been used, sources which often include patients' joyful testimony of the medicine's efficacy.[148] Regardless of whether these individuals were actually real, their statements must have been sufficiently believable to contemporaries, or else they would not have succeeded in persuading readers into making a purchase. Other useful sources are ballads, one-sheet rhyming tales set to well-known tunes, which were commonly chanted in public places, and accessible to people of all social levels, including the destitute.[149] While such documents do not necessarily constitute a 'mirror of the tapestry of habits, attitudes, and beliefs' of the poor, it is likely that they held some resonance with their consumers, otherwise they would not have been so popular.[150] Further sources of value are printed miracle accounts, documents which describe the supernatural recoveries of patients from a variety of social backgrounds. Although we tend to assume that Protestants believed 'the age of miracles has ceased', Alexandra Walsham and Jane Shaw have shown that in fact such events continued to be reported in Reformed England.[151] These accounts provide insights into poor people's emotional responses to recovery. Joseph Warden, a sailor, expressed 'alacrity and heartiness' when 'all his pains were driven out' by the 'Irish stoker' Valentine Greatrakes (1629–83) in 1666.[152] Such testimonies, like those in the medical advertisements, were not written by patients themselves, but it is likely that authors made any extraneous detail as believable as they could in order to convince any sceptics of the veracity of the miracle.[153] Finally, it will be possible to draw upon the work conducted by historians who have used poor law records in their investigations of the medical care provided to the poor.[154]

Another area of representativeness to address is religious background. The majority of individuals in this study were Protestant, the official religion at this

---

[146] A particularly rich study of Old Bailey materials, which attempts to 'give the poor a voice', is Tim Hitchcock and Robert Shoemaker, *London Lives: Poverty, Crime and the Making of a Modern City, 1690–1800* (Cambridge, 2015).

[147] Patricia Crawford, *Parents of Poor Children in England 1580–1800* (Oxford, 2010), 27.

[148] On medical advertisements and their conventions, see Turner, *Disability*, 53–4; Diana Wales, 'Equally Safe for Both Sexes: A Gender Analysis of Medical Advertisements in English Newspapers, 1690–1750', *Vesalius*, 11 (2005), 26–32.

[149] Classic studies on ballad production/readership are Margaret Spufford, *Small Books and Pleasant Histories: Popular Fiction and its Readership in Seventeenth-Century England* (1981); Tessa Watt, *Cheap Print and Popular Piety 1550–1640* (Cambridge, 1991), 52. For a more recent, interdisciplinary approach, see Patricia Fumerton and Anita Guerrinia (eds.), *Ballads and Broadsides in Britain, 1500–1800* (Farnham, 2010).

[150] Alexandra Walsham, *Providence in Early Modern England* (Oxford, 2003, first publ. 1999), 36–7.

[151] Alexandra Walsham, 'Miracles in Post-Reformation England', in Kate Cooper and Jeremy Gregory (eds.), *Signs, Wonders, Miracles: Representations of Divine Power in the Life of the Church*, Studies in Church History, vol. 41 (Woodbridge, 2005), 273–306; Shaw, *Miracles, passim*.

[152] Valentine Greatrakes, *A brief account of Mr. Valentine Greatraks* (1666), 70. On this healer, see Peter Elmer, *The Miraculous Conformist: Valentine Greatrakes, the Body Politic, and the Politics of Healing in Restoration Britain* (Oxford, 2013).

[153] On the links between medical advertisements and miracle accounts, see Turner, *Disability*, 53.

[154] For example, Pelling, *The Common Lot*; Weisser, *Ill Composed*, ch. 6.

time, and of these, most were devout: just over half the male diarists, and almost 90 per cent of the sermon and conduct book writers, were ministers. Of the lay authors, almost all identified themselves as members of the 'godly' in society. Only occasionally do Catholics feature, which reflects in part the fact that diary-writing was a predominantly Protestant tradition.[155] Within this pious Protestant population, however, there is a fairly wide range of affiliations: about half the diarists and conduct-book authors were conforming Anglicans, and the other half, nonconformists, including puritans and Presbyterians.[156] While some were on the extreme ends, exhibiting Laudian ceremonialism or radical puritanism, the majority seems to have clustered in the middle, displaying reluctant conformity or moderate nonconformity.[157] For example, the Presbyterian minister Henry Newcome (*c.*1627–95) was ejected from his parish after the 1662 Act of Uniformity, and yet he had deplored the execution of the king, and welcomed the Restoration.[158] Likewise, the judge and author Matthew Hale (1609–76) was a royalist, but he respected the puritan dislike of ceremonies, and acted as justice of the court of common pleas in 1654 for Oliver Cromwell, thus betraying sympathy for nonconformity.[159] Such ambiguities support Walsham's warning that to distinguish too rigidly between confessional groups is to 'do violence to the unstable and amorphous nature of religious affiliation at this time'.[160] We will see that within this devout population, people at both ends of the Protestant spectrum interpreted recovery providentially, and were aware of the spiritual duties connected to divine deliverance. This argument fits with Alec Ryrie's assertion that, 'the division between puritan and conformist Protestants...almost fades from view when examined through the lens of...lived experience'.[161]

Although the study covers the spectrum of Protestants, there still is a bias towards what can be called those who were 'in earnest in the practice of that religion'.[162] Did people who were less committed to their faith experience recovery in the same spiritualized manner? Most would have been familiar with the idea that God was the ultimate healer—such a message was espoused widely through compulsory Sabbath sermons, and popular ballads about Christ's healing miracles.[163] Christianity was 'in the social air which everyone alike breathed', so perhaps we can suppose that the

---

[155] Much has been said about the link between Protestantism and diary-writing—for instance, Tom Webster, 'Writing to Redundancy: Approaches to Spiritual Journals and Early Modern Spirituality', *Historical Journal*, 39 (1996), 33–56.

[156] Many studies discuss the meanings of these terms. For a recent example, see Ryrie, *Being Protestant*, 6–9. In my book, 'nonconformist' and 'puritan' are used interchangeably to denote those who disliked certain stipulations of the Church of England relating to church governance, and whose piety tended to be particularly conspicuous.

[157] 'Laudian ceremonialism' refers to a style of religion associated with Archbishop William Laud, which favoured free will over predestination, and emphasized liturgical ceremony and clerical hierarchy. See Peter Lake, 'The Laudian Style', in K. Fincham (ed.), *The Early Stuart Church, 1603–1642* (Basingstoke, 1993), 161–85.

[158] Henry Newcome, *The Autobiography of Henry Newcome*, ed. Richard Parkinson, Chetham Society, vol. 26 (Manchester, 1852); Henry Newcome, *The Diary of Rev. Henry Newcome from September 30, 1661, to September 29, 1663*, ed. Thomas Heywood, Chetham Society, vol. 18 (1849).

[159] ODNB (entry by Alan Cromartie, accessed 20/10/17).

[160] Walsham, *Charitable Hatred*, 20.   [161] Ryrie, *Being Protestant*, 6.

[162] Ibid., 6, 9.   [163] Shaw, *Miracles*, 8–10.

experiences of the devout individuals in this study would not have been vastly different from those of other, less religious people.[164] If sermons are anything to go by—documents notoriously pessimistic about the piety of the 'vulgar masses'—even those people with reputations for immorality regularly underwent spiritual awakenings during serious disease.[165] Of course, there must have been some individuals who were 'atheist', a term which in this period referred both to people who did not believe in God, and to those who did believe, but who rejected other tenets of orthodox Protestantism, such as divine providence; for these individuals, recovery may not have evoked so much spiritual reflection.[166]

Besides the issue of representativeness, the other major challenge presented by the task in hand is the difficulty of accessing the personal experiences of people from the past. It is a truism that language does not adequately capture sensory or emotional experience.[167] Early modern patients admitted that 'Great Griefs, as well as mighty Joys, exceed all our Words, and Bitterness is not to be described'.[168] Even when individuals did muster up appropriate words, there is the danger that they may have said what they wanted to feel, or thought they should feel, as opposed to what they were really feeling.[169] For example, patients may have expressed thanks to God because they knew that it was required, while secretly harbouring other emotions. This is especially likely in published didactic sources, like autobiographies and sermons, which were supposed to teach readers appropriate responses to life events like recovery. Manuscript diaries are not necessarily free from this tendency either: Andrew Cambers has demonstrated that these forms of writing were frequently circulated between friends, or bequeathed to children, as moral exemplars.[170] In fact, no personal document was entirely 'private', since most Christian writers were aware that God saw everything.

Adding to the difficulty of accessing authentic experience is the challenge of disentangling sincere feelings from conventional formulae. The composition of every type of source was governed by a set of rules, which shaped how people described their emotions. In the case of diaries and letters, for example, authors may have

---

[164] Peter Laslett, *The World We Have Lost* (1965), 60.

[165] For examples see Chapter 4, pp. 140, 141–2.

[166] On the various meanings of atheism, see Michael Hunter, 'The Problem of "Atheism" in Early Modern England', *Transactions of the Royal Historical Society*, 35 (1985), 135–57. We can infer that some people doubted God's existence from the fact that a genre of religious literature was devoted to trying to convince such individuals of this existence—see Kenneth Sheppard, *Anti-Atheism in Early Modern England 1580–1720* (Leiden, 2015).

[167] On the difficulty of describing sensory experience, see Martin Jay, 'In the Realm of the Senses: An Introduction', *American Historical Review*, 116 (2011), 307–15, at 309; on interior sensations, see Pilloud and Louis-Courvoisier, 'The Intimate Experience of the Body', 455; on expressing emotions/pain, see Graham Richards, 'Emotions into Words—or Words into Emotions?', in Penelope Gouk and Helen Hills (eds.), *Representing Emotions: New Connections in the Histories of Art, Music and Medicine* (Aldershot, 2005), 36–49, at 49.

[168] Rogers, *Practical discourses*, 156.

[169] The term 'emotional work' could be used here, which refers to 'the act of evoking or shaping, as well as suppressing, feeling': Arlie Russell Hochschild, 'Emotion Work, Feeling Rules, and Social Structure', *American Journal of Sociology*, 85 (1979), 551–75, at 561.

[170] Andrew Cambers, 'Reading, the Godly, and Self-Writing in England, c.1580–1720', *Journal of British Studies*, 46 (2007), 796–825.

mimicked the styles set out in manuals like John Beadle's *The journal or diary of a thankful Christian* (1656) or William Fulwood's *The enimie of idlenesse* (1568). A comparison of two letters, one a model and the other real, exemplifies this difficulty. Which is which? The answer is given in the footnotes!

1) It is not possible for... the heart of man... to thinke, (my singular and perfect frende) what sorrow...I had [when I heard]...that you were grevously sick,...[:] I even felte your sicknesse, through the...love that I beare unto you...But...I have now inestimable joy, for that it is...affirmed unto me...that you have wholly recovered your health.[171]

2) [I]t is scarce imaginable with what horrour the first newes of your lordship's disaster struck mee...But now, my lord, seeing the first newes so happily & beyond expectation... is blown over & succeeded by a bright sunshine[,]... I hope your lordship will give mee leave to change my stile as well as my countenance to rejoice... & congratulate you upon occasion of this bless't issue.[172]

Thus, it can be hard to tell whether the joy expressed upon a friend's recovery was partly an epistolary convention. It is also worth remembering that these sorts of letters necessarily provide a rose-tinted picture of relationships, since one of their functions was to convey affection. Those individuals who did not have many friends were obviously less likely to receive such letters.

In the light of the above obstacles, historians of emotion have largely concluded that it is not possible to uncover the 'true' feelings of people from the past. The medievalist Barbara Rosenwein, for instance, states that although we can 'understand how people articulated, understood, and represented how they felt', we cannot know how 'a certain individual feels in a certain situation'.[173] In other words, there is a gap between the way emotions are described and felt; this idea has become known as the 'expression–experience dyad'.[174] To distinguish between the two, leading scholars in the history of emotions have coined special terms, such as 'emotionology', 'emotional communities', and 'emotional regimes'.[175] The precise meanings of these terms differ, but broadly speaking they refer to the attitudes and rules that govern the expression of particular emotions in past societies, as opposed to the 'real' experiences of emotions. While these are useful conceptual tools, I am

---

[171] Model letter: William Fulwood, *The enimie of idlenesse teaching the maner and stile how to... compose... letters* (1568), 51–2.

[172] Real letter: Paston, *The Whirlpool*, 165–7.

[173] Barbara Rosenwein, 'Problems and Methods in the History of Emotions', *Passions in Context*, 1 (2010), 1–33, at 11. See also, Fay Bound Alberti (ed.), *Medicine, Emotion and Disease, 1700–1950* (Basingstoke, 2006), xvii.

[174] For a discussion on this issue, see Nicole Eustace, Eugenia Lean, Julie Livingston, Jan Plamper, William M. Reddy, and Barbara H. Rosenwein, 'AHR Conversation: The Historical Study of the Emotions', *American Historical Review*, 117 (2012), 1487–531.

[175] On 'emotionology', see Peter Stearns and Carol Stearns, 'Emotionology: Clarifying the History of Emotions and Emotional Standards', *American Historical Review*, 90 (1985), 813–36. On 'emotional communities', see Barbara Rosenwein, *Emotional Communities in the Early Middle Ages* (2006). On 'emotional regimes', see William M. Reddy, *The Navigation of Feeling: A Framework for the History of Emotions* (Cambridge, 2001). For an introduction to these concepts, see Broomhall (ed.), *Early Modern Emotions*, 3–10.

inclined to agree with Monique Scheer, who contends that the divide between the outward expression, and inner experience, of an emotion has been overstated. She believes that the manifestations of feelings—through words and gestures—are inseparable from the emotions themselves, since expressions influence what one actually feels.[176] The same could be said of pain and other bodily sensations.[177] On reflection, perhaps these worries are unnecessary: in early modern England, the devout in society were deeply wary of expressing 'empty words'.[178] The unique advantage of spiritual memoirs from this period is authors' apparent honesty about discrepancies between what were called 'inward' and 'outward' affections.[179] Given these considerations, I think it *is* possible to gain insights into past feelings. The chosen method is to find out how people at the time defined and conceptualized their emotions and sensations, and to analyse the language, metaphors, and gestures they used to express such feelings. Through this work, I hope the book will inject a dose of optimism not only into our perceptions of early modern health, but also into our level of confidence about our capacity as historians to uncover past experiences.

[176] Monique Scheer, 'Are Emotions a Kind of Practice (and is that What Makes them Have a History)? A Bourdieuian Approach to Understanding Emotion', *History and Theory*, 51 (2012), 193–220, at 195–6.

[177] Jenny Mayhew, 'Godly Beds of Pain: Pain in English Protestant Manuals (ca.1550–1650)', in van Dijkhuizen and Enenkel (eds.), *The Sense of Suffering*, 299–322, at 299.

[178] Ryrie, *Being Protestant*, 4, 15, 70.   [179] See Chapter 4, pp. 154–5, for examples.

PART I

MEDICAL UNDERSTANDINGS

1

'Nature Concocts and Expels': Defeating Disease

In November 1675, the Essex vicar Anthony Walker 'grew very ill' from fever and pleurisy. His wife, Elizabeth, reported: he 'groan'd all Night', with 'tremblings, and a fumbling in his Speech[,] [which] bad Symptoms gave me fear of the sudden approach of Death'. She sent for doctors from London, who proceeded to let her husband's blood twice, but to no avail. After the second bleeding, Anthony 'stretched out [his] left Arm', and demanded, 'I would [like to] Bleed again'. His justification was that, 'I...bled at [the] Nose, [and] Nature indicated thereby what must relieve'. The physicians, initially reluctant to repeat the operation, consented, and to their patient's great satisfaction, 'Blood sprang out so abundantly, that they drew at least ten Ounces'. His symptoms quickly receded, and the next morning Anthony concluded, 'my last...Bleeding...saved my Life, without which...I could not have escaped; blessed be God, who put that Resolution into my Mind, and heard her [his wife's] earnest Prayers'.[1]

This account is taken from the jointly authored memoirs of Anthony and Elizabeth Walker, published in 1694. It raises questions about how dangerous disease was overcome in early modern understandings. Anthony implies that three parties had played a role: God, Nature, and physicians. How did these agents fit together and interact? What did Anthony mean by 'Nature indicated thereby what must relieve'? Why was the evacuation of fluids like blood deemed beneficial, and was it always necessary? Recovery in this period denoted the transition from disease to health, and it comprised two stages: 'the away-taking of the *Disease*', followed by the restoration of strength, or convalescence.[2] This chapter is concerned with the first part, the removal of disease. It explores the agents and physiological processes through which this occurred, taking the viewpoints of doctors and laypeople.

There exists a rich historiography on early modern theories of disease and treatment. Scholars have shown that illness was attributed to the imbalance or corruption of the body's 'humours', the four special fluids from which living creatures were composed, and medicine was designed to expel or correct these

[1] Elizabeth Walker, *The vertuous wife*, ed. Anthony Walker (1694), 59. I would like to thank *Social History of Medicine* for allowing me to reproduce in this chapter material from an article, '"Nature Concocts & Expels": The Agents and Processes of Recovery from Disease in Early Modern England', *SHM*, 28 (2015), 465–86.
[2] Galen, *Galen's method of physic*, trans. Peter English (1656), 189. For a fuller definition of recovery, see the Introduction, p. 15.

humours.[3] Treatments included oral and topical remedies, surgical procedures, and the regulation of the 'non-naturals', the six environmental and dietary factors that were thought to affect the body.[4] Such insights are valuable, but they do not constitute a comprehensive picture of early modern explanations of recovery. By concentrating on medical intervention, other important agents and mechanisms have been overlooked, most notably, the vital force mentioned by Anthony Walker, Nature. While much has been written on the broader concept of the physical world—also known by this term—the bodily agent of Nature has received only minor attention, despite the fact that it was ubiquitous in accounts of recovery throughout the period.[5] The reason for this neglect may be that the word 'nature' is so common in today's parlance that when it does crop up in early modern texts, it is barely noticed. If we do pause to consider the meaning of this word, we usually assume it refers to the bigger cosmos, or to some spontaneous process happening in the body. As will become apparent, however, such a reading is mistaken: in early modern England, 'Nature' denoted a specific bodily agent which acted intelligently to restore health.[6] Personified as both a hardworking housewife and a warrior queen, this agent removed disease by processes that resembled cooking/cleaning and fighting. We will see that Nature's role has vital implications for the history of early modern medicine and physiology—it was the fundamental principle upon which medical treatment hinged, central to understandings of how the body worked. The discussions are also pertinent to gender history: an examination of the complex power dynamics between female Nature and the male physician will yield fresh insights into broader cultural attitudes to womankind.

Nature's role in recovery has not gone entirely unrecognized, however. In 1926, the German scholar Max Neuburger investigated the healing powers of this agent from ancient times to the present day, taking the perspective of learned physicians.[7] By focusing on a shorter period, this chapter seeks to provide a more nuanced account, which encompasses the opinions of laypeople as well as doctors. More recently, Gianna Pomata has investigated the concept of 'male menstruation',

---

[3] See the Introduction, notes 16, 27, and 30 for this historiography.
[4] For historiography on the non-naturals, see Chapter 2, note 3.
[5] The historiography on the wider concept of Nature is vast. Here are a few examples: R. G. Collingwood, *The Idea of Nature* (Oxford, 1945); Carolyn Merchant, *The Death of Nature: Women, Ecology, and the Scientific Revolution* (1980); J. Torrance (ed.), *The Concept of Nature* (Oxford, 1992); Lorraine Daston and Katherine Park, *Wonders of the Order of Nature, 1150–1750* (New York, 2001); Lorraine Daston and Giana Pomata (eds.), *The Faces of Nature in Enlightenment Europe* (Berlin, 2003); Lorraine Daston and Michael Stolleis (eds.), *Natural Law and Laws of Nature in Early Modern Europe: Jurisprudence, Theology, Moral, and Natural Philosophy* (Aldershot, 2008). See also the literature on learned medicine and its relationship to natural philosophy, such as Ian Maclean, *Logic, Signs, and Nature in the Renaissance: The Case of Learned Medicine* (Cambridge, 2002); P. J. Van der Eijk, *Medicine and Philosophy in Classical Antiquity: Doctors and Philosophers on Nature, Soul, Health, and Disease* (Cambridge, 2005); John Bono, *Word of God and the Languages of Man: Interpreting Nature in Early Modern Science and Medicine* (Madison WI, 1995).
[6] On the intelligence of the body, see the Introduction, note 67.
[7] Max Neuburger, *The Doctrine of the Healing Power of Nature Throughout the Course of Time*, trans. Linn J. Boyd (New York, 1932, first publ. in German in 1926).

a phenomenon interpreted as 'the healing endeavour of nature herself'.[8] Building on Pomata's findings, this chapter identifies a greater range of mechanisms through which Nature eradicated disease. The agency of Nature has also featured in case studies of particular physicians. Barbara Duden's analysis of the medical practice of the eighteenth-century German doctor Johann Storch discusses the 'efforts on the part of nature…to restore the body to good health'.[9] In an English context, Andrew Wear and Andrew Cunningham have evaluated the theories of the seventeenth-century physician Thomas Sydenham, in relation to Nature's role, suggesting that his emphasis on this agent was especially pronounced.[10] Here, the views of a greater assortment of individuals are explored, through which it will become clear that the belief in Nature's healing power was widespread. Finally, some historians refer to 'nature' occasionally, but do not interrogate the meaning of this term.[11]

The majority of the medical texts cited in this research draw on the Hippocratic–Galenic tradition, which means they subscribed to the humoral theory of disease and treatment.[12] Nevertheless, in recognition that this type of medicine did face a degree of opposition in the period, a section of the chapter is devoted to the beliefs of the Helmontians, followers of the Flemish physician and chemist Jan Baptista van Helmont (1579–1644).[13] The purpose of this case study is to demonstrate just how deeply ingrained was the role of Nature in the early modern imagination. Despite rejecting many of the fundamental tenets of Galenism, Helmontians retained the precept that 'Nature is the healer of disease'. The comparison also suggests some new reasons for why ultimately Helmontianism failed to break the hegemony of Galenism, despite its promise to provide pleasant and effective remedies. The first part of the chapter identifies the agents of recovery, and explores their interrelationships; the second section investigates the processes through which illness was overcome; and the final part is a case study of Helmontian theory.

[8] Gianna Pomata, 'Menstruating Men: Similarity and Difference of the Sexes in Early Modern Medicine', in Valeria Finucci and Kevin Brownlee (eds.), *Generation and Degeneration: Tropes of Reproduction in Literature and History from Antiquity through Early Modern Europe* (2001), 109–52, at 136–40.

[9] Barbara Duden, *The Woman Beneath the Skin: A Doctor's Patients in Eighteenth-Century Germany*, trans. Thomas Dunlap (1991), 170–8.

[10] Andrew Wear, *Knowledge and Practice in English Medicine, 1550–1680* (Cambridge, 2000), 339–44, 451–61; Andrew Cunningham, 'Thomas Sydenham: Epidemics, Experiment, and the "Good Old Cause"', in Roger French and Andrew Wear (eds.), *The Medical Revolution of the Seventeenth Century* (Cambridge, 1989), 164–90.

[11] For example, Roy Porter and Dorothy Porter, *In Sickness and in Health: The British Experience 1650–1850* (1988), 258–9; Michael Stolberg, *Experiencing Illness and the Sick Body in Early Modern Europe*, trans. Leonhard Unglaub and Logan Kennedy (Basingstoke, 2011, first publ. in German in 2003), 71, 94, 107, 118, 134, 150, 154; Michael Stolberg, *Uroscopy in Early Modern Europe* (Aldershot, 2015), 63.

[12] See the Introduction, note 83, on this tradition.

[13] On English Helmontians, see P. R. Rattansi, 'The Helmontian-Galenic Controversy in Restoration England', *Ambix*, 12 (1964), 1–23; Antonio Clericuzio, 'From van Helmont to Boyle: A Study of the Transmission of Helmontian Chemical and Medical Theories in Seventeenth-Century England', *British Journal for the History of Science*, 23 (1993), 303–34. On Helmont, see Walter Pagel, *Joan Baptista van Helmont: Reformer of Science and Medicine* (Cambridge, 1982); Jo Hedesan ' "Christian Philosophy": Medical Alchemy and Christian Thought in the Work of Jan Baptista van Helmont (1579–1644)' (unpublished PhD thesis, University of Exeter, 2012).

AGENTS

Disease was removed by three agents, which formed a clear hierarchy. The first was the Christian God: 'it is the will and power of God, which causeth all diseases to come upon us', preached the Shropshire minister Edward Lawrence (d. 1695), and when 'Christ bids diseases *go,...they go*'.[14] God sent sickness as a punishment for sin or a test of faith, and revoked it when the patient had prayed and repented. This belief persisted across the early modern period, and was articulated by doctors as well as laypeople: little evidence has been found to support Ian Mortimer's assertion that 'After 1690...the religious framework to...cure had ceased to dominate attitudes to treatment'.[15] God's role in recovery was rooted in Scripture, and revealed in the numerous instances of healing performed by Christ and His disciples.[16]

The Lord removed disease either directly, through miracles, or indirectly, via 'second causes'. A miracle was defined as 'an operation immediately proceeding from God...in doing what Nature could not do'.[17] It might be expected that in Protestant England, miraculous recoveries would not have been reported—the Reformation sought to rid the Church of all 'monkish superstitions', including miracle cures.[18] However, work by Alexandra Walsham and others has shown that 'Protestantism continued to preserve room in the reformed universe for occasional events of this kind'.[19] Amongst the individuals featured in this study, a range of opinions was held on the matter. At one end of the spectrum, the Suffolk puritan minister Isaac Archer (1641–1700) decided he should no longer pray for recovery from his speech impediment, because 'miracles were ceased, and 'twould be a miracle to restore speech to a stammerer'.[20] By contrast, the royalist Yorkshire gentle-woman Alice Thornton (1626–1707) believed that her deliverance from 'desperate extremity' in 1666 was 'by A miraculous Power from heaven'.[21] This split in opinion did not always fall neatly along Anglican and nonconformist lines, although Jane Shaw has observed a higher incidence of miracle claims amongst dissenting

---

[14] Edward Lawrence, *Christ's power over bodily diseases* (1672, first publ. 1662), 24.

[15] Ian Mortimer, 'The Triumph of the Doctors: Medical Assistance to the Dying, c.1570–1720', *Transactions of the Royal Historical Society*, 15 (2005), 97–116, at 114. For examples of the continued use of prayer after 1690, see Hannah Newton, *The Sick Child in Early Modern England, 1580–1720* (Oxford, 2012), chs. 4, 6.

[16] On God's healing role, see Raymond Anselment, *The Realms of Apollo: Literature and Healing in Seventeenth-Century England* (1995), 27–9.

[17] James Welwood, *A true relation of the wonderful cure of Mary Maillard* (1694), 19.

[18] This view is associated particularly with Keith Thomas, *Religion and the Decline of Magic: Studies in Popular Beliefs in Sixteenth- and Seventeenth-Century England* (1991, first publ. 1971), 87–8, 146–51, though he does point out that sectarians continued to report miracles.

[19] Alexandra Walsham, *The Reformation of the Landscape: Religion, Identity, and Memory in Early Modern Britain and Ireland* (Oxford, 2011), 444. See also Jane Shaw, *Miracles in Enlightenment England* (2006); Peter Elmer, *The Miraculous Conformist: Valentine Greatrakes, the Body Politic, and the Politics of Healing in Restoration Britain* (Oxford, 2013); Stephen Brogan, *The Royal Touch in Early Modern England* (Woodbridge, 2015).

[20] Isaac Archer, 'The Diary of Isaac Archer 1641–1700', in Matthew J. Storey (ed.), *Two East Anglian Diaries 1641–1729*, Suffolk Record Society, vol. 36 (Woodbridge, 1994), 41–200, at 55.

[21] BL, Additional MS 88897/2, fols. 58v–59r (Autobiography of Alice Thornton).

Protestant sects.[22] Most people in the present study tended to fall between the two extremes, preferring to couch their views in more tentative terms. In 1663, Sir Charles Lyttelton told a friend, 'My poore wife has bine, *as if* by miracle, raised to life...when given over by her phizitians' (my italics).[23] By saying 'as if', pious individuals could maintain their truly Protestant identities without appearing to limit God's powers.[24]

One thing that everyone seemed to agree on, regardless of their views on miracles, was that God usually operated through natural means. This leads us to the second agent of recovery, Nature. As it does today, the word 'nature' held many meanings, but in the context of Galenic physiology, it denoted a divinely endowed power in the body.[25] Since the body was conceived as a microcosm of the world, the Nature in the body was seen as a miniature version of the wider Nature that maintained the order of the universe.[26] Conrade Joachim Sprengell, an early eighteenth-century physician and Fellow of the Royal Society, provided a typical definition:

> [B]y the word Nature, we are to understand an Intrinsick Agent, by which the Vital motions...absolutely necessary...to the Preservation and Restoration of human Bodies, are directed.[27]

Nature was responsible for carrying out all the basic functions of the body, including nutrition, growth, reproduction, and most importantly here, the removal of disease. Galen's famous text, *The natural faculties*, which formed the foundation to many a doctor's university education, confirms, 'Nature...nourishes the animal, makes it grow, and expels its diseases...she skilfully moulds everything during the stage of genesis; and she also provides for the creatures after birth'.[28] Without this agent, 'there is not a single animal which could live...for the shortest time', he

---

[22] Shaw, *Miracles*, 3, 52.

[23] Christopher Hatton, *Correspondence of the Family of Hatton being Chiefly Addressed to Christopher, First Viscount Hatton, 1601–1704*, ed. Edward Maunde Thompson, Camden Society, vols. 22–23 (1878), vol. 1, 29.

[24] It is tempting to dismiss the phrase 'as if' as a mere linguistic convention, but I do think it sheds light on Lyttelton's views of supernatural healing. Given the highly charged religious and political climate in the 1660s, Protestants at this time were especially aware of the connotations of their language choices in relation to their confessional identities. For an insightful discussion of the saying 'as if', see Joe Moshenska, *Feeling Pleasures: The Sense of Touch in Renaissance England* (Oxford, 2014), 38–9, which points out that this 'parenthetic phrase' was used to express uncertainty about the 'fit between the language that we use, and the state of affairs which we describe', or to show that something might be 'formally exact though practically right'.

[25] The OED lists 14 categories of definitions, and a total of 34 meanings (accessed 4/01/15). The idea that Nature was divinely endowed was standard—to give one example, see Levinus Lemnius, *The secret miracles of nature* (1658, first publ. 1559), 1–3.

[26] Robert Boyle, *A free enquiry into the vulgarly receiv'd notion of nature* (1686), 37–8.

[27] Conrade Joachim Sprengell, 'Natura Morborum Medicatrix: Or, Nature Cures Diseases', in Matthaeus Purmann (ed.), *Chirurgia Curiosa* (1706), 319–43, at 319.

[28] Galen, *Galen on the Natural Faculties*, trans. Arthur John Brock (Cambridge, 2006, first publ. 1916), 33. An abridged vernacular version of this text was available in early modern England, in *Certaine works of Galens...with an epitome...of natural faculties*, trans. Thomas Gale (1586, first publ. 1566). University-trained doctors would have read the full Latin version, *De naturalibus facultatibus*, trans. Thomas Linacre (1523). My thanks to Professor Vivian Nutton for this information.

concluded.[29] Nature's vehicles for performing her various functions were the 'natural spirits', highly rarefied, 'subtile and Arey' vapours, 'raised from the purer blood', and carried around the body in the veins.[30] Two further spirits were associated with Nature: the 'vital spirit', which 'resides in the *Heart* and *Arteries*', and was the animating force of the body, responsible for respiration and the pulse; and the 'Animal Spirit', which 'doth spring from the *Brain*', was carried in the nerves, and powered the five senses, motion, and the rational faculties.[31] In these three spirits 'consist all the force and efficacy of our Nature', declared the French surgeon Ambroise Paré (*c*.1510–90).[32] So strong was the connection between the spirits and Nature, the two were often regarded as synonymous.[33] In turn, the spirits were 'nourished' by what were known as 'radical moisture' (an oily substance), and 'innate heat' (a glowing warmth); life itself was thought to consist in these two special substances, which gradually depleted with age.[34]

Nature's role in recovery was summed up by the philosopher and chemist Robert Boyle (1627–91) in his critical exposition of mainstream views of this agent, published in 1686: 'Men are wont to believe, that there resides, in the Body of a sick Person, a certain Provident or Watchful Being, that...industriously employs itself... to...restore the distemper'd Body to its Pristine state of Health'.[35] This notion was rooted in the writings of Hippocrates, and his famous axiom, 'Natura est morborum medicatrix', translated as 'Nature is the healer of disease'.[36] Historians usually associate this idea with the 'New Hippocrates', Thomas Sydenham (1624–89), but it is evident from this research that it was, in fact, widely articulated in society, by laypeople as well as doctors.[37] For instance, the Leicestershire chaplain George Davenport (*c*.1631–77) wrote that his friend Mr Gayer 'began to be sick...last week...but nature stept in & relieved him'.[38] One might expect clerics like Davenport to have omitted Nature from their accounts of recovery, on the grounds that it detracted from the agency of the Lord. This does not seem to have been the

---

[29] Galen, *Galens art of physic*, trans. Nicholas Culpeper (1652), 8; Galen, *Galen on the natural faculties*, 127.

[30] Ambroise Paré, *The workes of that famous chirurgion Ambrose Parey*, trans. Thomas Johnson (1634), 25. For more information on the spirits, see Elena Carrera (ed.), *Emotions and Health, 1200–1700* (Leiden, 2013), 62, 90, 106–7, 113, 115, 117–18, 197, 223.

[31] Galen, *Galen's method of physic*, 266; John Harris, *The divine physician, prescribing rules for the prevention, and cure of most diseases, as well of the body, as the soul* (1676), 163.

[32] Paré, *The workes*, 26–7.   [33] For example, Harris, *The divine physician*, 163–4.

[34] James Hart, *Klinike, or the diet of the diseased* (1633), 299. On the effects of ageing on the radical moisture and innate heat, see Newton, *The Sick Child*, 34–5.

[35] Boyle, *A free enquiry*, 304. Boyle himself disagreed with this notion—his treatise refutes the existence of Nature as an entity, and instead attributes recovery to the divinely framed mechanical structures of the body. See the introduction to Michael Hunter and Edward Davis (eds.), *Robert Boyle: A Free Enquiry into the Vulgarly Received Notion of Nature* (Cambridge, 1996). Boyle seems to have been unusual in his views, and I have not found any other author who agrees, even amongst those who share his mechanical philosophy.

[36] Neuburger, *The Doctrine*, 6.

[37] For examples at either end of the time-period, see William Bullein, *Bulleins bulwarke of defence against all sicknesse* (1579), 7; Philip Woodman, *Medicus novissimus; or, the modern physician* (1712), preface.

[38] George Davenport, *The Letters of George Davenport 1651–1677*, ed. Brenda M. Pask, Surtees Society, vol. 215 (Woodbridge, 2011), 33. See also Archer, 'The Diary', 173.

case, however: the devout understood that Nature was 'God's immediate Commissioner', and therefore to attribute recovery to this agent did not negate the overarching role of providence.[39] In any case, it was always God, rather than Nature, to whom patients and families directed their thanks and praise, as will be shown in Chapter 4. Due to a shortage of direct evidence, it is more difficult to uncover the beliefs of poorer people, but second-hand accounts indicate that Nature's healing role was probably a cross-class phenomenon. The phrase 'Nature... is the Curer of Disease', according to Boyle, is 'so very frequently us'd by Men of all sorts, as well Learned as illiterate'.[40]

What was Nature like? An analysis of the personification of Nature introduces an important theme that runs through the rest of this chapter, gender. Nature was personified as a benevolent female who looked after the body. The Northampton puritan physician James Hart (d. 1639), stated, 'nature is... like a kinde and loving mother, being very solicitous and carefull of the life of man'.[41] She was also depicted as a charwoman, who 'scoured away' illness, 'sweeping every corner, [and] making the whole Body polite and trim'.[42] Nature's economic status varied: the astrologer-physician Nicholas Culpeper (1616–54) called her 'a plain homely woman in a beggarly comtemptible condition' whose 'wayes are very plaine[;] you may finde them in the darkest night without a Candle'.[43] But she was also titled 'Dame' or 'Lady Nature', and depicted as an elite gentlewoman who presided over the task of recovery as a mistress over her household servants.[44] In these descriptions, the body is envisaged as a house, and disease as dirt, or an unruly guest, which needed to be washed away, or turned out.[45] It made sense to depict Nature as female, because the majority of her roles fell into the category of women's work—as well as tending the sick, she was responsible for nourishment and reproduction, tasks in which even elite ladies were expected to have some expertise.[46]

The female personification of Nature is not as simple as it seems, however: whilst using feminine pronouns, authors sometimes deployed masculine metaphors. 'Dame Nature', declared Culpeper, 'iss like a Prince in the body... she can expell her enemy out of her dominions'.[47] She is 'a wise and faithful consul, in a Civill and intestine war... to cast forth the disease', echoed the Dutch physician Levinus Lemnius (1505–68).[48] In these statements, disease is portrayed as an enemy, and

[39] On providence see Alexandra Walsham, *Providence in Early Modern England* (Oxford, 1999).
[40] Boyle, *A free enquiry*, 62.   [41] Hart, *Klinike*, 4.
[42] George Thomson, *Ortho-methodoz itro-chymike, or the direct method of curing chymically* (1675), 112.
[43] Nicholas Culpeper, *Semeiotica uranica: or, an astrological judgement of diseases* (1651), 173.
[44] Everand Maynwaringe, *The catholic medicine, and soverain healer* (1684), 13.
[45] For a discussion of the use of metaphors in early modern medicine, see Margaret Healy, *Fictions of Disease in Early Modern England: Bodies, Plagues and Politics* (Basingstoke, 2001), ch. 1. On the dirt metaphor, see Jennifer Vaught (ed.), *Rhetorics of Bodily Disease and Health in Medieval and Early Modern England* (Farnham, 2010), 1, 6, 11. The washing metaphor is discussed in the next section on 'Processes'.
[46] Sara Mendelson and Patricia Crawford, *Women in Early Modern England, 1550–1720* (Oxford, 2003, first publ. 1998), 256–9, 269, 301, 303–4.
[47] Culpeper, *Semeiotica*, 189.   [48] Lemnius, *The secret miracles*, 88.

the body as a battlefield.[49] It may seem surprising that such metaphors were used to describe the actions of a female agent—the violence of warfare was generally regarded as incompatible with femininity.[50] However, there was one context in which female aggression *was* legitimate: when women perceived members of their households to be in danger.[51] Garthine Walker has shown that during the Civil Wars, tales abounded of courageous wives who defended their homes from attack by enemy troops.[52] Plays and histories valorized selfless mothers for 'venturing on Swords, and rushing through the flames to save their Darlings'.[53] So powerful were these models that ordinary women invoked them in court to justify their acts of violence.[54] Since Nature was represented as the body's mother, it is understandable that this agent assumed the role of brave fighter during disease. The gender paradox may have also been rendered less problematic by the permeation of imagery of female warriors in early modern culture, derived from classical mythology and Christian scripture.[55] The same can be said of Elizabeth I's iconic status as a warrior queen following the defeat of the Spanish Armada.

Nature was blessed with many qualities. Quoting Aristotle, the Durham physician and minister William Bullein (c.1515–76) declared, 'Nature doth nothing in vain'.[56] She was imaginative, 'the best artist', who 'invents...certain extraordinary ingenious aid[s]' for recovery.[57] Nature was full of knowledge, 'discreete, sober, and wise', wrote John Cotta (c.1575–1627), a physician from Coventry.[58] She was also caring and diligent, 'very solicitous' for the well-being of her hosts. Such high praise was a mark of respect to God, the 'author of Nature'. Many of these traits were prized attributes in females—women were entreated to be wise, discreet, and kind.[59] Given all these qualities, it might be expected that Nature was an infallible agent. But this was not the case: her ability to remove disease was by no means

[49] On this metaphor, see Sabine Kalff, 'The Body as a Battlefield: Conflict and Control in Seventeenth-Century Physiology and Political Thought', in Helen King and Claus Zittel (eds.), *Blood, Sweat and Tears: The Changing Concepts of Physiology from Antiquity into Early Modern Europe* (Leiden, 2012), 171–94. Military metaphors have also been explored in other chronologies—e.g. Brendon Larson, Brigitte Nerlich, and Patrick Wallis, 'Metaphors and Biorisks: The War on Infectious Diseases and Invasive Species', *Science Communication*, 26 (2005), 243–68. On the broader use of metaphors in the modern day, see George Lakoff and Mark Johnson's classic study, *Metaphors We Live By* (Chicago, 2003, first publ. 1980).

[50] Anna Whitelock, 'Woman, Warrior, Queen? Rethinking Mary and Elizabeth', in Anna Whitelock and Alice Hunt (eds.), *Tudor Queenship: The Reigns of Mary and Elizabeth* (Basingstoke, 2010), 173–90, at 173.

[51] Garthine Walker, *Crime, Gender and Social Order in Early Modern England* (Cambridge, 2003), 86–9.

[52] Ibid., 93.   [53] John Shirley, *The illustrious history of women* (1686), image 13.

[54] Walker, *Crime, Gender and Social Order*, 88–9.

[55] Ibid., 87; Whitelock, 'Woman, Warrior, Queen?'

[56] William Bullein, *The government of health* (1595, first publ. 1558), 8. On Aristotle's use of this proverb, see Mariska Leunissen, *Explanation and Teleology in Aristotle's Science of Nature* (Cambridge, 2010).

[57] Galen, 'On the Causes of Symptoms I', in Ian Johnston (ed. and trans.), *Galen on Diseases and Symptoms* (Cambridge, 2006), 203–35, at 248.

[58] John Cotta, *A short discoverie of the unobserved dangers of...practisers of physicke* (1612), 117.

[59] The qualities of females are described in defences of women, as well as conduct books—for example, Shirley, *The illustrious history*; Hannah Wooley, *The gentlewomans companion* (1670).

guaranteed, but depended on her strength. The Scottish physician John Macollo (*c.*1576–1622) explained:

> [T]he original of Prognosticks doth consist in conferring the spirits with the sickness; for if Nature be strong enough to overcome the disease, then the Patient shall escape; but if she be so weak that she cannot obtain the victory, death then of necessity must follow.[60]

Illness was a tug-of-war between Nature and the disease, and the outcome was all down to strength. As Macollo implies, Nature's strength was determined by the condition of her instruments, the spirits (natural, vital, and animal), together with the innate heat. Nature was strong when the spirits were 'many' and 'lively', and the heat 'strong'; conversely, she was weak when the spirits were 'dissolved and overthrown', and the heat 'feeble' or 'extinguished'.[61]

The fallibility of Nature provided the justification for the third agent in the hierarchy of healers, the medical practitioner. The role of this agent was expressed through the proverb, 'the physician is nature's servant'. Derived once more from the writings of Hippocrates, this epithet is cited in most medical treatises across the period.[62] The physician's 'chief office' as Nature's servant was to 'underprop [her] when she fails', a situation which arose when she became 'exhausted or overwhelmed' during her encounter with the disease.[63] Practitioners were supposed to act as Nature's 'faithfull friend[s]', 'needfully assisting, helping, and comforting her' against the 'furious mercilesse' illness.[64] In these statements, doctors drew on popular gender stereotypes to justify their interventions, depicting themselves as romantic heroes who rescued 'languishing Nature', the damsel in distress.[65] Since chivalry was one of the few contexts in which male subservience to a female was culturally acceptable, physicians may have been invoking this language as a way to maintain their masculine identities in what might otherwise have been a demeaning situation.[66] After all, early modern society was deeply patriarchal, and the position of 'Nature's servant' overturned the traditional gender order.[67]

Patients and their relatives, as well as physicians, recognized the need to assist Nature. The nonconformist minister Henry Newcome (*c.*1627–95) wrote in his memoirs, 'It is our duty when we are sick, to make use of such means as are proper

---

[60] John Macollo, *XCIX canons, or rules learnedly describing an excellent method for practitioners in physic* (1659), 43.

[61] Lemnius, *The secret miracles*, 43; Hart, *Klinike*, 241; Macollo, *XCIX canons*, 44.

[62] Examples from either end of the period include A.T., *A rich store-house, or treasury for the diseased* (1596), preface; Nicholas Robinson, *A new theory of physic* (1725), 193.

[63] Lemnius, *The secret miracles*, 97.   [64] Cotta, *A short discoverie*, 118.

[65] Culpeper, *Semeiotica uranica*, 72, 167.

[66] Mendelson and Crawford, *Women*, 356. On anxieties about loss of patriarchal authority, see Anthony Fletcher, *Gender, Sex, and Subordination in England, 1500–1800* (1995), *passim*; Elizabeth Foyster, *Manhood in Early Modern England: Honour, Sex and Marriage* (1999), ch. 4. On the persistence of chivalry in the early modern period, see Jennifer Wollock, *Rethinking Chivalry and Courtly Love* (Santa Barbara CA, 2011), chs. 9, 10.

[67] Susan Amussen, *An Ordered Society: Gender and Class in Early Modern England* (Oxford, 1988), *passim*.

to help nature'.[68] The famous diarist and naval officer Samuel Pepys (1633–1703) recorded, 'I…keep to my bed…[and] will assist nature' through taking remedies advised by the apothecary, Mr Battersby.[69] Female patients and practitioners may have felt a special affinity with Nature, as fellow female healers. This was implied by the prominent London surgeon John Woodall, who commended the 'old wifes medicament' because 'she wrestleth not with Nature as great masters doe, and Nature[,] pleased with her milde and simple meanes is appeased, and by divine providence the disease often easily made whole'.[70] The gentle treatments associated with women practitioners were seen as more acceptable to Nature.

The power balance between Nature and the practitioner was supposed to rest firmly with the former: a lowly servant, the practitioner was entreated to 'act in subserviency to [Nature's] Designs', imitating her methods when treating the sick.[71] So inferior was his position, that in many cases, he was not needed at all. The Ordinary Professor of Anatomy at Utrecht, Ysbrand van Diemerbroeck (c.1609–74), commanded, 'leave Nature to do her own business, in regard she does it better of her own accord then the Physitians can do by Art'.[72] Even when armed with 'all his art, Method, Simples, compounds, Antidots,…Catharticks, Minoratives, Diaphoreticks, Coroboratives, [and] Anodynes' the physician 'is but a servant, and all his doings but the service unto the inward Physician', averred the bishop John Abernethy (d. 1639).[73] In practice, however, the power balance between Nature and the doctor could be reversed, with the latter taking on the dominant role. Cotta stated, 'it is requisite in a co[m]petant Physition, that he be truly able…to be unto nature a governor…to preserve her, to conserve her, behoofefully to…guide her'.[74] The physician was expected to restrain Nature when she became 'exorbitant', and 'rouse her' into action if she grew lazy or forgetful.[75] This inverted relationship was encapsulated by the saying, 'nature must play the physitian in curing of the disease', which suggests that it was Nature who was imitating the doctor.[76]

How can this contradictory power balance be explained? Essentially, it sprang from experience: practitioners observed that without physic, patients sometimes recovered, and sometimes remained ill or died. Such instances signified that

[68] Cited in David Harley, 'The Theology of Affliction and the Experience of Sickness in the Godly Family, 1650–1714: The Henrys and the Newcomes', in Ole Peter Grell and Andrew Cunningham (eds.), *Religio Medici: Medicine and Religion in Seventeenth-Century England* (Aldershot, 1996), 273–92, at 279.

[69] Samuel Pepys, *The Diary of Samuel Pepys*, ed. Henry B. Wheatley (1893), Project Gutenberg, managed by Phil Gyford, <http://www.pepysdiary.com/archive/1663/02/09/> (accessed 11/02/17).

[70] John Woodall, *The surgions mate…[and] the cures of…diseases at sea* (1617), 154–5.

[71] Boyle, *A free enquiry*, 325; Brice Bauderon, *The expert physician: learnedly treating of all agues and feavers* (1657), 49; *The aphorismes of Hippocrates*, trans. S.H. [possibly Stephen Hobbes] (1655), 3.

[72] Ysbrand van Diemerbroeck, *The anatomy of human bodies…To which is added…several practical observations*, trans. William Salmon (1694, first publ. in Utrecht in 1664), 33.

[73] John Abernethy, *A Christian and heavenly treatise, containing physicke for the soule* (1630, first publ. 1615), 15.

[74] Cotta, *A short discoverie*, 118.

[75] M. Flamant, *The art of preserving and restoring health* (1697), 46; John Pechey, *The store-house of physical practice* (1695), 318.

[76] Hart, *Klinike*, 164.

Nature's judgement was not always reliable, an observation that fitted with contemporary ideas about 'the very imbecility' of females, and their need 'to be always directed and ordered by others'.[77] One way to understand this ambivalent relationship is to look to the wider political context. For early modern society, the power balance between the physician and Nature may have brought to mind the case of female monarchs, most notably, Elizabeth I. Like Nature, the queen was divinely ordained to rule, and deserved unquestioning obedience from her subjects; and yet, the inferiority and weakness of her sex warranted the intervention of her ministers, and frequently, their flagrant disobedience, especially during warfare.[78] A more mundane, but equally powerful analogy concerns the roles of husbands and wives in the household. In his best-selling conduct book, *Of domesticall duties* (1622), the London clergyman William Gouge (1578–1653) declared, 'it is the wives... dutie to... *governe the house*' in such matters as 'nourishing and instructing children... adorning the house, [and] ruling maidservants'. However, the husband has 'a general oversight of all, and so [may] interpose his authority' whenever he perceives that something 'unlawfull or unseemly... [is] done by his wife'.[79] These two metaphors—of wife and monarch—may have acted as a model for the Nature–physician relationship.

Together, the three agents of God, Nature, and the medical practitioner were responsible for recovery. But ultimately the Lord was in charge: without His blessing and forgiveness, the efforts of the other agents were futile, a view shared by physicians as well as clergymen.[80]

PROCESSES

Having established who removed disease, we can ask how these agents went about this task. The focus will be on the physiological processes rather than the spiritual ones.[81] Through exploring the mechanisms involved, it will be possible to observe in more concrete terms the complex relationship between Nature and the medical practitioner. The discussions also contribute to debates about the conceptualization of disease, and uncover bodily processes that have rarely been explored.

Put simply, disease was removed by the removal of the cause of disease. The Dean of the Medical Faculty of Reims, Nicholas Abraham de La Framboisière (1560–1636), confirmed, 'while the [cause] is present, the Disease remains; but when it is remov'd,

[77] Richard Hooker (1554–1600) cited in Fletcher, *Gender, Sex, and Subordination*, 70.

[78] Much has been written on the relationship between queens and male advisers. A recent example is Carole Levin and Robert Bucholz (eds.), *Queens and Power in Medieval and Early Modern England* (Lincoln NE, 2009). On the disobedience of Elizabeth I's generals, see Whitelock, 'Woman, Warrior, Queen?', 182–4.

[79] William Gouge, *Of domesticall duties* (1622), 292, 367–8.

[80] Harris, *The divine physician*, 122; Thomas Cogan, *The haven of health, made for the comfort of students* (1634, first publ. 1584), 36; Culpeper, *Semeiotica uranica*, 164; Timothy Rogers, *Practical discourses on sickness & recovery* (1691), 36.

[81] The root cause of disease was sin; the chief spiritual processes through which sin was removed were prayer and repentance, discussed in Chapter 4.

the Disease ceases'.[82] Disease was defined in Galenic theory as a 'condition contrary to nature which impedes function', arising from the 'distemperature' of the four 'primary qualities' of heat, cold, moisture, and dryness.[83] All the faculties of the body and mind were thought to be driven by the special mixture of the aforementioned qualities, and therefore when this state changed, 'perceptible impairment' occurred.[84] Since Nature presided over bodily functions, it made sense to regard anything that hindered these faculties as 'contrary' to this internal agent.[85] In turn, the state of the primary qualities was dictated by the quantity and conditions of the humours, the four constituent fluids of living creatures, each of which contained a different amount of heat and moisture.[86] Hence, disease resulted when the humours altered in their proportions, or grew 'morbid'.[87] While historians have long recognized that disease was defined as imbalance, the other vital component—impairment of faculties—is often forgotten.

Given that disease was caused by the malignant alteration of the humours, it followed that the physiological mechanisms through which it was removed involved the rectification of these substances. Upon the command of God, Nature achieved this rectification through two main processes, the first of which was 'concoction', a concept rarely explored in this context.[88] It denoted 'the reduction [i.e. restoration] of the peccant humor in the body to a right temper and frame': the humours were to be altered in their temperatures, moisture levels, flavours, and consistencies, so that they could be safely reabsorbed into the body.[89] Concoction was carried out 'by nature it selfe, by meanes of naturall heat', the innate warmth of living creatures—the Latin *concoct* means 'to boil together'.[90] Just as raw food was rendered edible by cooking, doctors thought that the application of heat would purify the putrid humours. It made sense that Nature used this method,

---

[82] Nicholas Abraham de La Framboisière, *The art of physick made plain & easie*, trans. John Phillips (1684; originally publ. in Latin, 1628), 103.

[83] Galen, 'On the Causes of Symptoms I', 184. This is the standard definition—e.g. Macollo, *XCIX canons*, 12–13.

[84] Galen, *Galen's method*, 26; Galen, *Galen on the natural faculties*, 197; Framboisière, *The art of physick*, 16.

[85] For a discussion of the meaning of 'contrary to nature', see *De sanitate tuenda*, cited by Ian Johnston in his edition, *Galen on Diseases and Symptoms*, 29.

[86] Lemnius, *The secret miracles*, 86.

[87] Stolberg has pointed out that historians usually assume it was the altered quantities—i.e. balance—of the humours that caused disease; by contrast, he has found that in practice it was more often the qualities that were blamed: disease was caused by 'morbid matter' or humours: *Experiencing Illness*, 85–9, 95.

[88] The concoction of bad humours has only been explored occasionally—for example, by Fabiola I. W. M. van Dam, 'Permeable Boundaries: Bodies, Bathing and Fluxes', in Patricia Baker, Karine van't Land, and Han Nijdam (eds.), *Medicine and Space: Body, Surroundings and Borders in Antiquity and the Middle Ages* (Leiden, 2012), 117–48; Stolberg, *Uroscopy*, 55–6, 63. More, however, has been written about the digestion of food, breastmilk, and generative seeds, processes also known as 'concoction'—for example, Michael Schoenfeldt, *Bodies and Selves in Early Modern England: Physiology and Inwardness in Spenser, Shakespeare, Herbert, and Milton* (Cambridge, 1999), 25–33; Ken Albala, *Eating Right in the Renaissance* (Berkeley CA, 2002), 54–62.

[89] Hart, *Klinike*, 276. See also Galen, *Galens art of physic*, 118; Galen, *Galen on the Natural Faculties*, 179.

[90] Hart, *Klinike*, 277; OED (accessed 2/02/17).

since it fitted with her identity as a diligent housewife, who attended to the nutritional needs of the body. Indeed, this agent's method for digesting food was also called concoction, as historians are well aware—it was a 'species of alteration—a transmutation of the nutriment into the proper quality of the thing receiving it'.[91] In the same way, Nature was able to 'alter and tra[ns]mute morbid states' of the humours, turning them into the substance of the body.[92] The historian Fabiola van Dam believes this was *the* central node in Aristotelian thinking about all forms of natural change.[93]

Understandings of concoction influenced how patients were managed during serious illness. This process was thought to be most arduous and painful, both to Nature and to the patient: a Hippocratic aphorism states, 'Whiles filthy and corrupt matter is digesting, pains and Agues do…happen'.[94] Given the great labour involved, physicians 'command[ed] long quiet and rest to the patient' during concoction, so that all Nature's powers could be devoted to this task.[95] Macollo warned that under no circumstances should this agent be 'diverted or hindered' from her 'office & work' by such chores as eating or exercise.[96] The consequences of neglecting this advice could be grave, as the eminent surgeon William Clowes (1543/4–1604) confirmed. One male patient of his, sick of fever, had been fed an apple by a kindly, but ignorant, nurse: 'So soon' as the man had 'devoured all and every peece' of this foodstuff, 'nature left the disease to digest the apple, which was too hard to do…[;] at length, his Feaver…was now much worse'.[97] Poor at multi-tasking, Nature could only manage to digest 'thin' foods during illness, like broths.[98]

Nature's proficiency at concocting the noxious humours depended on their quantities and qualities. The medical writer from Suffolk, Phillip Barrough (d. 1600), noted that if there was only a small amount of 'grosse blood' in the body, 'nature will get the upper hand in digesting…the humour', and the disease will not last long.[99] But, when the illness is caused by 'diverse humours', Nature 'hath need to employ much time' in concoction, and the disease would endure for longer.[100] The consistency of the humours also had an impact: 'choler doth ever cause quick diseases', wrote Macollo, 'because it is easily resolved by its subtility', whereas 'Melancholy is the most viscous of all the humours, and makes the longest accesses, because it is dry, cold and thick'.[101] Of all diseases, cancers and plague were caused by the most 'grevous and pernicious' humours: 'by reason of the grossenes' and

[91] Galen, *Galen on the Natural Faculties*, 139–41. For the concoction of foods, see note 88 in this chapter.
[92] Ibid., 179.
[93] Van Dam, 'Permeable Boundaries'.   [94] *The aphorismes of Hippocrates*, 38.
[95] Philip Barrough, *The methode of phisicke* (1583), 187.
[96] Macollo, *XCIX canons*, 89. The danger of distracting Nature continued to be articulated in the 1700s and 1800s, as Martin Edwards has kindly informed me. Rather than referring to this agent's 'spirits', however, physicians used the term 'nervous force'. See for example, Richard Quain (ed.), *Dictionary of Medicine* (1894), 653; Peter Hood, *A Treatise on Gout* (1885), 123–4; Henry Bennet, 'On the Treatment of Pulmonary Consumption: pt. 2', *Lancet*, 88 (1866), 352.
[97] William Clowes, *Aprooved practice for all young chirurgians* (1588), image 7.
[98] Bullein, *The government of health*, 27. See Ken Albala, 'Food for Healing: Convalescent Cookery in the Early Modern Era', *Studies in History and Philosophy of Science Part C*, 43 (2012), 323–8.
[99] Barrough, *The methode*, 186.   [100] Macollo, *XCIX canons*, 65.   [101] Ibid., 49–50.

'untameable malignity' of the matter, 'nature is so irritated...that it can no way digest it'.[102] Ultimately, these humoral characteristics determined whether the disease would prove curable, chronic, or fatal.

Another major factor that influenced Nature's ability to concoct the humours was the strength of the innate heat, a variable determined partly by the patient's constitution, age, and sex. Macollo explained:

> Youth hath great strength to withstand a disease, because he hath store of natural heat, requisite to the concoction...of the evil humours: contrarily, old age is not able to resist, because of the defect of strength, not having much natural heat... [hence when] sickness...arrive[s] to old people, [it often] conveys them to their graves.[103]

Children's concocting capacities were rather more ambivalent: their bodies abounded in moisture, a characteristic that made all their bodily faculties—including their ability to concoct—less powerful, and yet, they benefited from strong natural heat, a key property in concoction.[104] Practitioners mentioned these factors in their casebooks. Van Diemerbroeck recorded that his sixty-year-old patient, 'troubled with a vehement *Asthma*', could not be cured, because 'crude, cold and phlegmatic Humors in old men, do not admit of Concoction, by reason of the Debility of the Concoctive Faculty; which in them is feeble, because of their cold Constitution'.[105] Gender also had an impact: women fared less well than men because, like children, they were full of moisture, and like the elderly, they were comparatively cold.[106]

What was the role of medical practitioners in concoction? Hart declared, 'if nature be feeble[,]...and [her] heat not in a due proportion answerable, it is then the Physitians part...to supply this defect'.[107] If Nature struggled to muster up the required heat, doctors could help by 'rais[ing] up' the temperature, so that this agent was empowered to concoct the matter. The easiest way to do this was to pile on extra blankets or stoke up the fire. Alternatively, practitioners could manipulate the non-naturals: for example, Hart suggested that 'in some diseases', the passion anger 'may be beneficial', because it 'stirreth up naturall heat'.[108] When Nature was very weak, however, practitioners opted to actively transform the humours themselves, effectively doing this agent's work for her. The use of the term

---

[102] Barrough, *The methode*, 274; Paré, *The workes*, 861. On perceptions of cancer, see Alana Skuse, *Constructions of Cancer in Early Modern England: Ravenous Natures* (Basingstoke, 2015).

[103] Macollo, *XCIX canons*, 45. The following historians also mention that the coldness of the old body was thought to be less suited to digestion and concoction, though they are speaking about nutrition rather than recovery: Daniel Schäfer, 'More than a Fading Flame: The Physiology of Old Age between Speculative Analogy and Experimental Method', in King and Zittel (eds.), *Blood, Sweat and Tears*, 241–66, at 250, 255–6; Albala, *Eating Right*, 53.

[104] Galen, *Galen on Diseases*, 295.   [105] Van Diemerbroeck, *The anatomy*, 93.

[106] This is mentioned by Stolberg, though in relation to the concoction of food rather than bad humours: Michael Stolberg, 'A Woman Down to Her Bones: The Anatomy of Sexual Difference in the Sixteenth and Early Seventeenth Centuries', *Isis*, 94 (2003), 274–99, at 294.

[107] Hart, *Klinike*, 277.

[108] Ibid., 391. On the beneficial effects of anger, Elena Carrera, 'Anger and the Mind–Body Connection in Medieval and Early Modern Medicine', in Elena Carrera (ed.), *Emotions and Health, 1200–1700* (Leiden, 2013), 95–146, at 136–43.

'concoction' to denote a medicinal drink indicates most obviously this role of physic: practitioners prescribed medicines, or regulated the non-naturals, in such a way as opposed the qualities of the offending humours, thereby transforming them out of their malignant state.[109] This strategy was called 'allopathic healing' or 'cure by contraries', terms familiar to medical historians. Barrough explained:

> Every distempure is corrected and amended by his contrary. Therefore you must coole a hote distempure, and heat a cold distempure: also moisten a dry, and dry a moist distempure.[110]

Medicinal ingredients were classified according to their 'degrees' of heat and moisture, so that they could be matched appropriately to the particular disease. For example, cucumbers were 'in the seconde degree, very moist and colde', and therefore 'The seedes be good to be given in hote sicknesses', such as acute fevers.[111] It is worth noting that there is some contradiction between the above methods: since concoction was driven by heat, it was necessary to warm the patient to promote this process. At the same time, however, if the noxious humours were excessively hot, it was essential to cool the patient in order to transform the humours into their 'natural temper'. Medical authors did not comment on this contradiction.

When describing their own involvement in concoction, physicians referred not to the imagery of cooking mentioned above, but to subjugation and taming. Barrough stated that by prescribing his drug, 'choler [will be] concoct[ed], & as it were tamed & made myld [and] is made so obedient'.[112] For doctors, such language may have brought to mind the taming or breaking in of a young horse, a practice with which they would probably have been familiar, since most practitioners travelled on horseback to visit their patients.[113] The language also carries connotations of subduing a headstrong child or a shrewish wife, popular tropes in early modern culture.[114] It is likely that physicians' choice of language was partly informed by the patient's gender and behaviour, as is implied in John Hall's casebook: he treated a seventeen-year-old girl called Edith Staughton, who was 'miserably afflicted' with a womb-related illness. Hall recorded she was 'very easily angry with her nearest Friends'; upon the administration of certain medicines, 'the Humor was rendred more obsequious', which presumably referred to the girl's demeanour as well as her humours.[115] Perhaps, by using this language rather than imagery of cookery, physicians like Hall could enhance their masculine identities as firm patriarchs when treating their patients.

---

[109] Walter Bruele, *Praxis medicinae, or, the physicians practice* (1632), 44.
[110] Barrough, *The methode*, 80.   [111] Bullein, *The government of health*, 44.
[112] Barrough, *The methode*, 7.
[113] Irvine Loudon, 'Medicine Before the Motor Car', *Journal of the Royal Society of Medicine*, 102 (2009), 219–22. See Peter Edwards, *Horse and Man in Early Modern England* (2007), on the prevalence of horse-ownership, and practices of breaking in.
[114] Fletcher, *Gender, Sex, and Subordination*, 107–9; David Underdown, 'The Taming of the Scold: The Enforcement of Patriarchal Authority in Early Modern England', in Anthony Fletcher and John Stevenson (eds.), *Order and Disorder in Early Modern England* (Cambridge, 1985), 116–36.
[115] John Hall, *Select observations on English bodies*, trans. James Cooke (1679, first. publ. 1657), 174–5.

Concoction was central to prognosis as well as treatment. Doctors believed it possible to predict the outcome of disease from signs of concoction in the bodily fluids. Macollo explained:

> The co[n]c[oc]tion of the humour appearing in the Excrement of the Patient, signifies the... conflict to be speedily in assurance of health; but the crudity denotes, that... the Patient is mightily troubled, or that the disease shall be longer... or finally, that death shall follow upon it.[116]

The more closely the excrements resembled their state in times of health, the more complete the concoction process, and the more 'sure' the recovery.[117] To make this judgement, doctors could activate all five of their senses, though in practice, few were prepared to taste bodily fluids![118] Likewise, any of the body's excrements could be analysed, but in everyday life it was most often the urine that was chosen, as the easiest fluid to access.[119] Michael Stolberg has investigated the changing fortunes of urine inspection, known as 'uroscopy', showing that as the period progressed, physicians became increasingly wary of basing their prognoses solely on the state of the urine. He interprets this trend as an attempt by physicians to disassociate themselves from the practices of quacks, the so-called 'piss-prophets'.[120] No such concern was expressed by laypeople, however, who continued to see the urine as a fairly reliable window into how well Nature was doing in her concocting duties.[121] The Essex clergyman Ralph Josselin (1617–83) recorded in 1648, 'my water brake very ragged [by which]...I conceive a remainder of ill humours in mee...that nature was concocting'.[122] There was a slight difference, however, between patients' and physicians' interpretations of the expelled fluid—the former tended to take a positive reading whatever its state. For example, when the urine was 'turning pale as in health', recovery was signified,[123] but if the expelled matter was 'vicious, green and black', they were equally relieved, because it meant the humour was no longer damaging the body.[124]

After concoction, the second mechanism for removing disease could occur: 'the expulsion...of humors which are troublesome, either in quantitie, or quallitie'.[125]

[116] Macollo, *XCIX canons*, 60.   [117] Ibid., 60–1.
[118] On historiography on senses in diagnosis, see Chapter 3, note 15. On physicians' dislike of tasting the excrements, see Stolberg, *Uroscopy*, 128–30.
[119] For examples of various bodily fluids, see *The aphorismes of Hippocrates*, 8–9, 23, 178–9; John Symcotts, *A Seventeenth Century Doctor and his Patients: John Symcotts, 1592?–1662*, ed. F. N. L. Poynter and W. J. Bishop, Bedfordshire Historical Record Society, vol. 31 (Streatley, 1951), 312; Framboisière, *The art of physick*, 119. On the practical reasons why urine was used more than other excrements, see Stolberg, *Uroscopy*, 64, 76–9.
[120] Michael Stolberg, 'The Decline of Uroscopy in Early Modern Learned Medicine', *Early Science and Medicine*, 17 (2007), 313–36.
[121] Stolberg acknowledges the continued popularity of uroscopy amongst laypeople in *Uroscopy*, *passim*.
[122] Ralph Josselin, *The Diary of Ralph Josselin 1616–1683*, ed. Alan Macfarlane (Oxford, 1991), 117.
[123] Samuel Jeake, *An Astrological Diary of the Seventeenth Century: Samuel Jeake of Rye*, ed. Michael Hunter (Oxford, 1988), 143.
[124] Walker, *The vertuous wife*, 95. See also James Clavering, *The Correspondence of Sir James Clavering*, ed. Harry Thomas Dickinson, Surtees Society, vol. 178 (Gateshead, 1967), 158.
[125] Paré, *The workes*, 37.

Evacuation was the fate of those humours which had retained a degree of malignancy in spite of concoction, or else were simply too voluminous. Although historians are aware of the role of evacuation, its full complexity is yet to be explicated. For a start, doctors believed it should not take place until certain preparative steps had occurred. Macollo explained:

> [B]efore the body be purged, it must be prepared and the humours must be made fluxible, otherwise the purgation will not be without great pain;...wherefore...all the passages of it are to be opened, and the gross humours within are to be made liquid.[126]

Thus, it was necessary to alter the consistency of the humours, so that they could more easily flow out of the body. Imagery of food preparation and cooking was used in this context: Nature 'chopped' and 'melted' the thick humours, and physicians could assist by giving 'Bitter' medicines to 'devide, [and] extenuate' the 'grosse and clammy humours'.[127] Readying the body for expulsion—making it 'fluxible'—was dirty work, conjuring up images of disgusting, stinking matter being scrubbed and washed. Lemnius observed, 'the filth and rubbish of the humours stick no lesse to...mens bodies, than the lees and dregs do to vessels, which must be soked with salt water...and rub'd...to make them clean'.[128] This imagery suited Nature's personification as a charwoman or housewife, who cooked and cleaned in the body. Laypeople as well as physicians understood the necessity of preparing the body in this way. Van Diemerbroeck recorded that one Nicholas of Rostock, 'by the Advice of an old Woman,...swallowed twice or thrice a day, the quantity of an Acorn of new Butter...to smoothen the Urinary Vessels, and render the Passages slippery'.[129]

Once the body was fluxible, the humours could begin their journey towards the bodily exits. Nature drove the matter outwards, from the interior 'noble parts' (the most important organs, the brain, heart, and liver), to the exterior 'ignoble parts' (the less vital regions, such as the skin).[130] Galen explained that the humours moved from the stronger, to the weaker, organs, until eventually they arrived at the body's orifices:

> [T]he strongest part deposits its surplus matter in all the parts near to it; these...parts are weaker; these next into yet others; and this goes on for a long time, until the superfluity, being driven from one part to another, comes to rest in one of the weakest of all...Thus the tendency of the eliminative faculty is step by step.[131]

---

[126] Macollo, *XCIX canons*, 107–8. The word 'concoction' was also used to denote the process of making the body fluxible.

[127] Hart, *Klinike*, 277; A.T., *A rich store-house*, preface.

[128] Lemnius, *The secret miracles*, 97. See Wear, *Knowledge and Practice*, 90.

[129] Van Diemerbroeck, *The anatomy*, 95.

[130] Lemnius, *The secret miracles*, 109; *The aphorisms of Hippocrates*, 135. On the skin, see King and Zittel (eds.), *Blood, Sweat and Tears*, Part 3; Jonathan Reinarz and Kevin Siena (eds.), *Medical History of Skin: Scratching the Surface* (2013).

[131] Galen, *Galen on the natural faculties*, 297.

This outward motion was regarded as an 'inherent power' of Nature, which she used also in nutrition to remove waste products from the body.[132]

Once more, practitioners could assist Nature by diverting the humours from the noble organs, and drawing them towards the exterior: common methods included giving warm drinks, laying a 'red cloth...next to the Skin', or lighting a fire.[133] Alternatively, doctors could tie bands ('ligatures') to the feet and wrists, or rub or scarify these parts, so that the humours would be attracted to the inflamed outer regions. Bruele stated that in cases of apoplexy, 'there must...be used strong and painfull ligatures of the extreme parts, that...Nature being provoked by the vehemency of those pains, may drive out those ill humors...[from] the braine'.[134] This medical intervention is an example of the physician rising above the status of servant: he was cajoling Nature into doing what he thought was necessary, by giving a painful treatment. Perhaps such thinking was informed by patriarchal ideas about the role of husbands in family life: heads of the households were expected to administer 'sharp reproofes' to their subordinates as corrections for faults—male practitioners may therefore have conceived the use of such treatments as one of their duties as good patriarchs.[135] Given the value of painful ligatures in moving the humours, it would be tempting to agree with earlier generations of historians who painted deeply negative pictures of early modern medicine, suggesting that taking a remedy was like 'leaping out of the frying pan into the fire'.[136] This interpretation, however, does not take into account the caveats that were placed on the use of painful medicines. If the patient was very young, old, or weak, such treatments were to be avoided, on the grounds that the 'grief and pain' of the medicine would further 'sink' and 'annoy' Nature, so that she would not be able to 'resist the *Disease*'.[137] In these circumstances, it was necessary for the physician to abstain from using painful treatments, and instead 'bend all' his efforts to 'eas[ing] the pain of the *Disease*'.[138]

Medical authors believed it was possible to track the outward movement of the humours by the appearance of certain visible signs. One of the Hippocratic aphorisms states, 'swelling and redness arising on the brest of him who have a Squiancie [tonsillitis] is good, for the disease inclineth outwards'. An anonymous commentator explained, 'Hippocrates *shews that it is good to have all sores and diseases of the body to come from the noble and inward parts to the ignoble and outward ones*'.[139] Thus, if new symptoms or diseases developed in the outward parts, the patient could rest assured that such things, although inconvenient, were '*not dangerous,*

[132] Ibid., 61.

[133] J.S., *Paidon nosemata; or childrens diseases* (1664), 63; François Mauriceau, *The diseases of women with child*, trans. Hugh Chamberlen (1710, first English edn. 1672), 358.

[134] Bruele, *Praxis medicinae*, 81.

[135] John Dod and Robert Cleaver, *A godly form of household government* (1621, first publ. 1598), image 27.

[136] Lucinda Beier, *Sufferers and Healers: The Experience of Illness in Seventeenth-Century England* (1987), 107; Porter and Porter, *In Sickness and in Health*, 105; Guy Williams, *The Age of Agony: The Art of Healing, c.1700–1800* (1975).

[137] Galen, *Galen's method*, 258.   [138] Ibid.   [139] *The aphorismes of Hippocrates*, 36–7.

but rather conducing to health.[140] Conversely, the disappearance of these signs indicated that the humoral movement had been reversed, with the matter 'striking in', resulting in the exacerbation of illness, and sometimes, death. The physician of the royal household, Tobias Whitaker (d. 1664), warned that in smallpox,

> [A] retraction of the matter in motion from the circumference to the centre...[is] an almost irrecoverable disorder in natural motion, and very few upon such accidents do escape death.[141]

Laypeople agreed, as is poignantly revealed in the correspondence of the D'Ewes family from Suffolk. In 1641, Anne D'Ewes, aged 28, fell ill of smallpox while at her mother-in-law's home. On the third day of the illness, she was moved to another building, to prevent the spread of infection in the household. The 'woefull issue' of this action was her death: her husband Simonds wrote angrily to his mother, bewailing, 'the violence of her removal...without all question lost her her life'. He explained that her 'tender and delicate' body was exposed to 'the open air', which caused the humours to be 'driven in', so that they 'soone seized on the noble and blessed hearte of my dearest comforte'.[142] Thus, the reversed motion of the humours resulted from 'taking cold' from exposure to outdoor air.

At last we have reached the point at which the humours left the body. Lemnius marvelled at the variety of exits ordained for this purpose:

> God that made the body of man hath not in vain created so many wayes and passages to purge forth the humours. So the head purgeth it self by the Nostrills [and] Ears[;] the Palate, [by]...[s]neesing and spitting; The...Lungs by...coughing; the Stomach... by vomit...; The Intestines...by the belly...; The Reins...by the urinary passages...; all...sweat through the skin that is full of holes.[143]

Expulsion was carried out by Nature during what was known as the 'crisis of disease' or 'critical expulsion'. In Galenic texts, the crisis was defined as the 'swift and suddain' evacuation of humours at the height of illness, in the form of sweating, urination, vomiting, diarrhoea, haemorrhage, the bursting of pustules, or other emission.[144] It was regarded as the turning point in illness, 'whereby the sick is either brought to recovery, or death'.[145] In the mid-1600s, Van Diemerbroeck visited a young man, who had become ill after 'violent Exercises of Tennis,...and hard drinking of Wine'; on 'The seventh day the Measles [pustules] came out all over his Body by way of Crisis', and the disease 'quite vanished'.[146] Unlike in the case of concoction, this mechanism was described in masculine language, commonly linked to combat: the 'healthfull crisis', wrote Cotta, is 'the victorie of

---

[140] Ibid., 53.

[141] Tobias Whitaker, *An elenchus of opinions concerning the cure of the small pox* (1661), 34.

[142] Simonds D'Ewes, *The Autobiography and Correspondence of Sir Simonds D'Ewes, Bart.*, ed. J. O. Halliwell, 2 vols. (1845), vol. 2, 286.

[143] Lemnius, *The secret miracles*, 344.

[144] Culpeper, *Semeiotica uranica*, 17. On sweating crises, see Michael Stolberg, 'Sweat: Learned Concepts and Popular Perceptions', in King and Zittel (eds.), *Blood, Sweat and Tears*, 503–22.

[145] Framboisière, *The art of physick*, 117.

[146] Van Diemerbroeck, *The anatomy*, 38.

nature in the masterie of her enemie the disease'.[147] It was depicted as the decisive battle between Nature and the illness, upon which the outcome of sickness depended; such imagery was appropriate given the personification of this agent as a virago fighter. Sabine Kalff has shown that this metaphor was so entrenched that it was appropriated by political thinkers to justify military decisions.[148]

Descriptions of the crisis shed light on how disease was conceptualized. Although in theory the evacuated humour was the cause of disease rather than the disease itself, practitioners often elided the two. Culpeper, for instance, states 'nature labours to expell the humour that causeth the disease', but in another place, writes, 'nature did the best she could to expell the disease'.[149] Laypeople made similar inferences. Speaking of his friend Mr Hill's 'Touch of a Feaver', the antiquary William Clarke (1695–1771) noted that the 'opening of a Vein intirely remov'd it'.[150] By suggesting that the humours constituted the material basis of disease, such statements challenge the widespread historiographical notion that disease was conceived non-ontologically in Galenic thinking.[151] This research thus supports Michael's Stolberg's view that disease was thought of as an entity in the early modern period.[152] Another striking implication of the crisis theory is that it gave the impression that diseases characterized by evacuative symptoms cured themselves. 'Vomiting [is] cured with vomiting, and purging with purging', declared Whitaker.[153] It is probable that this notion brought comfort to patients: they could reassure themselves that however unpleasant the crisis, it might lead to their recovery. Doctors and laypeople waited for the crisis, and longed for it to occur. The country gentleman James Clavering (1680–1748) received a letter from his brother-in-law about the condition of his young son James, who was suffering from a lung illness: he said, 'I wish this humour wou[l]d grow and swell more to a head and then burst, as there is no hopes left without an extraordinary evacuation somewhere'.[154]

Nonetheless, an evacuation of humours did not guarantee recovery. The outcome of disease hinged on whether Nature was able to bring about a 'perfect crisis': Macollo stated, 'a perfect Crise is that which evacuates all the vicious matter, and an imperfect Crise is that which evacuates but some part of it; the former is sure, but the latter is not to be trusted'.[155] In turn, Nature's ability to achieve this complete evacuation depended on her strength, together with the location, volume, and quality of the offending humours. If the humours were situated in regions of the body which did not have easy access to one of the exit points, the disease usually became chronic. Gout was a case in point: Nature was able to push the matter to the joints of the hands and feet, but these regions lacked any 'convenient passage'

---

[147] Cotta, *A short discoverie*, 18; Whitaker, *An elenchus*, 22–3.

[148] Kalff, 'The Body as a Battlefield', 171.

[149] Culpeper, *Semeiotica uranica*, 163, 168. See also Clowes, *Aprooved practice*, 105.

[150] St John's College Library, Cambridge, Miscellaneous CL3, letter 1 (Letters of William Clarke, 1724).

[151] See Mary Lindemann, *Medicine and Society in Early Modern Europe* (Cambridge, 2010, first publ. 1999), 9.

[152] Stolberg, *Experiencing Illness*, 24–7. This idea is also expressed by Skuse, *Constructions of Cancer*.

[153] Whitaker, *An elenchus*, 82.   [154] Clavering, *The Correspondence*, 158, 160–1.

[155] Macollo, *XCIX canons*, 75.

to the exterior, and as a result, it was 'not wont to have *Crises*'.[156] Conversely, death occurred when the humours were so 'dire and potent', and 'furious and swelling', that Nature could not manage to expel them all, or else, she was 'so irritated by the untameable malignity of the matter, that it can no way digest it, but is forced by any meanes to send it away crude as it is'.[157] Whether or not the evacuation was deemed perfect depended largely on how patients felt in its wake: if they felt much better, then it was usually pronounced complete. There was a special word for this feeling, 'euphoria', which denoted the sense of physical and emotional ease that followed a successful crisis.[158] The fact that distinctions were drawn between perfect and imperfect crises contradicts the notion that individuals at this time equated evacuation with recovery.[159]

The patient's age and gender were important variables in the process of evacuation. The Parisian obstetrician François Mauriceau (1637–1709) wrote in his best-selling midwifery manual, 'Infants are not in so great danger as elder Persons, in as much as...they...have a thinner and softer Skin, thro which this Matter is easier expel'd, than thro theirs that is harder, and whose Pores are less open'.[160] Young men were especially proficient at evacuating humours through nosebleeds, since the upward motion of the blood required heat, and this age and sex was the hottest.[161] Women also enjoyed certain advantages: the vagina constituted an additional avenue through which humours could be removed, and for those of reproductive age, menstruation functioned as a useful purge.[162] Paré confirmed in 1634, 'women, by the benefit of their menstruall purgation, escape and are freed from great, pestilent, and absolutely deadly diseases'.[163] The sudden onset of menstruation during illness was regarded as Nature's method of cure.[164] According to Gianna Pomata, these monthly evacuations rendered 'the female...exemplary from a therapeutic point of view'.[165] Nonetheless, Nature did not let men down: she invented alternative ways to remove bad humours from males, most notably, haemorrhoids.[166] Speaking of putrid fever, the French physician Brice Bauderon (c.1540–1623) wrote, 'if the Patient...have the Haemorrhoids...or [in women]

---

[156] Boyle, *A free enquiry*, 222.   [157] Paré, *The workes*, 861; Hart, *Klinike*, 284.

[158] See Chapter 3, pp. 96, 107 on euphoria.   [159] See the Introduction, note 30.

[160] Mauriceau, *The diseases of women*, 357.

[161] Culpeper, *Semeiotica uranica*, 189. Male youth was described as the 'hot office': see Alexandra Shepard, *Meanings of Manhood in Early Modern England* (Oxford, 2006, first publ. 2003), 24.

[162] Wendy Churchill, *Female Patients in Early Modern Britain: Gender, Diagnosis, and Treatment* (Farnham, 2012), 151–2; Michael Stolberg, 'The Monthly Malady: A History of Premenstrual Suffering', *Medical History*, 44 (2000), 301–22, at 316–17. Stolberg argues that by the 1600s, 'the majority of learned physicians' no longer believed menstruation served a useful purging function, but this does not seem to have been the case in the English medical texts examined in my study: *Uroscopy*, 93.

[163] Paré, *The workes*, 863.

[164] For instance, Thomas Willis, *Willis's Oxford Casebook (1650–52)*, ed. Kenneth Dewhurst (Oxford, 1981), 134. For other examples, see Churchill, *Female Patients*, 152 (William Petty writing in the 1640s and Richard Wilkes in the 1740s).

[165] Pomata, 'Menstruating Men', 138. Others disagree; for a summary of the debate, see Lisa Smith, 'The Body Embarrassed? Rethinking the Leaky Male Body in Eighteenth-Century England and France', *Gender & History*, 23 (2010), 26–46.

[166] Lisa Smith argues that in the 1700s, male forms of bleeding were recast as pathological, rather than as cathartic: 'The Body Embarrassed?'

the Courses appearing, then the whole business is to be committed to Nature'.[167] The haemorrhoids resembled menstruation, because it 'sometimes keeps a Lunar Motion like the Feminine Sex', explained John Archer (*fl.* 1660–84), court phys- ician to Charles II, in his book of medical secrets.[168] Patients' occupations might also affect their evacuative capabilities. When tending the soldiers at the 'campe at *Amiens*', Paré noticed that many of these men 'purged forth...blood' by stool: the reason was the 'excessive heat of the summers sunne, and the minds of the enraged souldierss', which produced 'great quantity of acride and cholericke humour' that 'flowed into the belly'.[169]

The theory of the critical evacuation had implications for medical treatment. Namely, it was considered inadvisable to relieve the evacuative symptoms of ill- ness.[170] Speaking of diarrhoea, Barrough insisted, 'you must suffer and watch, till nature hath bestowed all her care', warning, 'to stoppe the fluxe, it causeth a worse and greater disease'.[171] This idea was expressed by laypeople as well as physicians, and persisted into the eighteenth century.[172] It was feared that if the evacuations were stopped prematurely, the humours would be 'turned backe' into the interior, where they would harm the noble organs.[173] Rather than stopping the evacuations, the practitioner's role was to monitor, and when required, promote such emissions. In theory, the latter intervention was only judged necessary when Nature seemed to be struggling to produce an evacuation.[174] Van Diemerbroeck reported that one Monseiur de Guade, a French captain, was taken with nausea and a great desire to vomit, but 'he [could] not Vomit up very much'; the doctor administered a 'good draught of the Decoction of Barley', and the result was that he was able to vomit 'a great quantity'.[175] De Guade's nausea was a sign that Nature wanted the patient to vomit, and indicated that the practitioner should assist by administering an emetic. On the other hand, had this patient been already vomiting profusely, there would have been no need to promote the evacuation, since Nature was clearly coping on her own.[176] Given that practitioners were only supposed to prescribe evacuative treatments when their patients 'desired' that evacuation, early modern medicine begins to appear less barbaric than it has been conventionally portrayed.[177]

On those occasions when it *was* necessary for the practitioner to administer an evacuative treatment, he was instructed to consider the 'inclinations of Nature'. This meant choosing the type of evacuation that this agent seemed to be attempting.[178] Such a strategy, which endured into the 1700s, exemplifies the subservient position

---

[167] Bauderon, *The expert phisician*, 79–80.
[168] John Archer, *Secrets disclosed of consumptions* (1684), 42.   [169] Paré, *The workes*, 864–5.
[170] Historians are aware of this—for instance, Stolberg, *Experiencing Illness*, 91, 94; Schoenfeldt, *Bodies and Selves*, 14.
[171] Barrough, *The methode*, 95. See also Symcotts, *A Seventeenth Century Doctor*, 19.
[172] Rachel Russell, *Letters of Rachel, Lady Russell*, 2 vols. (1853, first publ. 1773), vol. 2, 67; Benjamin Rogers, *The Diary of Benjamin Rogers Rector of Carlton, 1720–71*, ed. C. D. Linnell Symcotts, Bedfordshire Historical Record Society, vol. 31 (Streatley, 1951), 88.
[173] Paré, *The workes*, 1027.   [174] For example, Hart, *Klinike*, 284.
[175] Van Diemerbroeck, *The anatomy*, 77.
[176] *The aphorismes of Hippocrates*, 19; Hart, *Klinike*, 236.   [177] See note 136 in this chapter.
[178] Van Diemerbroeck, *The anatomy*, 27; Maynwaringe, *The catholic medicine*, 5–6.

of physicians.[179] How could practitioners discern Nature's inclinations? Thinking back to Anthony Walker, he had demanded to be blood-let on the grounds that he had suffered a nosebleed, a sign that Nature wished to purge his body of blood.[180] Each evacuation was signalled by a particular sign—sweating, for example, was suggested through 'moystnesse of the skin', while diarrhoea was hinted by 'gripings… [and] murmuring… of the guts'.[181] Doctors warned that to fail to follow Nature's intentions would 'move or irritate' this agent so that she would 'greedily keep back' the humours, and refuse to cooperate with the practitioner.[182] Such language implies disapproval on the part of physicians for Nature's recalcitrant response, despite the fact that it was really their fault for failing to obey her inclinations.

There was, however, an important caveat to the rule of following Nature's inclinations, which provided practitioners with an opportunity to rise above the status of servant: her inclinations were not always trustworthy. Sprengell commented, 'she… *Errs* now and then in selecting *improper Organs*, and attempting her… *Excretions* through incongruent… Passages'.[183] Typical examples included the use of 'the Nipples, the Mouth, or the Eyes' for the voiding of blood, situations in which practitioners sought 'to oblige *Nature* to alter Her Purpose'.[184] The fact that doctors distinguished between different passages of the body, and considered some more appropriate than others for the evacuation of humours, contradicts the historical view that the early modern body was depicted as a hollow container, within which fluids could move around freely and unconstrained.[185]

Evacuative treatments worked in different ways. 'Issues' (incisions to the skin) allowed the continual draining of fluids in the form of pus: a pip was usually placed in the wound, so that it would not close. Phlebotomy—blood-letting—was performed using a lancet, scarification, or leeches. The suppuration of pustules, together with sweating, were induced by plasters, hot baths, piling on more bed-clothes, or taking simples 'somewhat hot and drie', like china root.[186] Evacuation by urine was provoked by 'hot and dry' medicines called 'diureticks', which, 'by their attractive faculty', drew the 'thinnest serositie… into the bladder'.[187] Vomiting was induced by giving 'naucous and vomitory' medicines which, through their bitter taste and smell, caused the stomach to 'rid itself' of the matter.[188] Finally, purges worked by drawing the noxious humours to themselves, and then thrusting the mixture outwards.[189] Laypeople seem to have been familiar with these ideas. The poet and Dean of St Paul's Cathedral, John Donne (1572–1631), wrote that purging physic 'drawes the *peccant humour* to it selfe, that when it is gathered together, the weight of it selfe may carry the humour away'.[190] Of course, the exact mechanisms were not always known: medics acknowledged that 'every kinde' of

[179] William Vickers, *An easie and safe method for curing the King's evil* (1711), 17–18.
[180] Walker, *The vertuous wife*, 59.   [181] Paré, *The workes*, 861–2.
[182] Bauderon, *The expert physician*, 59; Lemnius, *The secret miracles*, 129.
[183] Sprengell, 'Natura Morborum Medicatrix', 333.   [184] Boyle, *A free enquiry*, 333–4.
[185] This conception of the body was first proposed by Duden, *Woman Beneath the Skin*, 109, 123–30.
[186] Hart, *Klinike*, 291.   [187] Ibid., 311.
[188] Paré, *The workes*, 1032.   [189] Lemnius, *The secret miracles*, 260–1.
[190] John Donne, *Devotions upon emergent occasions and severall steps in my sicknes* (1624), 243.

medicine 'hath that secret vertue' or 'inexplicable quality', which physicians 'cannot by any reason finde out... but only [know] by experience'.[191]

Thus far, it has been implied that recovery always involved evacuation, a view which many medical historians would support.[192] However, this was not the case—on some occasions, the opposite process was required, retention. One of the Hippocratic aphorisms states, 'Diseases which are bred of satiety... are cured by evacuation and those which proceed from emptiness are cured by fulness.'[193] Almost completely overlooked in the historiography, retention meant the termination of evacuative symptoms, and the replenishment of lost humours. It was required when the crisis had been too violent, or when the disease itself had been caused by a shortage of humours.[194] Often, Nature was to blame—in keeping with her female identity, she was inclined to be 'exorbitant' with her evacuations, removing too great a quantity of the humours. Boyle observed satirically, 'Physicians oftentimes... employ their best Skill... to suppress... the inordinate Motions... that... *Nature* rashly begins to make'; so far 'from taking *Nature* for his Mistress', the physician spends 'a great Part' of his time 'hinder[ing] her from doing what She seems to Design'.[195] In this situation, the power balance between Nature and the doctor is overturned.

The process of retention was the reverse of the process of evacuation: the humours had to be made *in*fluxible. Barrough suggested that this could be achieved 'by cooling [the humour], or by thickening it, or else... by shutting & occluding the... wayes wherby it would flow out'.[196] Physicians sometimes administered orally what might usually be regarded as inedible substances to congeal the humours. Van Diemerbrock recorded that when the French army was taken with dysentery, the physicians 'took white Wax... cut... very small', and boiled it in milk 'till the Wax was perfectly melted', and then 'gave their Patient that Milk... hot... to drink'. As the wax cooled in the body, it would set, thereby thickening the humours.[197] Other methods included placing physical barriers at the exit points, such as 'Tents of new Cloth' in the nostrils to staunch nosebleeds, or inducing alternative evacuations in the hope that a new emission would stop the original one.[198] A typical example was to administer a laxative to a patient who was vomiting—the humours would be 'turne[d] out... at the back-door', and diverted from the stomach to the bowels, where they could be expelled more safely.[199] Finally, retention could be achieved by replacing the lost humours: Barrough stated that 'in them which have the convulsion caused by emptiness, the dyet must be moist', such as 'soupinges & fat brothes', and 'wyne that is thinne and watery, which maye quickly be dispersed into all partes of the body'.[200] Bathing was also

---

[191] A.T., *A rich store-house*, preface; Paré, *The workes*, 1032–3.
[192] For example, Gianna Pomata, *Contracting a Cure: Patients, Healers, and the Law in Early Modern Bologna* (1998, first publ. 1994), 133.
[193] *The aphorismes of Hippocrates*, 26.   [194] Barrough, *The methode*, 108.
[195] Boyle, *A free enquiry*, 228, 325, 332.   [196] Barrough, *The methode*, 215.
[197] Van Diemerbroeck, *The anatomy*, 73.   [198] Hall, *Select observations*, 57.
[199] Lemnius, *The secret miracles*, 18; Culpeper, *Semeiotica*, 162.
[200] Barrough, *The methode*, 33.

useful—'through the moisture' of a 'bath of sweete water', the patient 'may recover the hum[i]ditie that is lost'.[201]

Laypeople as well as practitioners attempted retention, thus indicating once again their shared understanding of the mechanisms through which disease was removed. Domestic recipe books are replete with remedies for the 'staunching of fluxes'. The collection associated with the gentlewoman Elizabeth Okeover (b. 1644), for instance, suggests taking a powder of burnt bacon in posset to 'stop a laxe or bloody Flux'.[202] Letters provide more moving insights into the experiences of family members as they strived, and sometimes failed, to restrain Nature's evacuations. In 1647, the Buckinghamshire politician Ralph Verney (1613–96) wrote to his uncle about the diarrhoea of his eight-year-old daughter Pegg: despite giving 'Asses Milke', a thickening agent, 'wee can by noe means stay it, nor thicken the Humours, [for]…she comonly goes to stoole 16, 18, or 20 times in 24 howors'. He concluded his letter with the mournful words, 'I am soe full of affliction that I can say no more but pray for us'.[203] Although it is harder to uncover the practices of lower socio-economic groups, second-hand evidence suggests they too sought to end violent evacuations. The Huntingdon physician John Symcotts (c.1592–1662) recorded in his casebook that in 1639, a certain 'cook-maid' staunched the nosebleed of the thirteen-year-old daughter of her Mistress, Lady Cotton. The maid 'boldly took a cloth wet in cold water', and made the girl 'sit upon it, and so [it] was stayed'.[204] Popular medical lore taught that there was a connection between the nose and womb; since the girl was at the age of menarche, it is possible that the cook was trying to divert the blood from the nose to the womb through this treatment, where it could be safely evacuated through menstruation.[205]

Age had an impact on how the patient fared when it came to retention. The elderly did well because their skin was dense and impermeable, making it more difficult for the humours to escape.[206] On the other hand, however, their comparative dryness meant that they were especially vulnerable to diseases caused by depletion, and they could afford to lose a smaller volume of humours before they became unwell. Children, by contrast, had very weak powers of retention—the sphincters encircling the orifices of the body were saturated with fluid, so they had more trouble keeping the exits shut, and yet their high levels of moisture meant that retention was not usually so urgent in this age group, as they had reserves.[207] In short, disease was removed through processes of concoction and expulsion or

[201] Ibid., 174.
[202] WL, MS.3712/71, fol. 71r (Elizabeth Okeover). See also from the WL, MS.160/36, fols. 28v–29r (Anne Brumwich); MS.3009/37, fol. 42r (Elizabeth Jacob); MS.4338/43, fol. 56v (Johanna Saint John).
[203] BL, M.636/8; no folio numbers (a letter from Ralph Verney to Dr Denton, dated 13 October 1647).
[204] Symcotts, *A Seventeenth Century Doctor*, 71.
[205] Holly Dugan, *The Ephemeral History of Perfume: Scent and Sense in Early Modern England* (Baltimore MD, 2011), 117.
[206] Mauriceau, *The diseases of women*, 357.
[207] Galen, *Galen on Diseases*, 295–6; W.S., *A family jewel, or the womans councellor* (1704), 66. See Newton, *The Sick Child*, 56–61.

retention, with the power balance between Nature and the physician varying in accordance with how successfully the former was thought to be performing the mechanisms.

One gap in the above account is the powerful role of the imagination and passions in the removal of disease.[208] Quoting Galen, the medical writer and cleric John Harris (1667–1719) averred, '*confidence doth more good then Physick*': when patients 'erroniously concev[e] things better then…they really are', the imagination 'causeth a vehement passion of hope, wherewith followeth' feelings of joy:

> [T]wo passions [which] awake and rouse up the…Spirits, and unite them together,…
> which thus…do most effectually…strengthen her [Nature] in the performance of
> any Corporal action…[in this case] the mastery and expulsion of noxious humours.[209]

Thus, the hope and joy evoked by the expectation of recovery strengthened the spirits, Nature's instruments, so that she could go about the task of removing disease more powerfully. This thinking was articulated when justifying the use of placebos, and it explained doctors' emphasis on the need to 'nourish' cheerful passions in their patients.[210] It was also invoked in medical advertisements for panaceas or cure-alls, and defences of these 'universal medicines': doctors insisted that such treatments worked by strengthening the spirits, so that Nature was empowered to fight whatever disease she faced.[211] Such an explanation made more credible the notion that one remedy could combat any distemper.

HELMONTIANS

To demonstrate the pervasiveness of the tripartite model of the agents of recovery, this final section examines the beliefs of a group of physicians who rejected many of the other key features of Galenic medicine, the Helmontians. Helmontians were supporters of the Flemish doctor and chemist Jan Baptista van Helmont, who in turn had been strongly influenced by the Swiss medical reformer Paracelsus (1493–1541). This movement was part of the development of the 'new science', which repudiated the learning of the ancients; it was also deeply religious—Helmont

---

[208] More attention has been given to the negative, than the positive, impact of the imagination and passions; much of this work focuses on mothers' influence on their babies in the womb—see H. Roodenburg, 'The Maternal Imagination: The Fears of Pregnant Women in Seventeenth-Century Holland', *Journal of Social History*, 21 (1988), 701–16; David Turner, *Disability in Eighteenth-Century England* (Abingdon, 2012), 44–5; Philip Wilson, *Surgery, Skin and Syphilis: Daniel Turner's London (1667–1741)* (Amsterdam, 1999), ch. 6. On the role of the imagination in causing disease, see David Gentilcore, 'The Fear of Disease and the Disease of Fear', in William Naphy and Penny Roberts (eds.), *Fear in Early Modern Society* (Manchester and New York, 1997), 184–208; Y. Haskell (ed.), *Diseases of the Imagination and Imaginary Disease in the Early Modern Period* (Leiden, 2011). There are several scholars, however, who have examined the positive impact of emotions on health—see Chapter 2, notes 165, 175.

[209] Harris, *The divine physician*, 150–1.

[210] Ibid., to the reader. See also Hart, *Klinike*, 357–8; Timothy Nourse, *A discourse upon the nature and faculties of man* (1686), 99–100.

[211] For example, see Francis Anthony, *The apologie, or defence of…a medicine called aurum potabile* (1616), 13–16.

believed that Galenism's roots were pagan, and was convinced he had been sent by God to bring a truly Christian form of medicine into the world. In England, the influence of Helmontianism peaked in the 1660s, when thirty-five physicians nearly succeeded in establishing a Society of Chemical Physicians.[212] In the end, however, this brand of medicine failed to topple Galenism: by the close of the seventeenth century, it had been largely absorbed into humoral medical practice.[213] Through comparing Galenic and Helmontian explanations of the removal of disease, it will be possible to arrive at a better understanding not just of why the agency of Nature proved so resilient, but also the likely reasons for the Helmontian failure.

Helmontians agreed with Galenists on the roles of God, Nature, and the physician in recovery. Helmont affirmed 'that thing *Hippocrates* so long agoe smelt out...that Nature alone...is the Physitianess of Diseases, but the Physitian the Minister or Servant'.[214] There were, however, differences in vocabulary: Helmontians usually substituted the term 'Nature' with the word 'Archeus', a term defined as 'the Arch Preeminent Author of Health'.[215] Like Nature, the Archeus carried out all the body's basic functions, including digestion, reproduction, and the removal of disease. Helmontians used the terms 'Nature' and 'Archeus' interchangeably, and on occasions made it clear that the two were synonymous. In his popular chemical treatise, the physician Thomas Cock (b. 1630), referred to 'Nature, i.e. [the] *Archeus*', and in another place spoke of the '*Archeus* or Nature'.[216] In dictionaries these two concepts are merged.[217] Nevertheless, the Archeus and Nature were distinguished in their sex—the former was male, although, as we will see below, he was described using feminine imagery. A possible reason for favouring the male Archeus over the female Nature was its lack of heathen connotations: Carolyn Merchant has shown that the female identity of this agent is age-old, dating back to pagan times.[218] The resemblance between these agents in their physiological functions indicates that the Archeus was not such a novel invention as has sometimes been implied by historians.[219]

While agreeing about the agents of recovery, Helmontians and Galenists diverged in their understanding of the causes of disease. Helmont asserted, 'a Disease is not a certain distemperature of elementary qualities,...as hitherto the *Galenists* have dreamed', but rather, 'it is a strange Image...out of the Archeus'.[220] Dismissing the humours as 'frivolous...fictions', human bodies were instead composed of just

---

[212] Wear, *Knowledge and Practice*, ch. 8; Anselment, *The Realms of Apollo*, 34–7.

[213] Wear, *Knowledge and Practice*, ch. 9.

[214] Jean Baptiste van Helmont, *Van Helmont's works containing his most excellent philosophy, physick, chirurgery, anatomy* (1664), 524.

[215] Thomson, *Ortho-methodoz*, 64.

[216] Thomas Cock, *Kitchin-physick: or, advice for the poor* (1676), Part 1, 41, Part 2, 6.

[217] Steven Blankaart, *A physical dictionary* (1684), 28.

[218] Merchant, *The Death of Nature*, xix, xxiii.

[219] For example, Peter Elmer (ed.), *The Healing Arts: Health, Disease and Society in Europe 1500–1800* (Manchester, 2004), 123.

[220] Helmont, *Van Helmont's works*, 552.

two elements: water and 'Ferment', an 'active, brisk, aetherial substance'.[221] Helmont taught that after the Fall, the Archeus had been 'pierced or defiled' by innumerable 'diseasie ideas'.[222] Compared to the seeds of plants, these immaterial ideas were like blueprints for every sort of disease: in health, they lay dormant, but as soon as the Archeus began to think about them, they 'hatched', 'spread[ing] into various Branches, and Fruits', and harming the organs.[223] The Archeus began to dwell on these ideas when it became 'sorrowful, angry, ... [or] vexed', a description which implied this agent was like an enraged woman who had become 'violent and disobedient'.[224] Such notions were informed by the belief that females had particularly powerful imaginations, and were prone to anger.[225] Helmont's deep religiosity, and his belief in the sinful state of mankind, also shaped this theory. In sum, whereas Galenists regarded disease as a state of malfunctioning caused by the alteration of the humours, Helmontians defined it as a 'strange idea' fashioned by the Archeus or Nature herself.[226]

In the light of these contrasting ideas about disease causation, it followed that Galenists and Helmontians held different views about how recovery occurred. As we saw earlier, for Galenists, the processes involved rectifying the humours; by contrast, Helmontians taught that illness was overcome by removing 'the ... Idea of the Disease in the *Archeus*'.[227] There were two ways to do this. The first was to strengthen the Archeus, so that it was better able to resist the disease ideas. Helmontians used 'sympathetic' remedies: the opposite to Galenic allopathic treatments, these were medicines which 'have Similtude' with the Archeus, such as highly purified minerals. It was believed that, 'seeing Like doth readily unite with Like', the Archeus and medicine would 'embrace each other intimately', whereby the 'Spirits', the instruments through which the Archeus worked, 'in a moment [are] encreased' and strengthened.[228] By depicting the Archeus and medicine as close friends, Helmontians hoped to make their remedies appealing to their patients.

The second method for removing disease was to 'pacify and gratify' the Archeus, so that it 'layeth aside' its rage.[229] This was achieved through giving 'exquisite', 'delectable' medicines, of 'grateful smell and taste'.[230] The leading English Helmontian, George Thomson (1619–77), imagined the medicine would be 'Conducted into the very Bed-Chamber' of the body, where its beauty would be shown in a 'Looking-Glass' to the Archeus; the contrast between 'the ugly shape of the Disease', and the beautiful medicine would be so great that the Archeus

---

[221] Ibid., 1, 30–1; William Bacon, *A key to Helmont* (1682), 3.

[222] Helmont, *Van Helmont's works*, 491, 535, 548; Thomson, *Ortho-methodoz*, 18, 21.

[223] Thomson, *Ortho-methodoz*, 19.

[224] Helmont, *Van Helmont's works*, 548; Thomson, *Ortho-methodoz*, 12, 21.

[225] Helmont, *Van Helmont's works*, 505. On women's proneness to anger, see A. Ross, *Arcana microcosmi or the hidden secrets of man's body* (1652, first publ. 1651), 86; Linda Pollock, 'Anger and the Negotiation of Relationships in Early Modern England', *The Historical Journal*, 47 (2004), 567–90, at 570. On women's imagination, see Fletcher, *Gender, Sex, and Subordination*, 71–3.

[226] Thomson, *Ortho-methodoz*, 20.

[227] George Thomson, *Galeno-pale: or, a chymical trial of the Galenists* (1665), 99; Thomson, *Ortho-methodoz*, 62, 117.

[228] Thomson *Ortho-methodoz*, 64–6.   [229] Ibid., 106.   [230] Ibid., 66, 86.

would 'Repent of Former Errors', and end its diseasie thoughts.[231] Rather than using language of warfare and housework, Helmontians deployed imagery of light, beauty, and feasting. Medicines were 'beautiful objects' that 'send forth Lively Illustrious Beams' into the body, 'scatter[ing] those black clouds of mischievous Idea's [*sic*]'.[232] Physic was a 'Dainty Morsel for the Archeus to Banquet on . . . feasting upon [it] with admirable delight'.[233] Light was the emblem of Helmontianism, chosen for its religious associations—Christ 'is the truth, the life, the light', who had enlightened Helmontians to understand the true art of curing.[234] The references to beauty tap into popular gender stereotypes, namely the vanity of women, and their penchant for pretty things like jewellery.[235] In these descriptions, the personalities of the Galenic Nature and the Helmontian Archeus seem very different: the antithesis of the hardworking cleaner, the Archeus was a spoiled queen. Given that Helmontian physic sounds far more pleasant than Galenic medicine, it might seem incongruous that the latter remained more popular. Andrew Wear suggests that people were so accustomed to the notion that the 'medicine must be as bitter as the disease', that to take a medicine of pleasing smell and taste would instantly have raised doubts about its efficacy.[236]

Why did Helmontians retain the precept that 'Nature is the healer of the disease', whilst rejecting other fundamentals of Galenism? One vital reason was that it offered valuable opportunities for anti-Galenic propaganda. Helmontians sought to undermine the very foundation upon which Galenic physic rested by accusing its practitioners of failing to fulfil their roles as Nature's servants. 'Far from assisting . . . Nature', the Galenic doctor 'becomes a *hindrance* . . . to her', declared Thomson.[237] Helmontian attacks centred on the effects of evacuative treatments, which they believed 'are pernicious to . . . Nature, destroying more then ever the Sword'.[238] Essentially, Galenic intervention exacerbated the cause of illness: it 'enrage[s] the Archeus, stirring up Storms . . . in the Microcosm', thereby encouraging this agent to dwell even more on the 'diseasie ideas'.[239] Rhetorically, it was useful that Nature was personified—it made for a more emotive argument: this fragile female was 'fretted, gall'd, or opprest with . . . *disgusting* medicines'; she was 'betrayed', 'worried by a Disease, and thrown flat on [her] . . . back . . . by cruel Phlebotomy, [and] poisonous Purgations'.[240] In short, the agency of Nature was preserved by Helmontians because it was simply too useful to relinquish—they could fight Galenists at their own game by undermining their mission as physicians.

CONCLUSION

In early modern England, disease was believed to be removed by the combined efforts of three agents: God, Nature, and the practitioner. While scholars are familiar

[231] Ibid., 117.   [232] Ibid., 106.   [233] Ibid., 115.
[234] Wear, *Knowledge and Practice*, 377.   [235] Fletcher, *Gender, Sex and Subordination*, 21–4.
[236] Wear, *Knowledge and Practice*, 405–12.   [237] Thomson, *Galeno-pale*, 93–5.
[238] Ibid., 2.   [239] Thomson, *Ortho-methodoz*, 50.
[240] Thomson, *Galeno-pale*, 37.

with the roles of providence and medicine, the vital agency of Nature has been largely overlooked. Nature was the body's internal healing agent, the equivalent to the modern idea of the immune system. By drawing attention to this forgotten agent, the chapter has sought to transform our understanding of the rationale behind medical treatments at this time. As the physician Francis Anthony (1550–1623) explained:

> [N]ot the Medicine, but nature alone is the true physition, curing all infirmities... In all diseases the Physitions part is, to promote the indeavour of nature to expel the offending humors by those passages, which herselfe sheweth and directeth.[241]

Remedies were thus designed to do what Nature was already attempting. An awareness of this thinking helps us to overcome a pressing challenge faced in the history of early modern medicine: the urge to pass judgements on pre-modern medical practices. Whilst it is no longer acceptable in academic circles to ridicule early modern medicine, in the sphere of popular history, this attitude continues to dominate. By properly appreciating the rationale behind treatment, those medicines which might have initially appeared irrational—such as giving a laxative to a patient who is vomiting—are suddenly rendered more understandable. The significance of these findings extends beyond medical history, to the history of physiology more generally: Nature was responsible for carrying out all the body's basic functions, as is indicated by the word 'physis', which means 'nature' in Greek.[242] Nature's role also has implications for religious history: if we study what this agent *could* accomplish, we will be in a better position to understand events which were classed as *super*natural—above nature—such as miracle cures. This chapter has concentrated mainly on the relationship between Nature and physicians; it invites further studies on the interactions between God and Nature, as well as the host of other healthcare providers who attended the sick, such as nurses, female practitioners, and surgeons. Finally, it would be fruitful to consider how conceptions of recovery were influenced by the rise of 'medical specifics' and proprietary medicines, treatments designed to target particular diseases.[243]

A recurring theme in this chapter has been the complex gender and power dynamics between Nature and the physician. In theory, the latter 'is not directer and Master, but minister and servant' to Nature, but in practice the balance of authority was rather more ambivalent, with the physician frequently appearing like Nature's co-governor, or even the superior party.[244] These complexities

---

[241] Anthony, *The apologie*, 13. This is similar wording to that used by the thirteenth-century bishop and medical writer of Lincoln, Robert Grosseteste, in his treatise, *De artibus liberalibus*: 'Medicine is the assistant of nature, and helps nature to expel illness; and medicine does not heal, but rather nature assisted by medicine' (translation from the Latin). This is one of many medieval texts that demonstrate the longevity of ideas about Nature's role. My thanks to Prof. Anne Lawrence-Mathers for sharing the extract. I would also like to thank Dr Martin Edwards for informing me that Nature's role continued to be acknowledged in the 1700s and 1800s by European physicians, though the strength of this agent's power was located in the body's 'nervous energy' or force rather than in the spirits; see note 96 for examples.

[242] OED (accessed 2/10/13).   [243] On medical specifics see the Introduction, note 64.

[244] Anthony, *The apologie*, 16.

reflect wider cultural paradoxes surrounding womankind: female Nature was benevolent and caring, but also impetuous and weak. This fallibility legitimized the interventions of the practitioner, and in so doing provided opportunities for gender construction: the doctor could see himself as a gallant hero who rescued the swooning Nature, or as a wise patriarch who restrained her 'outrageous' acts. In one sense, it was entirely appropriate that Nature was female—concoction was akin to cooking, and expulsion resembled washing. And yet recovery was also described in masculine language: it was a battle between a princely Nature and the enemy disease. Contemporaries may have reconciled this gender paradox by considering that Nature, like a loving mother, would fight to the death to protect her child, the human body.

The removal of disease was 'chiefly busied about [the] Humours': the morbid matter had to be corrected through processes of concoction and expulsion or retention.[245] Historians are more familiar with expulsion than with the other two processes, but I hope to have shown that the former was rather more complicated than has been recognized. People pictured the 'thicke grosse' humours being chopped and scrubbed by Nature, and pushed outwards from one organ to the next, until at last they arrived at the bodily exits. These lucid imaginings demonstrate the importance of the organs and vessels in early modern bodily understandings, a finding that supports the recent 'body in parts' historiographical approach, which challenges the entrenched notion that such structures hardly featured in concepts of the body at this time.[246] The research also contributes to debates about illness, concurring with Michael Stolberg that disease could be envisaged ontologically in the early modern period.

This study has supported Wendy Churchill's thesis that early modern medicine recognized multiple differences between individuals, which included the variables of age and sex.[247] We have seen that women and the elderly, in contrast to the young and men, were cold, a quality that hindered concoction. On the other hand, females benefited from an extra mechanism for the ejection of humours, menstruation, and old people had better powers of retention, useful in diseases caused by depletion. Such contradictory notions reflect contemporary tensions in attitudes to these groups: women and the elderly were simultaneously venerated for their wisdom and piety, and denigrated for their decrepitude and weakness.

Finally, this chapter has compared Galenic and Helmontian ideas about recovery as a way to demonstrate how deeply ingrained the notion of Nature had become in early modern medicine. Helmontians rejected some of the core components of Galenic medicine, and yet they did not part from the precept that 'Nature is the healer of disease, and the physician but the servant'. This may have been because the axiom was flexible, and could be applied to any medical theory. A more important reason, however, was that the personification of Nature served as powerful propaganda upon which rival groups could promote themselves and denigrate their opponents. Helmontians accused Galenists of being cruel oppressors of 'sweet

---

[245] Galen, *Galens art of physic*, 118.   [246] See the Introduction, note 19.
[247] Churchill, *Female Patients*, 176, 178.

Nature', and depicted themselves as her 'kindly friends'.[248] In view of the competitive character of the 'medical marketplace' of early modern England, there was a great demand for this sort of emotive strategy.[249] Given that Helmontian medicine was probably more pleasant than Galenic physic, we might wonder why the latter continued to dominate in this period. A likely reason is that the Helmontian theory was emotionally less palatable than the Galenic one. Although Galenists also believed that humankind was responsible for disease—God brought illness as a punishment for sin—their version of Nature was not so explicitly culpable. Nature cured, rather than caused, disease. By contrast, the Helmontian Archeus appeared a sinister figure, who could at any moment bring disease simply by thinking about it. Nature's role was also attractive to patients—it gave them an excuse to abstain from medicines when they wished, on the grounds that their internal healer would do the job instead. The grocer and ironmonger William Stout (1665–1752) boasted that 'for therty years past', he had not consulted any physicians, 'but always let nature...worke a cure'.[250] Ultimately, however, the appeal of Galenic theory lay in its capacity to make illness seem less terrifying to the sick: it transformed the most painful part of illness—the crisis—into the method of cure.

---

[248] Maynwaringe, *The catholic medicine*, 6.
[249] On the 'medical marketplace', see the Introduction, note 21.
[250] William Stout, *The Autobiography of William Stout of Lancaster, 1665–1752*, ed. J. D. Marshall (Manchester, 1967), 178.

2

'She Sleeps Well and Eats an Egg':
Restoring Strength

In the mid-sixteenth century, the Dutch physician Levinus Lemnius (1505–68) provided a vivid picture of the patient after a serious illness. He likened him to a victim of highway robbery:

> [A] Traveller that is got out of Theives hands, he yet pants and trembles, and is not wholly restored from the great fear and danger of his life;...so a sick man, though...his disease is gone, and he begins to...find all things better with him, yet some footsteps of the disease stay...in his body...he is weak, feeble, exhausted, and of little force.[1]

Early modern patients and their families and physicians routinely observed that disease left the body weak and emaciated, full of the 'footsteps of disease', to use Lemnius' phrase. It was not until full strength and flesh had been restored, that the patient was pronounced back to health. Chapter 1 was about the removal of disease; this chapter turns to the second part of recovery, the restoration of strength, or 'convalescence'. It asks how doctors and laypeople measured the patient's growing strength after illness, and analyses the physiological processes through which this restitution was thought to occur. I argue that both the measures, and the mechanisms, for the restoration of strength were intimately connected to the 'non-natural things', the six dietary and life-style factors which were believed to affect the body—excretion, sleep, food, passions, air, and exercise.[2] Patients' sleeping patterns, appetites for foods, and emotions, along with other inclinations and behaviours that related to the non-naturals, were used to track their progression on 'the road to health'. Medical practitioners and the patient's family sought to regulate each non-natural in an effort to promote the body's restoration, and guard against possible relapse. It is suggested that this regulation, together with the meticulous monitoring of the patient's growing strength, constituted a concept of convalescent care, or to use the early modern term, 'analeptics'.

By uncovering the roles of the non-naturals in convalescence, this chapter responds to Sandra Cavallo and Tessa Storey's plea for more attention to be paid to

---

[1] Levinus Lemnius, *The secret miracles of nature* (1658, first publ. 1559), 243–4. My thanks to Manchester University Press for permitting in this chapter the use of material from my contribution, 'She Sleeps Well and Eats an Egg: Convalescent Care in Early Modern England', in Sandra Cavallo and Tessa Storey (eds.), *Conserving Health in Early Modern Culture: Bodies and Environments in Italy and England* (Manchester, 2017), 104–32.
[2] See note 3 for literature on the non-naturals.

these factors.[3] The discussions will deepen our understanding of these phenomena in two ways. Firstly, we will uncover the precise mechanisms through which these factors affected the body. Usually historians suggest that the non-naturals 'influenced the balance, movement, and evacuation of the body's humors', but here we will see that they also changed the condition of the 'spirits'.[4] Secondly, this chapter will show that the non-naturals played a crucial, hitherto overlooked, prognostic function, as each one could be used as a sign and measure of growing health.

Convalescent care has rarely been addressed in the historiography of early modern medicine, perhaps because scholars have assumed that it was a later, nineteenth-century invention. Indeed, the word 'convalescence' conjures up an image of Victorian gentlefolk at the seaside or in the mountains, an impression enhanced by the proliferation of convalescence homes from the mid-1800s.[5] This is deceptive, however, for the concept had far older origins—it was rooted in Hippocratic–Galenic medical traditions, appearing in discussions of what was known as the 'neutral body'. Seldom recognized outside the realms of intellectual history, the neutral body was a category of bodily states into which were placed all those patients who were deemed 'neither sick nor sound', such as the 'decrepit elderly', newly delivered mothers and their babies, and most importantly for our purposes, convalescents.[6] Tellingly, the words 'convalesce' and 'convalescent' *were* used in the early modern period, cropping up in dictionaries such as *Glossographia* (1656), by the London barrister Thomas Blount, which gives the definition of 'to wax strong, to recover health'.[7] However, such terms did not yet possess a monopoly over this health state—'convalescent' was used interchangeably with such phrases as 'the recoverer', 'the patient after illness', and the 'weak party'. We shall see that the treatment of convalescents was distinctive, differing both from the care provided to the sick and the healthy, a finding which expands our knowledge of the scope of early modern therapeutics.[8] Since convalescence occupied a liminal space, 'floating

---

[3] Sandra Cavallo and Tessa Storey, *Healthy Living in Late Renaissance Italy* (Oxford, 2013), *passim*. There have been some studies on this topic, however: Lelland Rather, 'The "Six Things Non-Natural": Origins and Fate of a Doctrine and a Phrase', *Clio Medica*, 3 (1968), 337–47; Saul Jarcho, 'Galen's Six Non-Naturals: A Bibliographic Note and Translation', *Bulletin of the History of Medicine*, 44 (1970), 372–7; Antoinette Emch-Deriaz, 'The Non-Naturals Made Easy', in Roy Porter (ed.), *The Popularization of Medicine, 1650–1850* (1992), 134–59; Luis Garcia-Ballester, 'On the Origin of the "Six Non-Natural Things" in Galen', in Luis Garcia-Ballester, Jon Arrizabalaga, Montserrat Calbre, and Lluis Cifuentes (eds.), *Galen and Galenism: Theory and Medical Practice from Antiquity to the European Renaissance* (Aldershot, 2002), 105–15; Olivia Weisser, *Ill Composed: Sickness, Gender, and Belief in Early Modern England* (2015).

[4] Weisser, *Ill Composed*, 21.

[5] On convalescence homes, see Michael Worboys, 'The Sanatorium Treatment for Consumption in Britain, 1890–1914', in John Pickstone (ed.), *Medical Innovations in Historical Perspective* (1992), 47–73; Helen Bynum, *Spitting Blood: The History of Tuberculosis* (Oxford, 2012); John Hassan, *The Seaside, Health and the Environment in England and Wales since 1800* (Aldershot, 2003).

[6] Important exceptions include Maaike van der Lugt, 'Neither Ill nor Healthy: The Intermediate State Between Health and Disease in Medieval Medicine', *Quaderni Storici*, 136 (2011), 13–46; Timo Joutsivuo, *Scholastic Tradition and Humanist Innovation: The Concept of Neutrum in Renaissance Medicine* (Helsinki, 1999). These scholars discuss the philosophical controversies surrounding the neutral body, particularly between Aristotle and Galen.

[7] Thomas Blount, *Glossographia, or, a dictionary* (1656), image 82. The Latin *convalescere* means to grow strong: OED, 'convalesce', verb (accessed 13/02/17).

[8] See the Introduction, note 23, on historiography relating to care of the healthy.

betwixt' health and disease, a discussion of this concept has the added benefit of shedding fresh light on the meanings of these other two vital concepts.

Of course, convalescence has not gone completely unnoticed. The food historian Ken Albala has written an article on convalescent cookery in early modern Europe: drawing on cookbooks and medical texts, he asserts that 'Despite major theoretical shifts in early modern nutritional theory…the form and structure of convalescent cookery remained remarkably constant throughout the era and…even down to the present'. He interprets this continuity as a sign that convalescent care is based on 'common sense intuition rather than theory'.[9] Anne Stobart has also briefly explored convalescent diets in her book *Household Medicine*: she argues that throughout the seventeenth century, easily digestible broths remained the staple food for recovering patients, though new exotic ingredients were introduced in the later 1600s.[10] While agreeing about the lack of change in the principles behind convalescent cookery, I argue that the treatment of these patients derived not from 'common sense', but from historically specific ideas about how the body regained strength. Through examining the roles of all six non-naturals—not just diet—this chapter seeks to provide a more complete view of convalescent care.

Another area of research which bears some relation to the present chapter is work on the care of newly delivered mothers, a group of patients also classified as 'neutral'. Leah Astbury, for example, highlights a gap between the therapeutic priorities of doctors and women after childbirth: whereas the former emphasized the need to purge the 'remnants of pregnancy', the latter were more intent on remedying the weaknesses that followed labour.[11] My chapter is chiefly about convalescence from illness rather than childbirth, but it does draw occasional parallels between the two, thereby revealing the shared thinking behind the care of various members of the neutral category. It is hoped such findings will promote a more coordinated approach to the history of these groups.[12]

The ensuing discussions focus on the dominant medical theory of the early modern period, the Hippocratic–Galenic tradition.[13] Unlike in Chapter 1, the views of Helmontian physicians will not be considered in detail, for the simple reason that they did not usually believe convalescence was necessary. William Walwyn (1600–81), a practitioner of Helmontian leanings, asked his readers to:

Heedfully observe the vast difference between those who recover out of any considerable sickness, having run the usual [Galenic] Tract of Physick, and those who are raised from the beds of sickness by these [his own] kindly Medicines: How pale, weak, and crazy the one, long languish[ing], liable to relapses upon every small occasion, . . . : Whilst the other [who

---

[9] Ken Albala, 'Food for Healing: Convalescent Cookery in the Early Modern Era', *Studies in History and Philosophy of Science Part C: Studies in History and Philosophy of Biological and Biomedical Sciences*, 43 (2012), 323–8, at 235.

[10] Anne Stobart, *Household Medicine in Seventeenth-Century England* (2016), 112–13. Stobart mentions one change over time, and that is the addition of exotic ingredients, such as china root and sassafras.

[11] Leah Astbury, 'Being Well, Looking Ill: Childbirth and the Return to Health in Seventeenth-Century England', *SHM*, 30 (2017), 500–19.

[12] See the Introduction, note 18 on the historiography on the medicine of children and the elderly.

[13] See Introduction, p. 17 for an explanation of the term 'Hippocratic–Galenic'.

have been treated with Walwyn's medicine] are no sooner discharged from their main
Distemper, but in a manner, immediately their Strength, Stomach, Courage, and countenance,
return at once without fear of any other inconveniences.[14]

Thus, Walwyn claimed that any weaknesses that followed illness sprung not
from the disease, but from the unwholesome medicines of Galenic physicians.[15]
Effectively, Helmontians believed that once the disease was gone, health should
return immediately, without any period of convalescence. To explain this idea,
disease was likened to a flame, which, once 'Extinguish't', was completely gone,
'leav[ing] nothing behind'.[16] As will become apparent below, Galenic doctors
depicted disease rather differently.

The first part of the chapter asks why the body was weak after illness, establishing
the need for convalescent care. The next part categorizes the convalescent within
early modern schemes of bodily states, and identifies the distinctive therapeutic
aims directed at each category. The rest of the chapter is structured around the
milestones or signs of increasing strength, each of which is associated with a particular non-natural or component of care.

WEAKNESS AFTER DISEASE

To understand why the body was weak in the wake of illness, it is necessary to go
back a step, and remind ourselves of how disease was removed in early modern
perceptions. As shown in Chapter 1, three hierarchical agents were thought to be
responsible: God, Nature, and medical intervention. 'Nature' was 'God's instrument', the 'intrinsic agent' and life force of the body, also responsible for nutrition,
growth, and generation.[17] Nature's vehicles for performing her functions were the
'natural spirits', highly rarefied, 'subtile and Arey' vapours, 'raised from the purer
blood', and carried around the body in the veins.[18] At the bottom of the hierarchy
was the medical practitioner, who was supposed to be 'an assistant and helper of
nature in time of neede'.[19] Nature removed disease by rectifying the bad humours
that had caused it: her chief methods were concoction (a form of internal cooking
which erased the malignant quality of the humours) and expulsion (the ejection
of superfluous humours through the 'crisis of the disease', the sudden evacuation
of body fluids at the height of illness, in the form of sweating, vomiting, or other
emission).[20] If Nature seemed to be struggling to produce these evacuations, the
physician stepped in, and administered evacuative treatments, such as emetics
and purges.

[14] William Walwyn, *Physick for families* (1669), 104.
[15] Andrew Wear, *Knowledge and Practice in English Medicine, 1550–1680* (Cambridge, 2000), 388.
[16] Walwyn, *Physick for families*, 54.
[17] See Chapter 1, pp. 37–8 for a definition of Nature.
[18] See Chapter 1, p. 38 on the spirits.
[19] James Hart, *Klinike, or the diet of the diseased* (1633), 358.
[20] See Chapter 1 for these processes.

When these processes were judged as successful—an assessment based on the patient's perception of feeling better, together with signs of concoction in the expelled excrements—the disease was said to have gone.[21] The patient was not, however, yet pronounced back to health, since the body was usually weak. The Wiltshire gentlewoman Grace Thynne told her daughter Frances in 1723, 'the gout is gone and I have nothing but the weakness left'.[22] Weakness was defined as the 'slowness' or 'imbecility' of the faculties of the body, caused by the 'dissipation' or 'decay' of the natural, animal, and vital spirits.[23] To recap, the natural spirits were Nature's vehicles for carrying out the body's basic functions. The other two types—the animal and vital spirits—drove the higher faculties of the body and mind: muscular movement, the senses, and rational powers (animal faculty), and breathing, the pulse, and the emotions (vital faculty).[24] In turn, all three spirits were 'nourished' by 'radical moisture' (an oily substance) and 'innate heat' (a glowing warmth): these were the substances in which 'life consisteth', which gradually depleted with age.[25] Crucially, the processes of removing disease consumed these substances: the heat of concoction dried out the radical moisture, and the critical evacuations removed all three types of spirits, along with the bad humours. Speaking of diarrhoea, the German physician Walter Bruele wrote: 'excrements ofentimes come downe with such force, that the spirits are also expelled with the humours: from whence [occurs]...a languishing of the strength'.[26] Patients and their families also recognized this cause.[27] Bereft of the requisite quantity of spirits, Nature was unable to carry out the body's operations with her usual vigour. This situation was described using military metaphors: Nature was exhausted from her battle with the disease, 'hardly [able to] recollect her forces...but recovers [them]... by degrees,...to reedifie and fortifie her batter'd walls'.[28] Such imagery is consistent with the finding in Chapter 1 that Nature was a warrior queen, and the body a battlefield.[29]

The effects of the loss of the spirits were multiple forms of weakness, each connected to the particular spirit that had been evacuated, and varying in accordance with the length and severity of the disease. The dissipation of the animal spirits

---

[21] The meaning of 'feeling better' is discussed in Chapter 3; on evidence of concoction in the excrements, see Chapter 1, p. 48.

[22] Frances Seymour, *The Gentle Hertford: Her Life and Letters*, ed. Helen Hughes (New York, 1940), 84. See also St John's College Library, Cambridge, Miscellaneous Box 7, FA2 (Letter from Thomas Fairfax to his grandfather, 1st Baron, 24 July 1637).

[23] Lemnius, *The secret miracles*, 43; Hart, *Klinike*, 241; John Macollo, *XCIX canons, or rules learnedly describing an excellent method for practitioners in physic* (1659), 44.

[24] Felix Platter, *Platerus golden practice of physick* (1664), 148; Ambroise Paré, *The workes of that famous chirurgion Ambrose Parey*, trans. Thomas Johnson (1634), 25–6.

[25] Paré, *The workes*, 26; Hart, *Klinike*, 299.

[26] Walter Bruele, *Praxis medicinae, or, the physicians practice* (1632), 223. See also Platter, *Platerus golden practice*, 149.

[27] For example, Ralph Thoresby *The Diary of Ralph Thoresby*, ed. Joseph Hunter, 2 vols. (1830), vol. 1, 124; Hampshire Record Office, Winchester, 44M69/F6/1/2, letter number 18, 26 April 1684 (Jervoise letters, 1683–6).

[28] Lemnius, *The secret miracles*, 99.

[29] See Chapter 1, pp. 39–40, 51–2, for a discussion of this imagery.

caused weak musculature,[30] slow mobility,[31] poor memory,[32] and dullness of hearing or eyesight.[33] The clergyman Thomas Brockbank (1671–1732) recorded that after smallpox, 'I was so weak that my back wo'd not bare my shoulders, and I co'd [not] go without supporters'.[34] By contrast, the loss of natural spirits brought about thinness, paleness,[35] hair loss,[36] and constipation,[37] footsteps of disease associated with the weakened nutritive faculty. The biographer of the controversial clergyman and historian Peter Heylyn (1599–1662) recalled:

> [W]hat strange alterations his sickness had wrought in him; for he was before a fresh lively *complexion*;...but now...of a pale *discoloured* countenance...his Cheeks fallen, his Eyes a little sunk within his *Temples*, and leanness of Face and whole Body.[38]

Finally, the loss of the vital spirits resulted in weaknesses associated with the heart, such as dizziness and faintness.[39] In 1652, Sir Thomas Hervey told his lover, Isabella May, 'When I rose in the morning, my head was light...as is common after great fits of sickness...[I] was [so] giddy as I was glad to throw my self upon the bed'.[40] Faintness of body was often accompanied by 'faint-heartedness', a term which denoted emotional anxiety or timidity, and was most frequently sparked by the anticipation of relapse.[41] Defined as 'the Return of a Disease cured, after a short time', relapse was likely because Nature, the agent responsible for preventing illness, was exhausted.[42] Later in the chapter, we will see that the restoration of strength was achieved by the replenishment of the three types of spirits, together with the innate heat and radical moisture.

The footsteps and weaknesses identified above were at a height immediately following the illness, after which point they usually began to recede, with strength increasing over time. The speed at which this process occurred ranged from minutes to years. In 1602, Lady Elizabeth Hunsdon (1552–1618) recorded that 'within the space of one halfe howre' her husband 'returned agayne to his former estate' after a 'sudden sicknes' which had temporarily deprived him of 'all sence and

---

[30] For example, Ann Fanshawe, *Memoirs of Lady Fanshawe*, ed. Richard Fanshawe (1829), 125; Izaak Walton, *The lives of Dr. John Donne, Sir Henry Wotton, Mr. Richard Hooker, Mr. George Herbert* (1670), 71.
[31] Lemnius, *The secret miracles*, 245.
[32] Henry Cuffe, *The differences of the ages of mans life* (1607), 125–6; Philip Barrough, *The methode of phisicke* (1583), 21; James Fisher, *The wise virgin, or, a wonderful narration of the various dispensations towards a childe of eleven years of age* (1653), 152.
[33] Sarah Savage, *Memoirs of the Life and Character of Mrs Sarah Savage*, ed. J. B. Williams (1821), 20; Samuel Jeake, *An Astrological Diary of the Seventeenth Century: Samuel Jeake of Rye*, ed. Michael Hunter (Oxford, 1988), 89–90; Platter, *Platerus golden practice*, 84.
[34] Thomas Brockbank, *The Diary and Letter Book of the Rev. Thomas Brockbank 1671–1709*, ed. Richard Trappes-Lomax, Chetham Society New Series, vol. 89 (Manchester, 1930), 37.
[35] Platter, *Platerus golden practice*, 514.
[36] For example, Brockbank, *The Diary*, 39; Francis Bacon, *The historie of life and death* (1638), 25.
[37] Platter, *Platerus golden practice*, 140–1.
[38] John Barnard, *Theologo-historicus, or, the true life of...Peter Heylyn* (1683), 279.
[39] Platter, *Platerus golden practice*, 148–50; John Pechey, *The store-house of physical practice* (1695), 187.
[40] John Hervey, *Letter-Books of John Hervey, First Earl of Bristol, vol. 1, 1651–1715* (Wells, 1894), vol. 1, 26.
[41] See Chapter 3, p. 111, on the fear of relapse.
[42] John Pechey, *A plain introduction to the art of physic* (1697), 99.

motion'.[43] At the other end of the spectrum, ten-year-old Hannah Martindale from Lancashire 'cannot stand upright' after her long palsy, though she 'gets some little strength every year', recorded her father.[44] These variations in timing were attributed, above all, to the length of the disease, as is revealed in one of the Hippocratic aphorisms:

> Bodies... wasted with long sickness, are to be restored... little by little, but those which have been brought low quickly and in short time, are sooner to be restored.

A commentator added, *'For in those who are wasted with long sickness, the flesh is wasted; in those who are quickly brought low, the spirits onely, which may sooner be restored'*.[45] Flesh took longer to rebuild than spirits, hence the lengthy convalescence of emaciated patients. The fastest of all recoveries were miracle cures—a defining feature of this type of healing was the rapid return of strength.[46] Of course, not everyone reached a state of perfect strength and health: some footsteps came to be regarded as permanent disabilities or disfigurements, such as scars, blindness, and lameness; these legacies of illness will not be discussed here.[47]

CATEGORIZING THE CONVALESCENT

Where did convalescents fit in contemporary bodily categorizations? Drawing on Galen's *Ars medica*, physicians usually envisaged three main bodily states: healthful (or sound), neutral, and unhealthful (or sick).[48] Healthful was defined as the balance of the 'primary qualities' (heat, cold, dry, and wet), together with the strong functioning of the faculties (animal, natural, and vital). Unhealthy was the opposite: individuals suffered the 'perceptible impairment' of the faculties, and the imbalance of the four qualities—this state included diseases, disabilities, and wounds.[49] Suspended between these two categories was the 'neutral body',

[43] Cecil Project, HMCS 94 87 V12 266; my thanks to Caroline Bowden for supplying this information.

[44] Adam Martindale, *The Life of Adam Martindale*, ed. Richard Parkinson, Chetham Society, vol. 4 (Manchester, 1845), 214.

[45] *The aphorismes of Hippocrates*, trans. S.H. [possibly Stephen Hobbes] (1655), 20.

[46] For instance, Mary Maillard, cured by miracle in 1693, 'at that very moment betook her self to Walking, and Leaping up and down the Chamber': James Welwood, *A true relation of the wonderful cure of Mary Maillard* (1694), 16. On this characteristic of miracle cures, see David Gentilcore, *Healers and Healing in Early Modern Italy* (Manchester, 1998), 187.

[47] For historiography on scars from smallpox, see Chapter 3, note 265. On other disabilities resulting from illness, see David Turner, *Disability in Eighteenth-Century England* (Abingdon, 2012), 44, 48–50, 117. Turner discusses the medical treatments and practical assistance available for those suffering from disabilities, including use of wheelchairs on pp. 50–5, 109–16.

[48] For a vernacular version of this text, see Galen, *Galens art of physic*, trans. Nicholas Culpeper (1652), 5, 8–10. Timo Joutsivuo states that 'Whether authentic or not, the *Ars medica* is nevertheless regarded as a summary of Galen's medical ideas', and was one of the 'main texts' for learning medical theory in the early modern period: *Scholastic Tradition*, 11, 19, 22–3.

[49] Galen, *Galens art of physic*, 13, 18, 105. This definition is cited in most medical texts across the period.

otherwise known as the 'crazie' or 'valetudinarie' body.[50] Defined by Galen as 'an exquisite medium between healthful and unhealthful Bodies', the neutral body was a melting-pot for all those individuals deemed 'neither perfectly whole, nor thoroughly sicke'.[51] This category has attracted only limited attention from historians, perhaps because it is no longer recognized in modern medicine.[52]

A number of groups of patients were encompassed within the neutral category, including people of 'sickly Constitution', who by 'Nativity...are born' this way; those individuals who were falling sick, though 'not yet fastned to their beds'; and most importantly for our purposes, patients who 'hath already discussed the disease...it selfe from it, yet is weak, feeble, exhausted, and of little force'.[53] Termed *neutra convalescens* in Latin, these were '*Persons recovering*, who recollect themselves from some Disease'.[54] Convalescents were no longer sick because the majority of the bad humours had been concocted and expelled, nor were they in health because the body was still weak; their bodies functioned, but they functioned slowly and weakly. By excluding the convalescent from the category of health, early modern doctors implied that this state was not just the absence of disease, but the presence of strength.[55] This subtle, but important, distinction has not been recognized in the historiography of early modern medicine.

Several other groups were sometimes added to the neutral category.[56] The historian Timo Joutsivuo confirms that in Renaissance gerontologies, 'the relationship between old age and convalescence was well known'.[57] Patients frequently compared themselves to the elderly. The Shropshire minister and prolific writer Richard Baxter (1615–91) complained that he 'continued...in languishing Pains and Weaknesses...just the same Symptoms as most men have about Fourscore [i.e. eighty] years of Age'.[58] Speaking of 'Feebleness...[of] voluntary Motion', the Swiss physician Felix Platter (1536–1614) noted that it occurs both in 'olde folks...who are...sluggish and presently tired', and in those 'recover'd of...Disease'.[59] Lying-in mothers also qualified for the neutral category, on the grounds that childbirth, like disease, exhausted Nature and dissipated her spirits.[60] As Leah Astbury has commented, the vaginal bleeding that commonly followed the delivery of the infant was similar to the critical expulsion.[61] Women as well as doctors recognized the

---

[50] Hart, *Klinike*, 270.   [51] Galen, *Galens art of physic*, 10.
[52] For the exceptions, see note 6 in this chapter.   [53] Lemnius, *The secret miracles*, 243.
[54] Galen, *Galens art of physic*, 9; Joutsivuo, *Scholastic Tradition*, 147.
[55] This contradicts Lucinda Beier's assertion that 'good health could apparently be defined as the absence of illness': *Sufferers and Healers: The Experience of Illness in Seventeenth-Century England* (1987), 242.
[56] Van der Lugt states that it was Avicenna who included infants and the elderly in the category of 'neutrum': 'Neither Ill nor Healthy', 26.
[57] Joutsivuo, *Scholastic Tradition*, 161, 192.
[58] Richard Baxter, *Reliquiae Baxterianae, or, Mr. Richard Baxters narrative of the most memorable passages of his life*, ed. Matthew Sylvester (1696), 10.
[59] Platter, *Platerus golden practice*, 58. He also mentions dim eyesight and weak hearing.
[60] François Mauriceau, *The diseases of women with child*, trans. Hugh Chamberlen (1710, first English edn. 1672), 57.
[61] Astbury, 'Being Well, Looking Ill', 7; see also Sara Read, *Menstruation and the Female Body in Early Modern England* (Basingstoke, 2013), ch. 7.

similarities between convalescence from illness and childbirth. The Buckinghamshire gentlewoman Brilliana Harley told her son in 1639, 'I am still so weake, and, I thinke, allmost as weake as after lyeing in of any of my chillderen'.[62] The final group in the neutral category were 'sucking infants' (breastfed babies): treatises devoted to the diseases of children describe this age group as 'weak' and 'tender', owing to the high level of moisture contained within their body parts.[63] Occasionally, convalescing patients compared their physical helplessness to the plight of infants, suggesting that they too suffered from 'childish' weakness.[64] As will become clear later in the chapter, convalescent care in some ways resembled the treatment of these other neutral groups.

The neutral category elicited considerable controversy amongst the medical and philosophical elite.[65] Although vernacular medical texts rarely discussed the details of the debates, they do allude to the key points of contention. *The art of physic made plain*, by the dean of the Faculty of Medicine in Reims, Nicholas Abraham de La Framboisière (1560–1636), contains an imagined disputation between a medical candidate and the dean:

DEAN: There is no such thing as a Neuter Body...I prove it thus...Sound and unhealthy are immediate Contraries, according to the Opinion of *Aristotle*: Therefore seeing Health and Sickness are diametrically opposite, there can be no middle Constitution between 'em.

CANDIDATE: I answer, Health and Sickness are immediately opposite according to *Aristotle*, but not according to the Physicians.[66]

Essentially, Aristotle's concept of health and disease was absolutist: disease was imbalance, and health the polar opposite, which made the existence of an intermediary state an intellectual impossibility. Most physicians, however, seem to have accepted Galen's notion that it was necessary to recognize the neutral category in order to accommodate the daily experiences of ordinary people. Lemnius expressed this view aptly, stating that 'though some...will not endure to heare of' the neutral body:

[S]uch a thing is determind by...daily use and custome...Hence proceed those answers of our friends..., if they aske how any man doth, what health he is in...[he will] answer in so many words; [']So so, indifferent, not very well, doubtfully, inclining, floting between both, instable, not sound, not as we could wish, or would have it['].[67]

---

[62] Brilliana Harley, *Letters of The Lady Brilliana Harley*, ed. Thomas Taylor Lewis (1853), 128, 82.

[63] See Hannah Newton, *The Sick Child in Early Modern England, 1580–1720* (Oxford, 2012), 34–6, 38–9.

[64] For example, John Donne, *Devotions upon emergent occasions and severall steps in my sicknes* (1624), 48.

[65] On this debate, see Van der Lugt, 'Neither Ill nor Healthy', at 6–9; Joutsivuo, *Scholastic Tradition*, especially 47–56, 90–1.

[66] Nicholas Abraham de La Framboisière, *The art of physick made plain & easie*, trans. John Phillips (1684; originally publ. in Latin, 1628), 6–8.

[67] Lemnius, *The secret miracles*, 244. See also Thomas Coxe, *A discourse wherein the interest of the patient in reference to physick and physicians is soberly debated* (1669), 187.

The neutral body was thus a necessity.

Each category of body—healthy, unhealthy, and neutral—required a different sort of therapy. The prominent Fellow of the Royal College of Physicians Francis Glisson (*c*.1599–1677) declared that the 'three Species' of body, 'are the subjects of the three kinds of Method to Practice': namely, 'a sound state indicateth the conservation of health…; a diseased state [requires] the removal of some affect' (the process described in Chapter 1 by which illness was taken away), and 'the *Neutral* state [needs] the caus[e] of the imminent malady…to be corrected least it break out into a Diseas[e]'.[68] Within the neutral category, further distinctions were drawn between sub-groups of patients. The Polish physician Johannes Johnstonus (1603–75) stated that whereas those who were falling sick required measures that would prevent the illness from taking hold, 'persons…recovering' require 'two things':

1. That they fal not back again into their sicknesses.
2. That they may soon recover their perfect health.[69]

Thus, the aims of convalescent care were to prevent relapse and restore strength. The term used to denote this special branch of physic was 'analeptics', which meant 'to cherish and renew the strength'.[70] The ensuing paragraphs show how these distinctive aims were fulfilled. Five components of analeptics are examined, each of which was connected to a particular non-natural, and acted as a measure of growing strength.

THE FINAL PURGE

The first component of analeptics relates to the non-natural excretion. After illness, patients and practitioners worried that the body might contain residues of malignant humours, 'left over' from the critical expulsion.[71] The concern was that these humours would grow in the body, and cause relapse. Convalescent care sought to prevent this from happening by giving a 'final gentle purge' to 'carry off' the remnant humour. The Scottish physician John Macollo (1576–1622) warned in his posthumously published medical canons, 'if the Crise [crisis] have been imperfect, it is the duty of the Physitian to purge [the] rest of the vicious humours, fearing lest by process of time, putrifying within the body, they renew the sickness'.[72] Colourful metaphors were used to explain the need for this treatment. Walwyn recorded in his casebook that a gentleman, aged 30, whose ague had been 'quite discharged'

---

[68] Francis Glisson, George Bate, and Assuerus Regemorter, *A treatise of the rickets being a diseas common to children*, trans. Philip Armin (1651), 277–8.

[69] Johannes Johnstonus, *The idea of practical physick*, trans. Nicholas Culpeper and W.R. (1657), 26.

[70] Stephen Blankaart, *A physical dictionary* (1684), 16. Analeptics has also been discussed by Joutsivuo, *Scholastic Tradition*, at 102, 191–2.

[71] Examples from either ends of the timeframe include Barrough, *The methode*, 19; Mauriceau, *The diseases of women*, 358–9. This idea is derived from *The aphorismes of Hippocrates*, 22.

[72] Macollo, *XCIX canons*, 111.

was informed by his doctors that 'the work...could not be perfect', and that the disease would 'return upon him...if he did not speedily take some fit Purgative to carry of the Relicks'. They likened disease to a dead dog: '[if] you kill a Dogg in your house, and you let him lie there, and [do] not quickly throw him out, hee'l soon make you weary of your Habitation', and therefore a final purge is necessary after illness.[73] The remnant humour was also compared to dirt, which must be 'swept clean' from the house to keep it free from 'future feares'.[74] Depicting the body as a house, and the humours as dirt or an animal, is common in early modern medical writings; it fitted with the identity of Nature as a 'homely woman', who kept the body 'polite and trim'.[75]

Laypeople as well as physicians advised giving 'a gentle purge when the distemper is over'.[76] Domestic recipe collections often contain instructions for making a 'very good purge for a weak constitution after feavour' or some other disease.[77] In hindsight, patients and their relatives attributed future illnesses to their failure to purge the body. The Lancashire-born Presbyterian clergyman Adam Martindale (1623–86) reminisced that after smallpox as a child in the early 1630s, he 'should have been soundly purged, but was not; which as I verily believe, caused a vehement fermentation in my bodie, which, after two or three yeares' space, [came] out in an ugly dry scurfe'.[78] The reason for failing to take the purge—besides the expense—may have been that patients were tired of physic, and wanted to give it up at the earliest opportunity.[79] The consequences could be fatal. Peter Heylyn's biographer claimed that 'the reliques of his long *quartane* Ague not purged out by *Physick*... threw' this man 'into a malignant Fever', of which he died.[80]

In theory, the convalescent's purge differed from those prescribed to the sick and healthy. Those who were still ill required stronger, and more frequent, evacuations, because their bodies contained larger quantities of bad humours. Conversely, 'those persons that be perfectlie in health ought not to take a[ny] *Purgation*[,] since they doe not abound with corrupt humours', wrote the anonymous author of a popular late sixteenth-century medical manual for the poor.[81] The reason it was wrong to purge the healthy was that these medicines, finding 'no excrements' in the body, would set upon 'solid and sound parts', and 'make a colliquation of good flesh'.[82] Of course, in practice many healthy people *did* take purges, because it was believed that those bodies which were 'inclined to fall' into sickness might also

---

[73] Walwyn, *Physick for families*, 54–5.   [74] Hart, *Klinike*, 284.

[75] See Chapter 1, pp. 39, 44–5, 49. On the use of animal imagery, see Alanna Skuse, 'Wombs, Worms and Wolves: Constructing Cancer in Early Modern England', *SHM*, 27 (2014), 632–48.

[76] John Magrath (ed.), *The Flemings in Oxford*, Oxford Historical Society, vol. 44 (Oxford, 1904), vol. 2, 214–15.

[77] WL, MS 1320, fol. 96v ('A book of physick', made in 1710). See also BL, Additional MS 45196, fols. 44v, 70v (Brockman Papers, 'Ann Glyd Her Book 1656').

[78] Martindale, *The Life*, 20.

[79] This was the case for Brilliana Harley's son Ned in 1641: in Harley, *Letters*, 128.

[80] Barnard, *Theologo-historicus*, 290.

[81] A.T., *A rich store-house, or treasury for the diseased* (1596), 'divers & sundrye Good instructions & Rules' (no pagination). This text went through eight editions by 1650.

[82] *The aphorismes of Hippocrates*, 35, 68; Hart, *Klinike*, 269.

contain some noxious matter.[83] It should also be noted that the convalescent's gentle purge was not exclusive to these patients: it was apposite for other members of the weak 'neutral' category too, such as 'big-bellied' or lying-in women, the elderly, and young children.[84]

After the final purge, it was necessary to comfort and strengthen Nature and the body, especially the 'noble organs'—the brain, heart, and liver. The Latin term *condita*, meaning preserve or restore, was used to denote these treatments: they were designed to 'strengthen the might' of the 'worthiest membres' of the body in those 'that begin to recover and waxe stronge'.[85] A variety of forms were recommended, including juleps and cordials (sweetened drinks and spirits), electuaries (powders mixed with honey or preserve), and topical remedies (plasters, baths, and ointments). A typical example is the surgeon Alexander Read's (d. 1641) '*Restorative for weak Convalescent persons after a long and tedious sickness*', made of pistachios, sugar, and fragrant spices.[86] Similar treatments can be found in domestic recipe books, which suggests that condita was a normal part of household medicine.[87] These drugs were thought to work through their effects on the spirits: once taken, they travelled to the noble organs, the 'seats' of the spirits, and proceeded to 'corroborate and strengthen...the vertues naturall, vitall, and animall' by expanding, comforting, and refreshing their respective spirits.[88] The forms of condita do not appear to have changed substantially over the early modern period, though it is possible that there was an upturn in the use of newly available ingredients, such as tea leaves, which were products of the expanding trade with the East.[89] It is also likely that as the period progressed, patients and their families were more likely to make use of 'ready-made' preparations, owing to the proliferation of apothecary shops.[90] Beyond the gentle purge and strengthening medicines, convalescents could 'bid farewell to Phisick'.[91]

SLEEPING THROUGH THE NIGHT

The next non-natural to discuss is sleep, a function defined as 'the rest of the whole body, and the cessation of the Animal faculty'.[92] Sleep was thought to occur when the stomach sent a 'certain vaporous, sweet, and delightsome humidity' to the

---

[83] Hart, *Klinike*, 270.

[84] Pechey, *The store-house*, 497; Astbury, 'Being Well, Looking Ill'; Newton, *The Sick Child*, ch. 2.

[85] Barrough, *The methode*, 292–3.

[86] Alexander Read, *Most excellent and approved medicines* (1651), 30–1.

[87] Examples of restorative physic in recipe books include WL, MS 1321, fol. 77v ('A book of receits, c.1675–1725') and MS 213, fol. 154v (Mrs Corylon, 'A Booke of divers medecines', 1606).

[88] Barrough, *The methode*, 291.

[89] On these introductions, see Patrick Wallis, 'Exotic Drugs and English Medicine: England's Drug Trade, c.1550–c.1800', *SHM*, 25 (2012), 20–46.

[90] Patrick Wallis, 'London Apothecaries and Other Medical Retailers, 1580–1702', in Louise Hill Curth (ed.), *From Physick to Pharmacology: Five Hundred Years of British Drug Retailing* (Aldershot, 2006), 13–27, at 23.

[91] John Hall, *Select observations on English bodies*, trans. James Cooke (1679, first. publ. 1657), 27.

[92] Paré, *The workes*, 24. For a fabulous new study of early modern sleep, see Sasha Handley, *Sleep in Early Modern England* (2016).

brain, which blocked the nerves, the routes through which the animal spirits travelled; the result was the temporary suspension of the powers of the animal faculty—movement, sensation, and understanding.[93] During serious illness, the special vapour evaporated, or became 'infected' with the bad humours: the result was 'unquiet' or interrupted sleep. Dr John Hall recorded that his patient, John Nason, a barber, 'had seldom any Sleep at night', which was a sign of the severity of his illness.[94] Patients themselves usually attributed sleepless nights to pain.[95] Upon recovery, however, sleep came more easily: the abatement of pain 'allured' the animal spirits to 'quiet rest', and the rectification of the humours restored the sleep-inducing vapour to its proper quality.[96] Throughout the period, doctors and patients regarded uninterrupted sleep as a 'good signe' of recovery.[97] George Davenport from Leicestershire, aged 31, told his former Cambridge tutor in 1662, 'I am like to do well... if I may ghess... by... [my] most profound sleep. I never waked in the night'.[98] The fact that continuous sleep was proof of growing strength seems to contradict the common assumption in the historiography that 'Western Europeans on most evenings experienced two major intervals of sleep bridged by up to an hour or more of quiet wakefulness'.[99] If unbroken sleep was a token of improving health—the norm to which most people aspired—it could be an indication that segmentation was in fact less widespread than has been acknowledged.

As well as signifying that the patient was on the mend, sleep was thought to play a crucial restorative role. This notion persisted across the period.[100] Lemnius stated in his popular book of secrets, '[he who] hath already discussed the disease... yet... is weak, feeble, [and] exhausted... may be restored by sleep'.[101] Sleep achieved this restoration by moistening the brain and body parts, thereby furnishing the 'whole man' with new radical moisture. Imagery of plant irrigation was used to describe this process—the organs were 'besprinkled' with a *mild and pleasant vapour*, just as overnight the plants and fields were rejuvenated by dew.[102] The spirits also benefited from sleep—exhausted from the disease, they were 'refreshed' and 'recruited' by 'soft Slumbers'.[103] Such language suggests that the spirits were capable of experiencing human feelings. The other function of rest was to nourish the lean body: digestion was best performed during sleep, since it was at this time

---

[93] Paré, *The workes*, 24. For more details, see Bill Maclehose, 'Fear, Fantasy and Sleep in Medieval Medicine', in Elena Carrera (ed.), *Emotions and Health, 1200–1700* (Leiden, 2013), 67–94, at 83.

[94] Hall, *Select observations*, p. 64.

[95] For examples, see Chapter 3, p. 103. Doctors agreed that pain was a major cause of wakefulness—see Robert Bayfield, *Enchiridion medicum: containing the causes... cures of... diseases* (1655), 162.

[96] John Kettlewell, *Death made comfortable* (1695), 212.   [97] Hart, *Klinike*, 336.

[98] George Davenport, *The Letters of George Davenport 1651–1677*, ed. Brenda M. Pask, Surtees Society, vol. 215 (Woodbridge, 2011), p. 89.

[99] Roger Ekirch, *At Day's Close: A History of Nighttime* (2005), 300–10.

[100] From both ends of the time-period, see William Bullein, *Bulleins bulwarke of defence against all sicknesse* (1579), 33–4; Joseph Browne, *Institutions in physick, collected from the writings of the most eminent physicians* (1714), 168–9, 226, 255.

[101] Lemnius, *The secret miracles*, 244.   [102] Hart, *Klinike*, 332.

[103] Kettlewell, *Death made comfortable*, 212.

that Nature was undistracted by other tasks, and could concentrate solely on fattening the patient.[104]

Medical authors prescribed different sleep routines for each bodily state. The puritan physician James Hart (d. 1639) wrote in his regimen that the sick should be 'suffer[ed] to sleep when[ever] they can', including the daytime, because it was 'often out [of] our power to accommodate it...to the right and proper time'.[105] By contrast, the healthy were told that 'the night should bee more convenient for sleepe than the day' because the sunlight of daytime would draw the body's innate heat in the wrong direction—outwards.[106] Convalescents fell in between: ideally, they should remain awake in the morning, but they were permitted to nap in the afternoon.[107] Special armchairs for daytime rest were emerging in this period, which may have been used for this purpose (see Figure 8, in Chapter 6).[108] Over the course of recovery, however, convalescents were instructed to let daytime sleep be 'lost by litle and litle', until at last they had acquired the 'accustomed order' of the healthy.[109] Daytime rest was also permitted for other groups within the neutral category, such as infants and the elderly: babies remembered sleeping in the womb, so required more rest after birth, while the dry constitutions of older people benefited from the moistening effects of sleep.[110]

FEELING HUNGRY

Sleep was rarely mentioned without reference to appetite, and together the two served as a litmus test for the state of the body. The first sign of approaching sickness was 'tast...inspid;...the appetite...dull'.[111] Once illness arrived in full, it was said that 'sick men loathe nothing so much as meate'.[112] The reason that the sick did not feel hungry was that Nature, the agent of appetite and nutrition, was not proficient at multi-tasking. During illness she was wholly occupied with the concoction and expulsion of the bad humours, and should not be 'diverted from her office & work' by the task of digestion.[113] Once the bad humours had been rectified, however, this agent had time once more to carry out the digestion of food; the result was the return of appetite, a widely recognized sign of growing strength. 'I praise God I am now in the way of recovery: I am able to...eate my meat with reasonable stomacke', wrote the Essex gentleman Henry Cromwell to

---

[104] Hart, *Klinike*, 332. On the nutritional purposes of sleep, see Maclehose, 'Fear, Fantasy and Sleep', 78–9.

[105] Hart, *Klinike*, 333.

[106] Thomas Cogan, *The haven of health, made for the comfort of students* (1636, first publ. 1584), 271.

[107] Afternoon naps for convalescents are mentioned in Cavallo and Storey, *Healthy Living*, 122–3, 125.

[108] On this development, see Chapter 6, note 45.

[109] John Banister, *A needefull, new, and necessarie treatise of chyrurgerie* (1575), 91.

[110] Robert Pemell, *De morbis puerorum, or, a treatise of the diseases of children* (1653), 20–1.

[111] Donne, *Devotions*, 26. See also the examples given in Chapter 3, pp. 101–3.

[112] Thomas Wright, *The passions of the minde* (1630, first publ. 1601), 13. Variations of this saying are common in medical and religious literature.

[113] See Chapter 1, p. 45.

his sister in 1630.[114] The loss or return of appetite was such an important measure of health that it became shorthand for sickness and recovery: a wigmaker from Manchester, Edmund Harrold, wrote in his diary in 1713, 'Very ill...Could not...eat', and in another entry, 'Better today. Could eat'.[115]

Although everybody required sustenance to stay alive, the dietary priorities differed in sickness, health, and convalescence. In sickness, the main purpose of eating was to help Nature remove the disease by correcting the humours. To this end, the patient was given an 'allopathic diet', which meant consuming foods and drinks of the opposite qualities to the malignant humours.[116] The healthy, by contrast, were entreated to preserve their humoral constitution by following a 'sympathetic' diet. The physician Thomas Cock (b. 1630), explained in his medical manual for the poor, 'When you are in perfect health and temper, eat and drink things temperate: and when distempered and sick, eat and drink things *contrary* to your distemper'.[117] However, in convalescence, the majority of the humours had already been rectified. As such, the aim of eating was less explicitly related to the balance of the humours, and more to do with the restoration of lost strength and flesh.

How were these goals achieved? There were many guidelines and hazards to bear in mind. The first was timing: Macollo warned, 'When the body is not clear, the more it is nourish'd the more it is hurt'.[118] It was believed that if nourishing foods were eaten before the final purge, they would be greedily 'licked up' by the residual humours, resulting in relapse. This idea derived from the Hippocratic aphorism, 'How much the more thou shalt nourish and cherish impure bodies, by so much the more thou shalt harm and hurt them'. A commentator explained, '*Because hard feeding whilst there be yet reliques of evil humors remaining in the body, increases the quantity of those evil humours, and so hinders their convalescencie*'.[119] Thus, the patient was to abstain from eating until after the final purge. The second factor to consider was the form of food. The Sussex physician Thomas Twyne (1543–1613), wrote in his regimen that for the first few days of convalescence, the 'Recoverer [should]...retain the same diet' that he had taken during illness, consuming only liquid foods. The reason was that 'it is not good to chaunge suddenly from that wherto a man is accustomed...because of custome'.[120] Twyne was referring to the proverb 'custom is a second Nature', which meant that habit was almost as vital to bodily functioning as Nature herself.[121] Liquid foods were advantageous because they could be quickly distributed around the body, despite being less nourishing than solid foods.[122] The best forms were jellies, possets, broths, and soups, in some ways resembling baby food; these meals were commonly served in 'posset cups' (see Figure 3).[123]

---

[114] Arthur Searle (ed.), *Barrington Family Letters, 1628–1632* (1983), 126.
[115] Edmund Harrold, *The Diary of Edmund Harrold, Wigmaker of Manchester 1712–15*, ed. Craig Horner (Aldershot, 2009), 91, 76.
[116] Hart, *Klinike*, 168.
[117] Thomas Cock, *Kitchin-physick: or, advice for the poor* (1676), 31–2.
[118] Macollo, *XCIX canons*, 96.   [119] *The aphorismes of Hippocrates*, 21, 31–2.
[120] Thomas Twyne, *The schoolmaster, or teacher of table phylosophie* (1583, first publ. 1576), sig. B2.
[121] N.R., *Proverbs English, French, Dutch, Italian, and Spanish* (1659), 24. Many more examples could be cited.
[122] Lemnius, *The secret miracles*, 118.   [123] Albala, 'Food for Healing', 327.

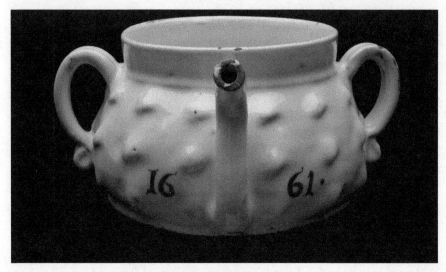

Figure 3. Posset cup, 1650–1700; Science Museum, Wellcome Images, reference: L0057146 (CC BY 4.0). Posset was a thick liquid food, commonly taken by convalescents and other 'weak stomached' patients; typically it was made from warm milk, curdled with ale/wine, and flavoured with sugar and spices. This pot is decorated with raised bumps, a technique known as repoussé. The bumpy texture, together with the handles, may have helped the weak convalescent to grip the pot; the spout facilitated drinking.

Another important consideration was liking. At the beginning of convalescence, it was vital to indulge the patient's dietary predilections. The Manchester physician Thomas Cogan (*c.*1545–1607) provided a justification in his regimen for sickly students:

> [L]iking causeth good concoction [i.e. digestion]. For what the stomacke liketh, it greedily desireth: and having received it, closely incloseth it about untill it bee duly concocted…wherein wee have great delight…it doth us more good.[124]

Personified as a fussy child, the weak stomach of the convalescent would more effectively digest foods which it desired. It was Nature who produced these cravings—she 'calls for that which is good for it self': the practitioner's role was simply to supply her with what she wanted.[125] The consideration of liking was less important in the other states of health. In acute sickness, patients rarely desired anything, even those foods which they normally enjoyed.[126] The merchant John Verney (1640–1717) complained that 'Those things' his feverish children Molly and Ralph 'love so very well in health as Sugar, Candy, Pruines, etc. they will not now

---

[124] Cogan, *The haven of health*, 201. See also Lemnius, *The secret miracles*, 17; Ken Albala, *Eating Right in the Renaissance* (Berkeley CA, 2002), 59.

[125] Roger North, *Notes of Me: the Autobiography of Roger North*, ed. P. Millard (Toronto, 2000), 80; see also Noah Biggs, *Mataeotechnia medicinae praxeos, or the vanity of the craft of physick* (1651), 200.

[126] For a comment on this, see Robert May, *The accomplisht cook, or the art and mystery of cooking* (1660), image 6.

touch'.[127] Conversely, the healthy were supposed to be sufficiently 'stronge stomacked' so as to be able to make a 'good digestion' of most foods, regardless of whether they were craved.[128]

The next priority was nourishment: it was essential to build up the convalescent's lean body by giving highly nourishing foods. In Galenic theory, the most nutritious foods were substances which resembled the human body: nutrition was a process of assimilation, with the ingested matter being transformed into the substance of the body.[129] Consequently, animals were deemed more nutritious than vegetables, because their 'fat and gluttonous substance has neerest affinity with mans radicall moisture'.[130] Likewise, flesh was considered to be superior to fish, since humans bore a closer resemblance to the former.[131] Given that life 'consisteth' in heat and moisture, it followed that foods richly imbued with these qualities would fatten and strengthen the body the most effectively.[132] Amongst non-aquatic creatures, further distinctions were drawn based on the animal's abilities and location: Hart averred that animals that could fly would 'affood the body a...subtill nourishment' because 'the wings of such fowles...are in perpetuall motion'.[133] By contrast, 'four-footed beasts', which lived on the ground, provided less wholesome nourishment. This view was informed by natural philosophical notions of the 'Chain of Being', the hierarchy of living things: Allen Grieco has shown that fowl and birds were deemed 'nobler' than quadrupeds and fish, because they were associated with the superior element of the air, whereas land- or ocean-bound creatures were analogous to the lower elements of earth and water.[134] The sky was closer to the heavens and to God, while the earth held connotations of death and hell.[135] Given this cultural backdrop, it is unsurprising that the most nutritious creatures were thought to be those which could fly.

As well as being nutritious, the convalescent's food had to be 'easie of digestion'.[136] Foods of this type were those that did not require much alteration from their present state. A classic example was the humble hen's egg, a staple ingredient in meals for the weak throughout the period.[137] In praise of eggs, the Wiltshire MP and physician Thomas Moffet (1553–1604) stated, 'They nourish quickly, because they are nothing but liquid flesh'.[138] In domestic recipe books, restorative broths typically contain between twelve and thirty eggs.[139] The clue to digestibility was colour: white, pale tones signified that the texture of the food was also light, and

---

[127] Frances Verney (ed.), *The Verney Memoirs, 1600–1659*, 2 vols. (1925, first publ. 1892), vol. 2, 376.
[128] Bullein, *Bulleins bulwarke*, 81.   [129] See Albala, *Eating Right*, ch. 2.
[130] Hart, *Klinike*, 173.   [131] Ibid., 182.
[132] John Harris, *The divine physician, prescribing rules for the prevention, and cure of most diseases, as well of the body, as the soul* (1676), to the reader.
[133] Hart, *Klinike*, 174.
[134] Allen Grieco, 'Food and Social Classes in Late Medieval and Renaissance Italy', in Jean-Louis Flandrin and Massimo Montanari (eds.), *Food: A Culinary History* (New York, 1999), 302–12.
[135] Alec Ryrie, *Being Protestant in Reformation Britain* (Oxford, 2013), 162.
[136] Hart, *Klinike*, 168.
[137] From either end of the time-period, see Barrough, *The methode*, 63; Pechey, *The store-house*, 187.
[138] Thomas Moffet, *Healths improvement: or rules...of preparing all sorts of food* (1655), 135. See also Hart, *Klinike*, 79; Platter, *Platerus golden practice*, 151.
[139] See WL, MS 1320, fol. 47v ('A Book of Physick, made in June 1710'); MS 1340, fol. 115r (Boyle Family, *c.*1675–*c.*1710); MS 7851, fol. 66v (English Recipe Book, late 1600s to early 1800s).

could be broken down with minimal effort.[140] For this reason, white meats such as chicken and partridges were pronounced best, whereas dark-coloured meats like beef and venison 'may not be allowed' because they are too heavy and dense.[141] These colour preferences, which endured throughout the period, may have been informed by religious ideas: light was a symbol of Christ, and darkness a metaphor for evil.[142] To make the foods easier to digest, practitioners recommended mashing or liquefying the ingredients; this would spare the patient from the 'unpleasant-nesse' of 'any mastication or chewing'.[143] Such a technique was used for other neutral groups too, like the elderly, 'whose teeth cannot be cheewing', as well as infants, who did not yet possess a complete set of teeth.[144] The cooking process could also help to make the foods more digestible: the best method was boiling, because it was most similar to Nature's own form of digestion in the stomach.[145] Over the course of convalescence, other cooking methods could be gradually introduced.[146]

The digestibility of the convalescent's food is one quality that overlapped with the diet of the diseased: doctors assumed the stomachs of the sick were even weaker than those of recovering patients. However, healthy individuals required the opposite. This is revealed in a regimen allegedly authored by the twelfth-century Italian physician Johannes de Mediolano, and published in English in 1650:

> For they that be strong and lusty, and exercise great labour must be dyeted with grosser meat because in them the way of digestion is strong, and so they ought not to use slender meats, as Chickens, Capons…or Kid, For those fleshes in them will burn, or be digested oversoon.[147]

The stomachs of 'sound persons' were depicted as fiery furnaces, which would combust simple food in a moment; these individuals therefore required much tougher meats, which would provide more sustained, slow-burning nourishment. As implied in the above extract, there was a link between social class and diet: labourers required foods which matched their rank—gross and unrefined—whereas the wealthy needed more delicate, 'fine' foods. The elites thus sought to reinforce their status through what they ate.[148]

Turning from the quality of food to the quantity, convalescents were advised to 'be temperate in eating and drinking…tak[ing] a little and often'.[149] Although moderation was important in all states of health, it was thought to be critical in convalescence, due to the residual weakness of the digestive faculty.[150] This advice sounds simple enough, but judging by doctors' reports, it was notoriously difficult

---

[140] Moffet, *Healths improvement*, 32–2. See also Albala, 'Food for Healing', 324–6, 328.

[141] Hart, *Klinike*, 79, 77–8, 173–4; Bruele, *Praxis medicinae*, 249.   [142] John 8:12.

[143] Hart, *Klinike*, 73; Barrough, *The methode*, 86.   [144] Bacon, *The historie of life*, 237.

[145] Hart, *Klinike*, 178.

[146] Ysbrand van Diemerbroeck, *The anatomy of human bodies…To which is added…several practical observations*, trans. William Salmon (1694, first publ. in Utrecht in 1664), 125.

[147] Joannes de Mediolano, *Regimen sanitatis salerni: or, the schoole of salernes regiment of health*, trans. Thomas Paynell (1650, first publ. in Latin in 1497, first English edn. 1541), 125. See also Moffet, *Healths improvement*, 94.

[148] Grieco, 'Food and Social Classes', 205–7, 311.   [149] Platter, *Platerus golden practice*, 159.

[150] Lemnius, *The secret miracles*, 244.

to follow. The young Oxfordshire physician Thomas Willis (1621–75), who would later become renowned for his theories on the nerves, noted that his patient, Abel Paine, 'for many days...had not tasted flesh [so] that [on the] day [of his recovery] he ate about half a roast chicken'. Three hours later, he was 'stricken with nausea, a signal loss of strength, and...difficulty in breathing'.[151] Physicians warned that the appetite is often 'sharp' after acute illness, which makes self-restraint especially challenging.[152] The social celebrations that were arranged to mark the person's recovery added to the danger, since they provided opportunities for overeating, along with other excesses. Lemnius complained:

> [W]hen men recover of their disease many witty merry companions come to see them, and they invite them to rejoyce, and make merry...Hence they eat, and drink healths...and commonly...they sing bawdy songs...To this I add the delicate and voluptuous meats, which the humours being augmented by, do stimulate and prick the obscene parts...and cause erection...[thus they] return to...gluttony, and profuse lusts.[153]

Lemnius implied that males were especially vulnerable to these vices because the first organ to regain strength after illness was the penis: directly connected to the liver, 'the nutriments are first carried' to the 'secret parts', so that 'upon the least lustfull thought, the Cods swell', hence 'such as recover are prone to venery'.[154] In this context, medical and religious concerns coalesce: gluttony for food and other sensual appetites would lead to the 'double relapse' of body *and* soul, as God used the natural consequences of immoderate eating to renew disease and punish the sinner.[155]

GROWING CHEERFUL

The next non-natural to consider is emotion, known in our period as the 'passions of the soul'.[156] While historians have paid considerable attention to the perceived impact of the passions on the body, much less work has been conducted on the influence of the body on the passions.[157] The following paragraphs illuminate both sides of the relationship.

---

[151] Thomas Willis, *Willis's Oxford Casebook (1650–52)*, ed. Kenneth Dewhurst (Oxford, 1981), 129. See also William Cockburn, *An account of...the distempers that are incident to seafaring people* (1697), 54.

[152] John Symcotts, *A Seventeenth Century Doctor and his Patients: John Symcotts, 1592?–1662*, ed. F. N. L. Poynter and W. J. Bishop, Bedfordshire Historical Record Society, vol. 31 (Streatley, 1951), 6.

[153] Lemnius, *The secret miracles*, 135.   [154] Ibid., 185.

[155] On the natural and divine causes of relapse, see Harris, *The divine physician*; Lemnius, *The secret miracles*, 135–6. Double relapse is discussed further in Chapter 4.

[156] For a definition of the passions, see the Introduction, pp. 17–18.

[157] On the effects of the emotions on the body, see Michael MacDonald, *Mystical Bedlam: Madness, Anxiety and Healing in Seventeenth-Century England* (Cambridge, 1981), 84, 72–3; David Gentilcore, 'The Fear of Disease and the Disease of Fear', in William Naphy and Penny Roberts (eds.), *Fear in Early Modern Society* (Manchester, 1997), 184–208; Andrew Wear, 'Fear, Anxiety and the Plague in Early Modern England: Religious and Medical Responses', in John Hinnells and Roy Porter (eds.), *Religion, Health, and Suffering* (1999), 339–63; Jan Frans van Dijkhuizen and Karl Enenkel (eds.), *The*

As with the other non-naturals, the passions provided clues into a person's state of health. The 'Messenger or forerunner' of illness was a creeping feeling of anxiety. Once illness had arrived in full, 'a horror... invades the sick', wrote the popular medical writer and astrologer Nicholas Culpeper (1616–54).[158] Patients routinely expressed grief and fear during illness.[159] Upon recovery, however, they began to grow cheerful. 'My mind is more cheerly, and I get strength', reported the Suffolk conformist clergyman Isaac Archer in 1679.[160] Laughter and cheerfulness were taken as clear signs of growing health.[161] Medical texts drew on the Aristotelian concept of the soul to explain these emotional responses. Hart averred:

> [A]lthough the substance of the soule and body differ much, God hath...tyed and united them so fast..., that there is no small...sympathy betwixt them: insomuch that either of them being affected, the other suffereth also.[162]

As Erin Sullivan has commented, the reciprocal influence between the body and soul seems to have been 'understood less as cause and effect and more as simultaneous happening'.[163]

Cheerfulness was not just a sign of recovery: it was also the means by which the weak body was restored to full strength. The author of *The sickmans rare jewel* (1674) states that this emotion 'recreates and quickens all the Faculties,...makes the Body to be better in liking, and fattens it'.[164] Sandra Cavallo and Tessa Storey have explored the perceived effects of cheerfulness in an Italian context, commenting that this emotion was understood to be a 'calm, tranquil happiness' which gently lifts and expands the spirits, 'thereby increasing the overall body heat and vitality'.[165] Since the strength of the body was synonymous with the quantity and liveliness of the spirits, the augmentation of these substances necessarily invigorated all the faculties of the body and mind.[166] This passion also helped the patient to put on weight, since the newly enlivened natural spirits would propel the digested aliment from the interior organs to the rest of the body, thereby facilitating the process of nutrition.[167] These ideas about the positive effects of cheerfulness continued throughout the period.[168]

Sense of Suffering: Constructions of Physical Pain in Early Modern Culture, Yearbook for Early Modern Studies, vol. 12 (Leiden, 2008); Elena Carrera (ed.), *Emotions and Health, 1200–1700* (Leiden, 2013); Cavallo and Storey, *Healthy Living*, ch. 6.

[158] Nicolas Culpeper, *Semeiotica uranica: or, an astrological judgement of diseases* (1651), 28–9.

[159] See Chapter 3, pp. 105–6.

[160] Isaac Archer, 'The Diary of Isaac Archer 1641–1700', in Matthew Storey (ed.), *Two East Anglian Diaries 1641–1729*, Suffolk Record Society, vol. 36 (Woodbridge, 1994), 41–200, at 162.

[161] See Chapter 3, pp. 109, 117–18.

[162] Hart, *Klinike*, 398. See also Thomas Walkington, *Optick glasse of humors* (1639, first publ. 1607), 8.

[163] Erin Sullivan, 'A Disease unto Death: Sadness in the Time of Shakespeare', in Carrera (ed.), *Emotions and Health*, 159–81, at 164.

[164] B.A., *The sick-mans rare jewell* (1674), 30.   [165] Cavallo and Storey, *Healthy Living*, 184.

[166] The link between the spirits and cheerfulness is evident in the use of the phrase 'high spirits' to denote a lively mood—see OED, 'cheerful' (accessed 17/02/17).

[167] Cavallo and Storey, *Healthy Living*, 185.

[168] For examples at either end of the timeframe, see Barrough, *The methode*, 6; Pechey, *A plain introduction*, 94.

Although cheerfulness usually accompanied recovery, it was not a universal response. As we saw earlier, one of the footsteps of disease was 'faint-heartedness' and anxiety.[169] Common causes included the traumatic memory of pain, and the fear of relapse.[170] What made these emotions all the more distressing for patients was the belief that they could precipitate the return of disease. The Essex puritan clergyman Ralph Josselin (1617–83) attributed the renewed illness of his eight-year-old daughter Jane in 1653 to her 'feare and griefe [at] see[ing] her mother so tormented...with a felon [boil] on her finger'.[171] Medical writers explained these effects by reference to the spirits: in motions of fear, these special vapours shrank and recoiled to the heart.[172] Since the spirits were the chief instruments through which Nature concocted and expelled bad humours, their sudden reduction in volume impeded her defence against the returning disease. These emotions also hindered nutrition: the centripetal direction of the spirits from the surface of the body to the heart starved the outer parts of nourishment—the result was the continuation of bodily wasting.[173]

In view of the divergent effects of cheerfulness and anxiety, convalescent care centred around the promotion of the former and the avoidance of the latter. The surest way to cultivate happy feelings was to surround the patient with 'merry company' and affectionate visitors. Speaking of her niece Kate in the 1650s, the Catholic nun Winefrid Thimelby wrote, 'I beleeve the company of her brothers and sisters will help much to her perfect recovery'.[174] Olivia Weisser has commented that the visits and letters of family and friends were found to be so therapeutic that they were called 'cordials', the term for medicines that strengthen the heart.[175] Indeed, patients often implied that these interactions were superior to physic. Robert Paston (1631–83), the First Earl of Yarmouth, told his wife Rebecca during his recovery from scurvy, 'your company will be the most soveraine remedye nature can apply'.[176] For children, play was encouraged during convalescence as a way to delight their spirits.[177] Alongside these positive measures, relatives and friends sought to protect the patient from anxiety by concealing bad news. In 1675, the Somerset gentlewoman Ursula Venner (1640–1710), warned her brother-in-law that although 'the danger is over', their father 'is soe extreamly we[e]ping at all kind of buisnesse that I would desire you to send him as little of ill news as possible'.[178] Of course, these forms of emotional support were unlikely to

---

[169] See p. 70 in this chapter.

[170] Timothy Rogers, *Practical discourses on sickness & recovery* (1691), 98.

[171] Ralph Josselin, *The Diary of Ralph Josselin 1616–1683*, ed. A. Macfarlane (Oxford, 1991), 297.

[172] Nicholas Coeffeteau, *A table of humane passions*, trans. Edward Grimeston (1621), 332.

[173] Hart, *Klinike*, 393.

[174] BL, Additional MS 36452, fol. 76r (Private letters of the Aston family, 1613–1703).

[175] Weisser, *Ill Composed*, 99, 107–8. In Latin, 'cor' means heart.

[176] Robert Paston, *The Whirlpool of Misadventures: Letters of Robert Paston, First Earl of Yarmouth 1663–1679*, ed. Jean Agnew, Norfolk Record Society, vol. 76 (2012), 311. For an example of the therapeutic effects of letters, see Henry Liddell, *The Letters of Henry Liddell to William Cotesworth*, ed. J. M. Ellis, Surtees Society, vol. 197 (Durham, 1987), 68.

[177] Fisher, *The wise virgin*, 146.

[178] Cited by Stobart, *Household Medicine*, 13 (SHC, DD/SF/3833: Sanford Family of Nynehead).

have been available to every convalescent: it was not always possible to hide bad news, nor did all convalescents enjoy such loving family relationships.

In contrast to some of the other aspects of convalescent care, cheerfulness was beneficial in all bodily states. Doctors agreed that 'nothing is more necessary for the Preservation of Health, than to live merrily'.[179] In sickness, cheerfulness was thought to 'rouse up and unite' the body's spirits, so that they were able to more 'effectively co-operate with Nature, and strengthen her in the performance of the...expulsion of the noxious humours', wrote the medical author and minister John Harris.[180] In fact, sudden joy could produce instantaneous healing: the sympathy between the soul and body was so great that the happiness of the soul might automatically bring health to the body.[181] Nonetheless, in practice it was difficult to provoke cheerfulness during sickness: the pain of illness, together with the 'true sorrow for sinne', conspired against these intentions.[182] Likewise, it was impractical to always promote cheerfulness in the healthy, since sorrow was an inevitable companion of life.[183] As such, the emotion of cheerfulness assumed a special status during convalescence: it was both a sign and a catalyst of growing strength.

SITTING UP TO GOING ABROAD

The final non-naturals to consider are exercise and air. Convalescence was basically a process of increasing physical exertion and exposure to the air. In acute sickness, the patient was usually confined to bed, breathing in warm indoor air—taking to bed, or 'decumbiture' as it was known, signified the beginning of sickness.[184] Once the illness was gone, however, the patient could begin to return to normal life, a trajectory that was marked by a number of key spatial movements. In 1666, fourteen-year-old Samuel Jeake from Rye in Sussex described his recovery from smallpox as follows:

21st July	I lay upon the bed all day.
22nd	Something better; but kept my bed till 27th then I rose.
28th	I went into my Study.
29th	Downstairs.
30th	into the garden.[185]

Each action and location signified a certain level of strength, which made them useful measures of a person's progress towards health. The final action, going outside,

[179] Pechey, *A plain introduction*, 95.
[180] Harris, *The divine physician*, 151.
[181] Hart, *Klinike*, 344. For a discussion of the curative effects of joy, see Weisser, *Ill Composed*, ch. 4; Olivia Weisser, 'Grieved and Disordered: Gender and Emotion in Early Modern Patient Narratives', *Journal of Medieval and Early Modern Studies*, 43 (2013), 247–73.
[182] Hart, *Klinike*, 395.
[183] See Chapter 5, pp. 177–8, for expressions on the sorrow of life.
[184] Culpeper admitted that this was not an infallible indicator of the beginning of illness because 'a lusty stout man...is longer before he takes his bed, then a puny weakly sickly man is': *Semeiotica uranica*, 28.
[185] Jeake, *An Astrological Diary*, 89–90.

or 'abroad' as it was usually known, was often used as a metonym for complete recovery. This can be seen in the correspondence of the MP William Fitzwilliam (1643–1719), who wrote in 1708, 'We are very glad to hear of Mrs Bull's being abroad again', implying she was better.[186] Such sayings indicate the vital, yet often overlooked, importance of place as a measure of health.[187]

Doctors believed that the exercise and exposure to air that accompanied the above physical movements contributed to the restoration of strength after illness. Hart explained, 'exercise… increase[s] the natural heat, [causes] a more speedy… distribution of the spirits…, and addition of strength to all the members therof'.[188] Pure, temperate air 'engenders both Vital and Animal Spirit', and 'opens the pores' of the skin, thereby enabling any remnant humours to escape, and preventing relapse.[189] Since the spirits shared the 'arey' consistency of the air, breathing was the most direct way to replenish these substances. Laypeople concurred about the strengthening effects of exercise and air, though they were less likely to describe the precise physiological processes involved.[190] The best air for the convalescent was fresh and fragrant mountain or country air, a preference which endured through-out the period. In 1598, the Countess of Shrewsbury, Elizabeth Talbot, urged her son-in-law and step-daughter to 'come into the cuntrye[,] [because] this eayre is better for you both than London, and especially… after your ague'.[191] Over a century later, the Northampton physician John Freind (1675–1728) advised his patient, Mr Hill, to 'go to Mount Cassel', in northern France, 'where the fresh air… will I hope not only recover, but mend his constitution'.[192] Perhaps this favouring of country air stemmed from the notion that the body's agent, Nature, felt most at home when in the wider, macrocosm of Nature—the hills and countryside.

The non-naturals of air and exercise were not without danger, however. Throughout the period, laypeople and doctors attributed relapse to the patient's premature activity or exposure to the air. The Dutch physician and professor Ysbrand van Diemerbroeck (1609–74), cited one patient of his, Henry Koelem, who, 'trusting too much to his strength' after a malignant fever in 1635, went 'abroad too soon', which sent him 'into a more dangerous Fever then [*sic*] his first… by reason of his strength debilitated by his former Sickness'.[193] Even apparently minor actions, such as sitting up in bed, could have significant consequences.[194] The reasons for these effects relate to Galenic ideas about the impact of cold air and exercise on

[186] William Fitzwilliam, *The Correspondence of Lord Fitzwilliam of Milton and Francis Guybon, His Steward 1697–1709*, ed. D. R. Hainsworth and Cherry Walker, Northampton Record Society, vol. 36 (1990), 271.

[187] Exceptions include Stobart, *Household Medicine*, 22–3; Alun Withey, *Physick and the Family: Health, Medicine and Care in Wales, 1600–1750* (Manchester, 2011), 127; Weisser, *Ill Composed*, 37, 113, 128.

[188] Hart, *Klinike*, 211.   [189] Galen, *Galens art of physic*, 91.

[190] John Buxton, *John Buxton, Norfolk Gentleman and Architect: Letters to his Son, 1719–1729*, ed. Alan Mackley, Norfolk Record Society, vol. 69 (Norwich, 2005), 99, 103.

[191] Lambeth Palace Library, MS 3205 f75; thanks to Caroline Bowden for this reference.

[192] RCP, ALS/F136 G (letters from John Freind to Henry Watkins). See also Rachel Russell, *Letters of Rachel, Lady Russell*, ed. Thomas Selwood, 2 vols. (1853, first publ. 1773), vol. 2, 4.

[193] Van Diemerbroeck, *The anatomy*, 72.

[194] Hervey, *Letter-Books*, 145.

weak bodies. Immediately after illness, when the body was frail and thin, Nature's main priority was nourishment; to force the body to exercise would therefore 'stop the Work of Nature so luckily begun', and delay the restoration of strength.[195] Exposure to cold air caused relapse by shutting the pores of the skin, thereby blocking the exits for the body's remnant humours, or causing them to putrefy.[196] Thomas Moffet recorded that one '*Harwood* of *Suffolk*, a rich Clothier, coming suddenly [into] an extream frost from a very hot fire into the cold aire' after an ague, 'his blood was presently so corrupted, that he became a leaper'.[197] Premature actions and air exposure were also common causes of illness amongst other 'neutral' patients, thus once again demonstrating the commonalities between these groups. Van Diemerbroeck complained that 'Child-bearing Women, in their Lyings in, frequently...trust themselves into the Air sooner than the time of their Lying in will permit; whence arise those dangerous Diseases'; he cited one acquaintance, who in the second week of her month, 'look[ed] to[o] soon after her House Affairs, and presuming to Combe her Head, fell into an Epilepsie'.[198]

Convalescent care sought to prevent these potential dangers by carefully 'ordering' the patient's progression through the actions, and ensuring they did not attempt anything too soon. Throughout the period, friends and family sent letters to recovering patients advising them to refrain from going abroad until they were quite ready 'to bear those journeys'.[199] Frances Seymour told her mother in the early 1700s, 'I am very sorry, dear Mama, that you are still so weak...and as much as I wish to see you[,] I would not have you venture on your journey...till you find yourself perfectly recovered'.[200] The clue as to when patients were ready to perform the actions was their sense of strength and ease. James Harrison, a lecturer and chaplain, wrote to Lady Joan Barrington about the condition of her husband in 1630: he told her that 'Mr Barrington [is] much better...but not yet so well as that he dares goe much abroad, but he finds most ease in being quiet within'.[201] Thus, the subjective experience of the patient was the best guide; this was because Nature made her wishes known through the patient's feelings.

Another tip for managing the progression through the actions was for convalescents to 'try their strength', and attempt everything gradually. It being 'so long a time since she had any use of her legs', eleven-year-old Martha Hatfield from Yorkshire, 'made [a] triall how she could go, and she went up and down the room', before embarking on a longer stroll around the house.[202] Patients like Martha, who had not walked for some time, might need help in weight-bearing; relatives supported their shoulders, or procured a crutch or staff for this purpose.[203] The patient's

---

[195] Van Diemerbroeck, *The anatomy*, 81.
[196] Symcotts, *A Seventeenth Century Doctor*, 45. On the shutting of the pores, see Cavallo and Storey, *Healthy Living*, 71–3.
[197] Moffet, *Healths improvement*, 27.   [198] Van Diemerbroeck, *The anatomy*, 62, 116.
[199] Hervey, *Letter-Books*, vol. 1, 335. For an early example, see a letter dated 15 May 1553 in the Cecil Project, reference: HMCS 15530515; thanks to Caroline Bowden for this reference.
[200] Seymour, *The Gentle Hertford*, 84.   [201] Searle (ed.), *Barrington Family Letters*, 159.
[202] Fisher, *The wise virgin*, 160–1.
[203] For example, Martindale, *The Life*, 214; Seale (ed.), *Barrington Family Letters*, 76–7; Brockbank, *The Diary*, 37.

exposure to the air, as well as exercise, had to be increased incrementally. Nicholas Abraham de La Framboisière suggested that, 'such [as] are newly recover'd from Sickness... must by degrees... accustom themselves to a more free and plentiful Air'.[204] The reason everything had to be done 'by degrees' is implicit in the common saying, 'Nature abhors all sudden change'.[205] When patients did decide to venture outdoors, they were advised to 'only stir abroad on warm days, and with very warm clothes to keep out the cold'.[206] Such measures, also recommended for lying-in mothers, would ensure that the pores of the skin remained open.[207] Patients themselves put in place special arrangements to help limit the hazards posed by exercise and air, such as delegating strenuous work to friends or colleagues, or securing comfortable transport for journeys.[208] Mary Cowper (1685–1724), Lady of the Bedchamber, recorded that her convalescing mistress had 'gone a walking' as far as Kensington, and 'the Coaches brought [her] back again'.[209] Walking only half the way was a sensible compromise, ensuring that exercise did not become 'excessive'. These arrangements were obviously dependent on the good will of relations and colleagues, as well as the occupation and financial position of the individual. Patients in low paid jobs, working under the authority of others, may not have been able to benefit from these sorts of flexible measures.

Advice about exercise and air differed for each bodily state. Hart cautioned that in acute illness, patients should 'not... use any exercise at all': such diseases were 'so violent and fierce' that Nature could not afford to divert her spirits from the vital tasks of concocting and expelling the humours.[210] Likewise, exposure to outdoor air was to be avoided in these illnesses, on the grounds that it would hinder the critical evacuation of the noxious humours, instead sending them inwards towards the 'noble organs'. Van Diemerbroeck confirmed that 'when... the Small Pox begin to appear, then the catching Cold will be the occasion of a great mistake, for that it detains the superfluity within, and carrys it to the Principal Members'.[211] The advice for the healthy was rather different: fresh air and 'vehement exercise' were 'so necessarie to the preservation of health' that without them 'no man may be long without sicknes', wrote the humanist and lawyer Thomas Elyot (*c*.1490–1546) in his best-selling regimen.[212] These non-naturals maintained the strength of the healthy body by stirring up the spirits and promoting the perspiration of superfluous humours. The convalescent's regimen was a transition between these two extremes, and involved some special exercises. The Bedfordshire doctor, John Symcotts (*c*.1592–1662), provides insights into these forms of exercise in a letter to his patient, Mistress Halford:

[E]xercise by degrees is requisite, otherwise the serous and watery moisture which abounds... will in you superabound. Which measure of exercise, because your weak

---

[204] Framboisière, *The art of physick*, 72.
[205] Galen, *Galens art of physic*, 202; Jane Sharp, *The midwives book* (1671), 89.
[206] Fitzwilliam, *The Correspondence*, 156.   [207] Paré, *The workes*, 916.
[208] Examples can be found in Fitzwilliam, *The Correspondence*, 125–6, 155.
[209] Mary Cowper, *Diary of Mary, Countess Cowper*, ed. John Murray (1864), 23.
[210] Hart, *Klinike*, 220.   [211] Van Diemerbroeck, *The anatomy*, 26.
[212] Thomas Elyot, *The castle of health* (1610, first publ. 1534), 72.

body will not admit of, you must…Let your upper parts, as neck, shoulder, arms, back and breast, be rubbed every morning before you rise with soft cloths, first more gently, after more strongly as you are able to bear it.[213]

Symcotts may have taken these ideas from Galen's *Method of physic*, which instructs, 'Whereupon the *Sick* being the better, he must…in the morning…be moderatly rubbed, till the whole body be warmed'.[214] The vibrations caused by this form of passive exercise restored strength by stirring the spirits, and cherishing the natural heat.[215] A more active type of exertion for 'weake people' was '*Slow* walking', which 'softens bodies exhaust[ed]…and purges them, by opening the Pores'.[216]

CONCLUSION

Thomas Saunders from Hertfordshire was told by his doctor in 1671 that 'the convulsions seem totally to have left' his young son, 'so that there remaynes cheefely to be attended, the universal weaknesse'. Saunders recommended that this deficiency could be remedied by a combination of 'gentle exercises', a diet of 'easy digestion' such as 'tostes…sopped in gravy', and 'strengthninge' medicines.[217] This chapter has shown that a concept of convalescence existed in early modern England: it denoted the gradual restoration of strength after illness, and was regarded as the second stage of recovery, which took place once the disease had been removed. Convalescents were considered worthy of their own special type of medical care, 'analeptics', which was designed to promote the patient's growing strength and guard against relapse. These aims could be achieved through the careful monitoring and management of the six non-naturals. Miss Kemey 'sleeps well and eats an egg and sits up for two or three hours', wrote the Bishop of Bath and Wells, Thomas Ken, in 1686, which he interpreted as signs and spurs of her growing strength.[218] Cheerful passions, an appetite for nutritious food, and the ability to 'walk abroad', signified that the patient was 'on the mending hand', while simultaneously helping to strengthen the body by expanding and enlivening the spirits, the instruments of bodily and mental functions. Personified to a high degree, the spirits were synonymous with the patient's own strength and well-being.

The discussions have concentrated on the roles of practitioners and the patient's family in convalescent care, but it should be pointed out that the other two healers identified in Chapter 1—God and Nature—remained crucial. It was the Lord who ordained the full restoration of health; His instrument was the body's internal agent, Nature, who set about strengthening the body by inducing certain inclinations and appetites in the patient, like a desire for tasty food and a breath of fresh air.

[213] Symcotts, *A Seventeenth Century Doctor*, 16.   [214] Galen, *Galen's method of physic*, 139.
[215] On passive exercise, see Cavallo and Storey, *Healthy Living*, ch. 5.
[216] Johnstonus, *The idea of practical physick*, 21.
[217] RCP, G62 (Letter from Francis Glisson to Thomas Saunders, Hertfordshire, 25 November 1671).
[218] Arthur Bryant (ed.), *Postman's Horn: An Anthology of the Letters of Latter Seventeenth Century England* (New York, 1946, first publ. 1936), 191.

She depended, however, on her 'servant', the patient's practitioner or relatives, to actually satisfy her cravings, and supply her with the things the body needed, such as an armchair for afternoon naps, easily digestible meals, and merry company. In the light of these interactions, it becomes clear as to why the non-naturals were known as *non*-naturals. The six dietary and life-style factors were *exterior* to the body's internal healing agent, Nature; she could induce appetites in the patient, but relied on the practitioner to satisfy the body's wants. Besides these insights, the discussions have shed fresh light on the meanings of health and disease, states which have often been equated with balance and imbalance; other crucial components were location and function: sickness was being in bed, unable to eat or sleep; health was being able to sleep, eat, walk, and go abroad. Health was not only the absence of disease, but the presence of strength.

While much work has been conducted on the gendering of bodies, far less has been written about bodily categorizations based on states of health.[219] We have seen that the convalescent was placed in the 'neutral' category of bodies, alongside other individuals who were deemed 'neither sick nor sound'. By resurrecting this forgotten category, the chapter has sought to expand our knowledge of early modern bodily classifications, and encourage comparative studies of groups within the neutral category. Much of the discussion of the neutral body is based on published medical literature, which raises the question of whether the wider populace also recognized this category. My impression is that while laypeople were less inclined to use the term 'neutrum' than physicians, they certainly were aware of the half-way state between sickness and health. This is evidenced by, as Levinus Lemnius put it, 'daily use and custome...Hence proceed those answers of our friends..., if they aske how any man doth, what health he is in...[he will] answer in so many words; "So so, indifferent, not very well, doubtfully, inclining, floting between both"'.[220]

An underlying question in this chapter has been to what extent the care of convalescents differed from the treatment of patients in the other bodily categories, health and sickness. The therapeutic intentions were clearly distinctive: the care of the sick centred on the removal of disease; the treatment of the healthy sought to preserve the current state; analeptics was devoted to the restoration of strength and the prevention of relapse. However, we have seen that there were some intersections between the three, since convalescence was a liminal state; over the course of recovery, the patient's regimen became increasingly similar to that of the healthy person. There were also some striking similarities between the care of groups within the neutral category, including the elderly, the newborn, and lying-in mothers. What all these patients had in common was weakness, although the causes and duration of their debility differed.

Little evidence has been found to show major change over time in the care or perception of the convalescent. The footsteps of disease—weakness, emaciation, and vulnerability to relapse—were reported consistently across the period. Likewise,

---

[219] See the Introduction, note 17, for a summary of this literature.
[220] See note 67 in this chapter.

the methods that were used to restore strength, such as nutritious and easily digestible food, plenty of sleep, and gentle exercise, went uncontested into the eighteenth century. Such continuity does not mean that convalescent care was based on ahistorical 'common sense', or was somehow divorced from medical theory. Rather, it reflects the endurance of the belief in the role of the spirits in the restoration of strength.[221] The majority of the examples cited in this chapter pertain to members of the middling and upper echelons of society; further research is required to find out if analeptics was also available lower down the social scale.

---

[221] On the endurance of the belief in the spirits between 1200 and 1700, see Carrera, *Emotions and Health*, 5, 99, 221, 224, 237–8.

PART II
PERSONAL EXPERIENCES

3

'O, How Sweet is Ease!'
Feeling Better

In 1682, the nonconformist minister Philip Henry (1631–96), recorded in his diary the words of his sick wife, Katherine (1629–1707), who was suffering from an acute fever. All through her illness, she could be heard crying out, 'sick, sick, never so sick'. However, 'by and by', this utterance was replaced by the welcome announcement, 'now I am better'.[1] These two little words, 'sick' and 'better', are ubiquitous in accounts of illness and recovery; they seem to have summed up perfectly what it was like to feel ill and well in early modern England. But what exactly did these feelings entail? What sensations constituted sickness and its mitigation? This chapter attempts to provide answers: it investigates the transition from feeling ill to feeling better, exploring the patient's physical and emotional experience of the abatement of bodily suffering, perhaps the most delightful aspect of recovery for many individuals.

While a considerable amount of research has been conducted on expressions and experiences of pain in the early modern period, the question of what it was like to be alleviated from suffering has rarely been addressed.[2] This is probably because it has been assumed that if anything, pre-modern medicine exacerbated, rather than eased, pain![3] The only work which has been undertaken on relief from suffering focuses on pharmaceutical breakthroughs in analgesics, rather than on the sensations of ease brought by these medicines.[4] Nor has much research been carried out on types of discomfort which today are not always classed as pain, and yet in the early modern era were considered to be notorious forms of suffering, common in many diseases, such as loss of appetite, nausea, and sleeplessness.[5] By examining how patients responded to the mitigation of all these varieties of suffering, the chapter seeks to illuminate not only what it was like to recover, but also to provide

---

[1] Philip Henry, *The Diaries and Letters of Philip Henry of Broad Oak, Flintshire, A.D. 1631–1696*, ed. M. H. Lee (1882), 315–17.

[2] See the Introduction, note 25 for this historiography.   [3] See Chapter 1, note 136.

[4] For example, Thomas Dormandy, *The Worst of Evils: The Fight Against Pain* (2006); Edmund Eger, Lawrence Saidman, and Rod Westhorpe (eds.), *The Wondrous Story of Anesthesia* (New York, 2014).

[5] In the health sciences, there is a growing awareness of these other 'neglected sensations'; for example, Christopher Eccleston, *Embodied: The Psychology of Physical Sensation* (Oxford, 2016). Nausea has been discussed in a nineteenth-century context by Rachael Russell, but we still lack an early modern history of this symptom: 'Nausea and Vomiting: A History of Signs, Symptoms and Sickness in Nineteenth-Century Britain' (unpublished PhD thesis, Manchester University, 2012); ch. 5 is devoted to the experience of nausea. My thanks to Jonathan Reinarz for alerting me to this thesis.

a more holistic picture of illness than is currently offered. I show that both 'feeling ill' and 'feeling better' were inherently sensory experiences: patients described their disease and ease by referring to the five senses, a tendency which has rarely been observed explicitly by historians. Ultimately, the decline of suffering was a double joy for patients, of their bodies and souls: they found that physical pain produced distressing emotions in their souls, and the eventual ease brought rejoicing. Through exploring these experiences, the chapter enhances our understanding of the body–soul relationship in early modern perceptions, whilst adding to the small, but growing, scholarship devoted to pleasurable sensations like euphoria.[6]

As well as analysing patients' experiences, this chapter examines the reactions of relatives and friends as they witnessed the sufferings and subsequent ease of their loved ones. Although valuable work has been undertaken on the practical roles of family members in the care and treatment of patients, the emotional and sensory experiences of these individuals have been largely neglected.[7] Amongst scholars of pain, there has been a surge of interest in the feelings of health professionals as they observed, or inflicted, pain, but very little has been said about the responses of relatives.[8] Even less research has been undertaken on families' reactions to the *mitigation* of the patient's suffering.[9] We will see that relatives and close friends shared the experience of the patient, a phenomenon known as 'fellow-feeling' in this period. So acute was their emotional distress upon observing their loved one's pains, they frequently claimed to feel something akin to the physical suffering itself; in the same way, the patient's ease was the source of intense emotional *and* physical relief in relatives. These findings support the thesis of the revisionist pain historian Jan Frans van Dijkhuizen, who has challenged Elaine Scarry's famous assertion that pain is an 'unsharable experience'.[10] Taking a new, sensory approach,

---

[6] For an intellectual history of euphoria, see Chris Milnes, ' "I am Better": A History of Euphoria' (unpublished PhD thesis, Birkbeck, University of London, 2014). Most of the historiography on pleasure focuses on erotic pleasure/pain; for example, John Wilson-Yamamoto, *Pain, Pleasure and Perversity: Discourses of Suffering in Seventeenth Century England* (Farnham, 2013); Sarah Toulalan, *Imagining Sex: Pornography and Bodies in Seventeenth-Century England* (Oxford, 2007), ch. 3.

[7] Here is a brief selection: Lucinda Beier, *Sufferers and Healers: The Experience of Illness in Seventeenth-Century England* (1987), ch. 8; Lisa Smith, 'Reassessing the Role of the Family: Women's Medical Care in Eighteenth-Century England', *SHM*, 16 (2003), 327–42; Lisa Smith, 'The Relative Duties of a Man: Domestic Medicine in England and France, ca. 1685–1740', *Journal of Family History*, 31 (2006), 237–56; Seth Stein LeJacq, 'The Bounds of Domestic Healing: Medical Recipes, Storytelling and Surgery in Early Modern England', *SHM*, 26 (2013), 451–68; Anne Stobart, *Household Medicine in Seventeenth-Century England* (2016). For a summary of women's roles in care, see Peter Elmer (ed.), *The Healing Arts: Health, Disease and Society in Europe 1500–1800* (Manchester, 2004), 34–7.

[8] On doctors'/surgeons' responses, see Lynda Payne, *With Words and Knives: Learning Medical Dispassion in Early Modern England* (Aldershot, 2007); Philip Wilson, *Surgery, Skin and Syphilis: Daniel Turner's London (1667–1741)* (Amsterdam, 1999), 52; for a later period, see Joanna Bourke, *The Story of Pain: From Prayer to Painkillers* (Oxford, 2014), ch. 8.

[9] I briefly consider this in *The Sick Child in Early Modern England* (Oxford, 2012), 137, 155. Olivia Weisser has also explored relatives' responses to illness/recovery in *Ill Composed: Sickness, Gender, and Belief in Early Modern England* (2015), 81, 87, 89, 94, 98–9. Weisser's focus is on medical ideas about how emotions affected health, rather than on the family's experience of recovery.

[10] Jan Frans van Dijkhuizen, *Pain and Compassion in Early Modern English Literature and Culture* (Cambridge, 2012); Elaine Scarry, *The Body in Pain: The Making and Unmaking of the World* (Oxford, 1985), 4. Bourke also believes pain is sharable, but her focus is a later period: *The Story of Pain*.

I argue that it was chiefly through the ears and eyes that relatives and friends came to share the patient's sufferings and eventual relief.[11] No longer hearing their 'mournful moans' or seeing their 'sad lookes' occasioned great joy.[12] These discussions shed fresh light on the meaning of the emotion of love: a 'signe…of true *Love*', wrote the French philosopher and theologian Nicholas Coeffeteau (1574–1623), was that 'friends rejoyce & grieve for the same things'.[13]

As implied above, this chapter engages with the flourishing field of sensory studies.[14] In the history of early modern medicine, work has been conducted on how the senses were thought to be involved in disease causation, diagnosis, and treatment.[15] Much less attention, however, has been paid to the sensory experience of illness itself.[16] As well as bringing us closer to what it was like to feel better, a sensory approach opens up opportunities for engagement with a vexed debate within the history of the senses: the question of how the five senses were ranked in early modern culture. Traditionally, this is the era in which society is said to have become ocular-centric—sight was elevated above the other senses, especially touch.[17] However, we will see that within the setting of the sickchamber, various different

[11] One exception is David Turner, who has explored strangers' emotional responses to the sights of disabled people in the 1700s, in *Disability in Eighteenth-Century England* (Abingdon, 2012), ch. 4.

[12] On the historiography of medicine and the senses, see note 15 in this chapter.

[13] Nicholas Coeffeteau, *A table of humane passions*, trans. Edward Grimeston (1621), 103–5.

[14] For a short introduction to the state of the field, and the 'styles' of sensory history, see Mark Smith, 'Preface: Styling Sensory History', in Jonathan Reinarz and Leonard Schwarz (eds.), 'Special Issue: The Senses', *Eighteenth-Century Studies*, 35 (2012), 436–627, at 469–72. On the challenges of this sort of history, see Mark Smith, 'Producing Sense, Consuming Sense, Making Sense: Perils and Prospects of Sensory History', *Journal of Social History*, 40 (2007), 841–58.

[15] On the role of the senses in diagnosis, see William Bynum and Roy Porter (eds.), *Medicine and the Five Senses* (Cambridge, 1993); Olivia Weisser, 'Boils, Pushes and Wheals: Reading Bumps on the Body in Early Modern England', *SHM*, 22 (2009), 321–39; Patrick Singy, 'Medicine and the Senses: The Perception of Essences', in Anne Vila (ed.), *A Cultural History of the Senses in the Age of Enlightenment* (2014), 133–53; Michael Stolberg, *Uroscopy in Early Modern Europe* (Aldershot, 2015); Ingrid Sykes, 'The Art of Listening: Perceiving Pulse in Eighteenth-Century Paris', in Reinarz and Schwarz (eds.), 'Special Issue', 473–88. On the role of bad smells in causing disease, see Jonathan Reinarz, *Past Scents: Historical Perspectives on Smell* (Urbana IL, 2014), ch. 6; Holly Dugan, *The Ephemeral History of Perfume: Scent and Sense in Early Modern England* (Baltimore MD, 2011), 97–125. On the therapeutic roles of the senses, see Carole Rawcliffe, '"Delectable Sightes and Fragrant Smelles": Gardens and Health in Late Medieval and Early Modern England', *Garden History*, 36 (2008), 3–21; Peregrine Horden (ed.), *Music as Medicine: The History of Music Therapy Since Antiquity* (Aldershot, 2000); Jennifer Evans, 'Female Barrenness, Bodily Access and Aromatic Treatments in Seventeenth-Century England', *Historical Research*, 86 (2014), 423–43. On the uses of the senses to decipher a drug's healing properties, see Andrew Wear, *Knowledge and Practice in English Medicine, 1550–1680* (Cambridge, 2000), 89–90, 397–8; Mark Jenner, 'Tasting Litchfield, Touching China: Sir John Floyer's Senses', *The Historical Journal*, 53 (2010), 647–70; Elaine Leong and Alisha Rankin (eds.), *Special Issue: Testing Drugs and Trying Cures*, Bulletin of the History of Medicine, 91 (2017), 167–8, 172. On the apparent decline in the use of the senses in disease diagnosis, causation, and cure, see David Howes and Constance Classen, 'Sensuous Healing: The Sensory Practice of Medicine', in their monograph, *Ways of Sensing: Understanding the Senses in Society* (Abingdon, 2014), 37–62.

[16] One notable exception is Reinarz's study of the sensory environment of the eighteenth-century hospital, which takes the perspective of visitors: 'Learning to Use their Senses: Visitors to Voluntary Hospitals in Eighteenth-Century England', *Eighteenth-Century Studies*, 35 (2012), 505–20.

[17] Exponents of this view include Walter Ong, *Orality and Literacy: The Technologizing of the Word* (1982); Norbert Elias, *The Civilizing Process* (Oxford, 1977–82); R. Jutte, *A History of the Senses: From Antiquity to Cyberspace*, trans. J. Lynn (Cambridge, 2005), 60–6; Constance Classen, *The Deepest Sense: A Cultural History of Touch* (Urbana IL, 2012), ch. 7.

hierarchies were in operation, which together confirm the revisionist position that there exist multiple rankings in any given situation.[18] Examples of 'intersensoriality', the interactions between individual senses, will also be presented.[19] The methodological challenges of accessing sensory and emotional experiences have been discussed in the Introduction, and so will not be repeated here.[20] The first part of the chapter examines the experiences of patients, and the second half turns to their families and close friends.

PATIENTS

Since the experience of feeling better was contingent on the preceding feeling of illness, it is first necessary to dissect, in some detail, what exactly sickness felt like. Often, patients found this hard to pinpoint. Seventeen-year-old Elizabeth Delaval (1649–1717), a royalist from Lincolnshire, lamented, 'what I now indure, it can scarcely be discribed', while suffering from worms in her gums.[21] For some patients, the only words that came close to encapsulating the experience of illness were 'misery', 'sick', or 'distress'.[22] The Quaker gentlewoman Mary Penington (*c*.1632–82) recalled that during a violent fever, 'I made my moan in these doleful words: "distress! distress! distress!"[,] finding these words comprehended all my feelings'.[23] Fortunately, these brief statements can be supplemented by more detailed descriptions of what it was like to feel ill. Despite considerable variation between diseases, three particular features recur with great frequency in accounts of serious physical illness: pain, nausea, and sleeplessness. These forms of suffering were sometimes classed as diseases in their own right, but doctors and patients also recognized that they accompanied many illnesses.[24]

Pain was thought to be the 'first *Symptom* of most diseases', and of all forms of bodily suffering, 'the most troublesome intruder upon the sick'.[25] Defined in

[18] Anne Villa highlights these multiple hierarchies in 'Introduction: Powers, Pleasures, and Perils of the Senses in the Enlightenment Era', in Anne Villa (ed.), *A Cultural History of the Senses in the Age of Enlightenment* (2014), 1–20, at 1–2. See also Mark Jenner, 'Follow Your Nose? Smell, Smelling, and Their Histories', *American Historical Review*, 116 (2011), 335–51. On the continued importance of touch in this era, see Joe Moshenska, *Feeling Pleasures: The Sense of Touch in Renaissance England* (Oxford, 2014).

[19] For an introduction to intersensoriality, see Herman Roodenburg (ed.), *A Cultural History of the Senses in the Renaissance* (2014), 6–10. Two recent intersensorial studies include Reinarz and Schwarz (eds.), 'Special Issue: The Senses', and Simon Smith, Jackie Watson, and Amy Kenny (eds.), *The Senses in Early Modern England* (Manchester, 2015).

[20] See the Introduction, pp. 28–30.

[21] Elizabeth Delaval, *The Meditations of Lady Elizabeth Delaval, Written Between 1662 and 1671*, ed. D. G. Greene, Surtees Society, vol. 190 (1978), 78.

[22] For example, John Donne, *Devotions upon emergent occasions: and severall steps in my sicknes* (1624), 177; Robert Harris, *Hezekiahs recovery. Or, a sermon, shewing what use Hezekiah did, and all should make of their deliverance from sicknesse* (1626), 35–6. The ubiquity of the word 'misery' is why the term appears in the title of this book.

[23] Mary Penington, *Experiences in the Life of Mary Penington Written by Herself*, ed. Norman Penney (1992, first publ. 1911), 66.

[24] My thanks to Elizabeth Hunter for her insights on the disorders of sleep. On the blurred boundary between disease and symptom, see Wear, *Knowledge and Practice*, 106–7.

[25] Everard Maynwaringe, *Pains afflicting humane bodies* (1682), 7.

Galenic medicine as the '*Molestation or trouble of the five Senses*', pain denoted any unpleasant sensory stimulus, including such things as bitter tastes and smells, harsh or loud sounds, and glaring lights.[26] Of all the senses, however, pain was associated particularly with touch. Galen confirmed in his treatise on the causes of symptoms, 'pain [is] inherent to all the senses, although clearly not to an equal degree, being least in that of vision, and most in that of touch'.[27] The full hierarchy is depicted in Figure 4; it is the reverse of the usual ordering of the senses in early modern culture.[28] Rarely recognized in the historiography, this sensory understanding of pain challenges the widespread assumption that pain was 'not a distinct medical phenomenon' at this time.[29]

When it came to putting pain into words, the use of figurative language was deemed indispensable.[30] Patients deployed a colourful variety of metaphors to describe pain, the most common of which referred to torture, warfare, animal attacks, temperature, storms, sharpness, and bitterness. Here, only the last two will be examined, as the others have been discussed elsewhere.[31] Henry Liddell (*c*.1673–1717), a coal-trader from North Yorkshire, told a friend he had endured 'a sharp tast[e] off [*sic*] an infirmity', toothache.[32] The nonconformist minister from Halifax, Oliver Heywood (*c*.1630–1702), complained in 1676 that his 'head akt very bitterly'.[33] Historians usually link the metaphor of sharpness with the instruments or weapons that produce these sensations, but I think its primary association would have been the sensory feeling itself: sharpness was defined as a bitter or sour taste, or a piercing and cutting tactile sensation.[34] Etymologically, the word 'bitter' comes from the Old English *biter*, which means 'biting, cutting,

---

[26] Felix Platter, *Platerus golden practice of physick* (1664), 187.

[27] Galen, 'On the Causes of Symptoms I', in Ian Johnston (ed. and trans.), *Galen on Diseases and Symptoms* (Cambridge, 2006), 203–35, at 220–1, 189. This text was available in Latin in the early modern period, translated from the Greek by Thomas Linacre as *De symptomatum differentiis et causis* (1524). For similar definitions in vernacular texts, see Platter, *Platerus golden practice*, 220; Coeffeteau, *A table*, 322.

[28] This ranking was developed in antiquity; it was based on the distance between the sensory organ and the object; the greater the gap, the 'nobler' the sense: Viktoria von Hoffmann, *From Gluttony to Enlightenment: The World of Taste in Early Modern Europe* (2016), 4–7.

[29] Jan Frans van Dijkhuizen and Karl Enenkel (eds.), *The Sense of Suffering: Constructions of Physical Pain in Early Modern Culture*, Yearbook for Early Modern Studies, vol. 12 (Leiden, 2008), 7–9. In the same volume, Stephen Pender does, however, acknowledge the sensory definition of pain in 'Seeing, Feeling, Judging: Pain in the Early Modern Imagination', 469–95; see also Roselyn Rey, *The History of Pain*, trans. Louise Elliot Wallace, J. A. Cadden, and S. W. Cadden (1998, first publ. 1993), 30–7.

[30] On the need for metaphors, see Bourke, *The Story of Pain*, ch. 3; Scarry, *The Body in Pain*, 15. Ariel Glucklich addresses the extent to which metaphors convey the actual experience of pain in *Sacred Pain: Hurting the Body for the Sake of the Soul* (Oxford, 2001), 42.

[31] See Newton, *The Sick Child*, 192–8; Weisser, *Ill Composed*, 133–9, 143–4; Bourke, *The Story of Pain*, 72–80; Mary Ann Lund, 'Experiencing Pain in John Donne's "Devotions Upon Emergent Occasions" (1624)', in Van Dijkhuizen and Enenkel (eds.), *The Sense of Suffering*, 323–45.

[32] Henry Liddell, *The Letters of Henry Liddell to William Cotesworth*, ed. J. M. Ellis, Surtees Society, vol. 197 (Durham, 1987), 115. See also Bulstrode Whitelocke, *The Diary of Bulstrode Whitelocke, 1605–1675*, ed. Ruth Spalding (Oxford, 1990), 690.

[33] Oliver Heywood, *The Rev. Oliver Heywood, B.A: His Autobiography, Diaries, Anecdote and Event Books*, ed. Horsfall Turner, 4 vols. (1883), vol. 3, 145.

[34] For example, Bourke, *The Story of Pain*, 62. See the OED definitions for 'sharp' (noun and adjective), which are based on early modern vignettes (accessed 1/10/16).

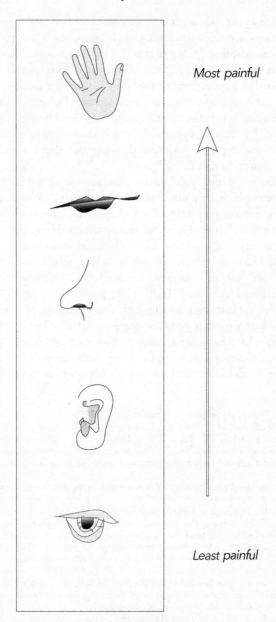

Most painful

Least painful

Figure 4. Hierarchy of the five senses in the context of pain; kindly created by Charles Shanahan for the author. This ordering is the reverse to the normal ranking associated with Aristotle.

sharp'; it also denotes acrid or sour tastes.[35] A biblical commentary on Hezekiah's 'bitter illness', by the Oxfordshire clergyman Adam Littleton (1627–94), provides some clues into why sensory language was used in accounts of pain:

> The sense of Taste... [is] that by which all *Animals* take in their food...; and therefore [it] has... a power to judge, what is... convenient to the nature of each kinde, what not. Now there is no gust the palate so much dis-relishes as the *bitter*;... Upon this score 'tis,... [the] usual *Metaphor* [for] everything that... is in any way afflictive to flesh and blood... [such as] grief, or pain.[36]

Littleton is alluding to contemporary nutrition theory, according to which the bitterness of the foodstuff signifies its perniciousness to the body; this notion made the quality apt for describing anything unpleasant, and rendered taste a much more powerful metaphor than it is today.[37] During illness, the association between taste and pain must have been accentuated by recent experiences of swallowing bitter-tasting medicines; this connection was so well known that allegorical paintings of this sense sometimes include a medicinal potion (see Figure 5).[38] Religion also contributed to patients' linguistic choices: theologians taught that pain was a 'bitter drink', ordained by God as a punishment for human sin.[39] This metaphor comes from John 18:11, where Jesus asks his disciple Simon Peter, just before his arrest, 'the cup which my Father hath given me, shall I not drink it?' Thus, patients associated pain most with touch and taste, the two 'lowest senses' in the traditional hierarchy of the senses.[40]

The second component of the feeling of illness to discuss is nausea, a term which denoted a cluster of symptoms relating to the nutritive faculty, including suppressed appetite, lost or depraved taste, and an inclination to vomit.[41] Reflecting on his recent illness in 1623, the poet and dean of St Paul's Cathedral, John Donne (1572–1631), recorded, 'In the twinckling of an eye... the tast[e] is inspid... the appetite... dull and desireless'.[42] Almost a century later, the Somerset teacher John Cannon (1684–1743) 'suddenly awoke with violent reaching' during smallpox.[43] So common were these symptoms in acute illnesses, the word 'sick' came to mean both the feeling of nausea, *and* illness in general, an obvious and yet strangely overlooked point.[44] Although patients recognized that these symptoms were part of the recovery process—nausea signalled that the body's healing agent, Nature, was gearing

[35] OED for 'bitter' (noun and adjective) (accessed 1/10/16); see also Edward Phillips, *The new world of English words* (1658), images 97, 119.

[36] Adam Littleton, *Hezekiah's return of praise for his recovery* (1668), 6–7.

[37] Ken Albala, *Eating Right in the Renaissance* (Berkeley CA, 2002), 82–3.

[38] On the rationale behind the bitter taste of medicines, see Chapter 1, p. 55.

[39] Rogers, *Practical discourses*, 156.

[40] Lucy Munro, 'Staging Taste', in Smith, Watson, and Kenny (eds.), *The Senses*, 19–38, at 20–1.

[41] For a definition of 'nausea', see Phillips, *The new world*, image 122.

[42] Donne, *Devotions*, 26.

[43] SHC, DD/SAS C/1193/4, p. 101 (Memoirs John Cannon, officer of the excise, West Lydford, Somerset).

[44] The OED states that 'sick' (adjective/noun) means 'Suffering from illness of any kind', and also 'Having an inclination to vomit, or being actually in the condition of vomiting' (accessed 2/10/16).

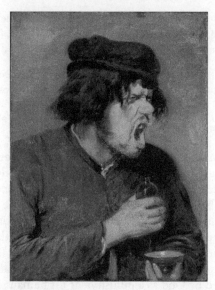

Figure 5. *The Bitter Potion* (*c.*1636–8), by Adriaen Brouwer; Städel Museum, Germany. The man's face is contorted in an expression of revulsion after tasting the bitter medicine; his grimace resembles the appearance of a person in pain.

up to expel the bad humours by vomiting—the feeling was nevertheless a deeply unpleasant one.[45] John Collinges (1623–91), an Essex clergyman, averred that 'there is nothing more...troublesome[e] to us [in sickness], than the sower recoilings of our stomack'.[46] Terms that occur frequently in patients' descriptions of nausea include 'disgustful', 'loathing', and 'distasteful', all of which suggest a sensation of deep repugnance towards edible substances.[47] This aversion was fundamentally sensory in nature: it was the texture, taste, and smell of a foodstuff or medicine that elicited these feelings. Speaking of texture, the sixteenth-century Suffolk surgeon Philip Barrough warned that 'those thinges that require much chewing, do cause unpleasantnesse' to the sick, while the London physician Thomas Moffet (1553–1604) observed that 'Weak stomacks...eschue' food of a slimy nature, such as 'fat, oily, and buttered meats'.[48] Purgative physic was obviously disgusting, since it was the 'loathsome savour' that provoked vomiting, but even ostensibly pleasant foods and medicines were found to taste and smell nasty.[49] This tendency was attributed to patients' inability to 'distinguish the true taste of any

---

[45] See Chapter 1, p. 54.

[46] John Collinges, *Several discourses concerning the actual Providence of God* (1678), 355.

[47] These words are used synonymously in the OED. See also Phillips, *The new world*, 41, 63.

[48] Philip Barrough, *The methode of phisicke* (1583), 86; Thomas Moffet, *Healths improvement: or rules...of preparing all sorts of food* (1655), 130.

[49] On how emetics work, see Chapter 1, p. 55.

food'.[50] Recalling a recent illness, the natural philosopher Robert Boyle (1627–91) observed that some of his remedies had been:

[S]weetened with as much Sugar, as if they came not from an Apothecaries Shop, but a Confectioners. But my Mouth is too much out of Taste to rellish any thing.[51]

The Galenic explanation for these altered perceptions was that the tongue 'is filled with some strange fluid' during illness, which mixes with the gustatory juice of the food, so that 'all things would seem salty to taste, or all bitter'.[52] So familiar was the experience of altered taste that religious writers found it a useful metaphor to invoke when describing the more abstract idea that sinners fail to relish wholesome spiritual counsel. The ejected Yorkshire minister Thomas Watson (d. 1686) wrote in his treatise on repentance, 'Tis with a sinner, as it is with a sick Patient[:] his pallat is distempered; the sweetest things taste bitter to him: So the word of God which is sweeter than honey-comb, tastes bitter to a sinner'.[53]

Besides suffering from pain and nausea, patients often found they 'could take noe Rest all Night', one of 'the uneasiest accidents that attend...sickness'.[54] Doctors attributed this tendency to the corruption or evaporation of the special sleep-inducing vapour in the brain, but patients were more likely to blame pain.[55] The politician and lawyer Bulstrode Whitelocke (1605–75), recorded that he 'slept not all night by his torment' from piles in 1665.[56] Those who did manage to fall asleep often reported 'terrible and amazing Dreams'.[57] The reason pain seemed worse at night was that the 'venerous virulency' of the bad humours was 'enraged by the warme bed', and patients' thoughts were more 'fixed upon the object of pain' due to a lack of distractions.[58] Language of labour and weakness was used to convey the experience of sleeplessness: the sick endured many *'wearisome nights'* of illness, which left them 'very weary and weak'.[59] A doctor from Kent, Everard Maynwaringe (b. 1627/8), observed that the nights and days seemed endless, accentuated by frequent waking: sleep stretched out, 'from *evening* to the fair

[50] Thomas Willis, *Willis's Oxford Casebook (1650–52)*, ed. Kenneth Dewhurst (Oxford, 1981), 131; Maynwaringe, *Pains*, 30.

[51] Robert Boyle, *Occasional reflections upon several subjects* (1665), 206–7.

[52] Galen, 'On the Causes', 215. For a chemical explanation, see Isaac Spon, *Observations on fevers*, trans. J. Berrie (1682), 90.

[53] Thomas Watson, *The doctrine of repentance* (1668). He is drawing on Proverbs 27:7.

[54] Brotherton Library, Leeds, Lt 50, fol. 152r: William Tipping's poem, which he composed when 'verie ill' in 1699; Boyle, *Occasional reflections*, 211.

[55] See Chapter 2, pp. 76–7, on the mechanism of sleep. On disturbed sleep in the context of night-time socializing, see Sasha Handley, 'Sociable Sleeping in Early Modern England, 1660–1760', *History*, 98 (2013), 79–104. Roger Ekirch mentions the effects of illness on sleep occasionally in *At Day's Close: A History of Nighttime* (2005), 13–14, 112–13, 288–9.

[56] Whitelocke, *The Diary*, 690. This diarist wrote in the third person.

[57] Rogers, *Practical discourses*, 151; see also James Clegg, *The Diary of James Clegg of Chapel-en-Frith 1708–1755*, vol. 1 (1708–36), ed. Vanessa Doe, Derbyshire Record Society, vol. 5 (Matlock, 1978), 114. On nightmares, see Bill MacLehose, 'Fear, Fantasy and Sleep in Medieval Medicine', in Elena Carrera (ed.), *Emotions and Health, 1200–1700* (Leiden, 2013), 67–94.

[58] Robert Bayfield, *Enchiridion medicum: containing the causes...cures of...diseases* (1655), 162.

[59] Edward Lawrence, *Christ's power over bodily diseases* (1672, first publ. 1662), 262; Clegg, *The Diary*, 116; Boyle, *Occasional reflections*, 209–10.

bright day, is now broken into pieces, and *subdivided*... the *night* before seemed *short* is now too *long*.[60] This strange sense of time is captured in a poem by the Norfolk gentlewoman Elizabeth Freke (1642–1714), written after a fever:

> I cannot Rest,
> My Midnight Torments call the Slugish Light;
> And when the Morning Comes,
> They woo the right.[61]

Those patients who were wealthy enough to own clocks measured the time by ticks and chimes, complaining they 'miss'd not hearing one stroke of the Clock all the Night long'.[62] Once more, sensory metaphors were used in accounts of suffering. During sickness, the 'downy bed presseth hard against the bones', wrote Maynwaringe, its usual softness turned into sharpness; patients were *'full of tossings to and fro'* in a vain attempt to get comfortable.[63] Many acute illnesses left the skin sensitive to touch, a state today known as allodynia; this acuity was what made the soft mattress seem hard.[64] In longer-lasting diseases, the exposure of the bones, through weight loss, contributed greatly to the apparent hardness of the bed.[65] Twelve-year-old Caleb Vernon, living in Battersea, was 'not able to endure so much as a... Gown upon him, his bones were so bare', reported his father in 1666: his thigh measured under four inches in circumference from a long consumptive illness.[66] These sensations may also have been the result of a change of mattress: patients were sometimes moved from their customary, feather mattresses onto ones stuffed with more absorbent, coarser materials, such as flock, sedge, or chaff, which could withstand the emission of sweat and other evacuations (see Figure 6). It was well known that, 'A downe bed is soft to lye on, but yet it soakes the bodie' in fevers.[67] Of course, lower down the social hierarchy, beds may actually have been uncomfortable: rather than sleeping on feather mattresses, servants and labourers were more likely to have rested on beds made from compacted straw.[68]

Thus, three of the most common components of the feeling of illness were pain, nausea, and sleeplessness, all of which were described using metaphors relating to the senses of taste and touch, the two which tended to be seen in other contexts as the least 'noble'. How did patients respond emotionally to this bodily suffering? Responses usually varied according to its severity: mild discomfort occasioned vexation. Sick of a bad cold on his birthday, Dudley Ryder (1691–1756), a London law student, wrote crossly, '[I] Had nothing of rejoicing on it',

---

[60] Maynwaringe, *Pains*, 26.
[61] BL, MS Additional MS 45718, fol. 82v (Commonplace book of Elizabeth Freke, 1684–1714).
[62] Boyle, *Occasional reflections*, 209–10, 214–15.
[63] Maynwaringe, *Pains*, 26. See also Richard Baxter, *A treatise of self-denial* (1675), image 15.
[64] Allodynia in the OED is defined as 'Pain resulting from a stimulus that does not normally cause pain' (accessed 3/05/17).
[65] See Chapter 2, p. 70, for examples of emaciation.
[66] John Vernon, *The compleat scholler; or, a relation of the life... of Caleb Vernon* (1666), 39.
[67] This was the case for bedwetting children, as Sasha Handley has shown in *Sleep*, ch. 4. My thanks to Sasha for sharing this with me before the book's publication. The quotation is from Nicholas Breton, *Wits private wealth stored with choise commodities to content the minde* (1612), image 14.
[68] Handley, *Sleep*, ch. 4.

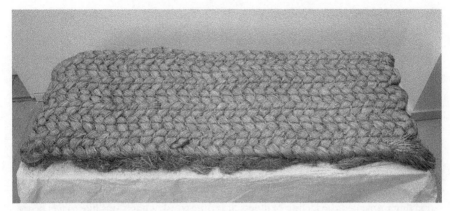

Figure 6. Carex mattress from Titchfield, Hampshire (1600s); Museum of English Rural Life (MERL), University of Reading, object no. 61/242. Carex/sedge mattresses were more absorbent than feather ones, and therefore may have been deemed apt for patients in acute sickness or childbirth, who were evacuating body fluids. After use, they would normally have been burnt; this one has survived because it functioned as loft insulation. My thanks to the curator at MERL, Dr Ollie Douglas, for this information.

but was in a 'very peevish, angry humour that everything that occurred made my blood rise within me'.[69] The reference to rising blood was not necessarily meant metaphorically—as the physician from Sheffield, Timothy Bright (c.1551–1615), explained in his book on melancholy, 'when we be moved to angrie passions...we sensibly feele an extraordinarie heate about our hearts', caused by the humour choler, which makes 'the bloud riseth'.[70] More severe suffering tended to elicit the stronger passions of grief and fear, responses implicit in the use of the adjectives 'grievous' and 'fearful' in descriptions of pain; indeed, the word 'grief' was a synonym for pain.[71] Recalling his 'strange and horrible Pains' in 1691, the Presbyterian minister Timothy Rogers (1658–1728) wrote, 'my Sorrows were beyond expression...all was hideous Darkness,...I was even stifled with Grief'.[72] This choice of imagery may have been informed by medical ideas: the humour melancholy, the bodily substance associated with grief, was thick and dark, and capable of causing suffocation when overly abundant.[73] In contrast to the passion of anger, sorrow caused the body's humours and spirits to move in a downwards direction, leaving the face pale and cold.[74]

To explain the tendency of physical suffering to elicit emotional suffering, contemporaries referred to the close relationship between the body and soul, the two

[69] Dudley Ryder, *The Diary of Dudley Ryder*, ed. William Matthews (1939), 38–9, 134.
[70] Timothy Bright, *A treatise of melancholie* (1586), 88.
[71] Newton, *The Sick Child*, 197–8. These terms denoted bodily pains as well as emotional suffering.
[72] Timothy Rogers, *Practical discourses on sickness & recovery* (1691), xxvi, 151–3.
[73] For a recent study of melancholy, see Erin Sullivan, *Beyond Melancholy: Sadness and Selfhood in Renaissance England* (Oxford, 2016), ch. 3. On drowning as an illness metaphor, see Lund, 'Experiencing Pain', 338.
[74] See Chapter 2, p. 85, on the physical effects of grief and fear.

constituent parts of the human being.[75] The theologian and cartographer John Norden (*c.*1547–1625) explained in his conduct book on affliction:

> [I]f the body be overmuch tormented with the grievousnesse of sicknesse, the soule cannot but feele, (through a mutuall love, which is between the soule and the body) a kinde of griefe.[76]

Thus, the body and soul were personified as close friends or relations, who loved one another dearly, and shared in each other's sorrows.[77] This idea was articulated throughout the period, which suggests that new theories of the soul advanced by the likes of the French philosopher René Descartes, exerted little impact on how most people understood the emotional effects of bodily suffering.[78] In short, 'the whole Man suffers' during illness, body and soul: sickness was a double misery.[79]

Having unpacked the feeling of illness, it is time to ask what it was like to feel better. The abatement of all three forms of suffering—pain, nausea, and sleeplessness—will be discussed together, since it usually happened simultaneously, and was described in similar terms. Patients' experiences varied greatly according to the severity of the preceding suffering, together with the speed at which the discomfort was removed. When suffering had been mild or short-lived, and its alleviation, incremental, the mitigation was hardly noticed. Galen explained that if healing 'occurs gradually, the return to what accords with nature will be unperceived'.[80] Since disease was defined as a condition 'contrary to Nature', the body's internal governor, recovery necessarily involved the return to conformity with this agent.[81] In these situations, patients did not usually express any positive feelings of relief, but instead noted that they could no longer sense or 'feel' their illness. Fifteen-year-old Samuel Jeake from Sussex (1652–99) recorded that over the course of two days, 'My Ague began to decrease', so that 'it could hardly be perceived'.[82] The abatement of minor illnesses, like colds, was also described in this way. The Essex clergyman Ralph Josselin (1617–83) wrote in his diary, 'my cold exceedingly abated, I can scarce feele it'.[83] The use of the word 'feel' suggests that Josselin conceived his experience as sensory, since touch was known as the 'sense of feeling' in this period.

The mitigation of more pronounced suffering was far more perceptible to patients, experienced as 'comfort' or 'ease'. Whitelocke wrote in 1650 that he bid 'farewell' to his 'violent fitts' of ague, 'to his great comfort'.[84] About forty years later, an anonymous female relative of Oliver Cromwell, in her thirties, recorded

---

[75] On the body–soul relationship, see Sullivan, *Beyond Melancholy*, 66–72.

[76] John Norden, *A pathway to patience in all manner of crosses* (1626), 78.

[77] Maynwaringe, *Pains*, 30.

[78] Examples from across the period include, William Folkingham, *Panala medica vel sanitatis et longaevitatis alumna catholica* (1628), to the reader; Jean-François Senault, *The use of passions*, trans. Henry Earl of Monmouth (1671, first publ. 1649), 480–2; Richard Allestree, *The art of patience and balm of Gilead* (1694, first publ. 1684), 12–13.

[79] Allestree, *The art of patience*, 13.   [80] Galen, 'On the Causes', 225.

[81] See Chapter 1 for definitions of 'disease' and 'Nature'.

[82] Samuel Jeake, *An Astrological Diary of the Seventeenth Century: Samuel Jeake of Rye*, ed. Michael Hunter (Oxford, 1988), 91.

[83] Ralph Josselin, *The Diary of Ralph Josselin 1616–1683*, ed. Alan Macfarlane (Oxford, 1991), 84.

[84] Whitelocke, *The Diary*, 253; see also James Fisher, *The wise virgin, or, a wonderful narration of the various dispensations towards a childe of eleven years of age* (1653), 158.

that after 'Being for the Space of a whole Day in Extremity of Payne the Lord was pleased to give me Ease'.[85] The adjective 'comfortable' denoted 'freedom from pain and trouble; at ease', 'gratifying to the senses', and carried connotations of a soft, wadded texture.[86] The word 'ease' held a similar meaning: it comes from the Old French *aise*, which means 'comfort, pleasure, well-being'.[87] This word encapsulated the experience of feeling better, and was the polar opposite to the feeling of illness, as is indicated by the fact it forms part of the word 'dis-ease'. Manuscript and printed collections of remedies confirm the importance of the patient's feeling of ease in experiences of recovery, since they frequently instruct the patient to take the medicine 'until you find ease' or similar wording.[88]

While relief from moderate suffering produced ease and comfort, the rapid abatement of severe discomfort was experienced as exquisite pleasure. Galen believed there was 'a correspondence in swiftness between the return to an accord with nature and the magnitude of the pleasure'.[89] Dudley Ryder would have agreed; he wrote in his diary in 1716:

> My arm pained me extremely. It [the pain] went off almost all of a sudden and I thought it was as great pleasure as I have felt a great while...It is almost worthwhile to be in pain a little while to feel the pleasure of going out of it.[90]

Pleasure was defined as 'a Passion *which proceeds from the sweetnesse which our senses receive from the objects which delight them*'.[91] It was a pleasant sensory experience, which could be felt by any of the five senses, though particularly in touch and taste. This word was used interchangeably with 'euphoria', a term which seems to have been associated especially with recovery: it denoted the feeling of relief that ensued after the 'critical evacuation' of bad humours.[92] In the 1650s, Mrs Hill, a widow of 60, sick of fever, took a purge which induced numerous stools, 'with great euphoria, and [she] completely recovered'.[93] Similar sensations were reported when patients were finally able to sleep or eat after periods of privation.[94]

---

[85] BL, Additional MS 5858, fol. 215v (Religious diary of a female cousin of Oliver Cromwell, 1687/90–1702).

[86] See OED definitions for 'comfort' and 'comfortable', which are based on early modern examples (accessed 1/10/16). On the material associations of comfort see John Crowley, *The Invention of Comfort: Sensibilities and Design in Early Modern Britain and Early America* (Baltimore MD, 2000).

[87] See OED definitions for 'ease', the noun; Online Etymology Dictionary: <http://www.etymonline.com/index.php?allowed_in_frame=0&search=ease> (both accessed 15/04/17).

[88] My thanks to the OUP reader who pointed this out. Here is a small a selection of examples which all refer to the patient's ease: WL, MS 1340/43, fol. 45r (Boyle Family, *c.*1675–*c.*1710); WL, MS 160, fols. 15v, 29v (Anne Brumwich, 'Booke of Receipts or medicines', *c.*1625–1700); Philiatros, *Natura exenterata: or nature unbowelled by the most exquisite anatomizers* (1655), 36; W.M., *The queens closet opened incomparable secrets in physick* (1659), 44–5, 46.

[89] Galen, 'On the Causes', 225–6.   [90] Ryder, *The Diary*, 301.

[91] Coeffeteau, *A table*, 247.

[92] Using a quotation from 1706, the OED defines euphoria as 'when the Patient finds himself eas'd or reliev'd' by the 'Operation of a Medicine' or spontaneous evacuation (accessed 4/04/17).

[93] Willis, *Oxford Casebook*, 103.

[94] Elizabeth Isham, *Diary and Confessions: Constructing Elizabeth Isham, 1609–1654*, Warwick University Online Editions, ed. Elizabeth Clarke, Nigel Smith, Jill Millman, and Alice Eardley, <http://web.warwick.ac.uk/english/perdita/Isham/index_bor.htm> (accessed 21/04/17), fol. 16r. See also Samuel Pepys, *The Diary of Samuel Pepys*, ed. Henry B. Wheatley (1893), Project Gutenberg, managed by Phil Gyford, <http://www.pepysdiary.com/diary/1663/02/11/> (accessed 30/05/17).

How were these delightful feelings explained? Fundamentally, it was the stark contrast between suffering and ease that made the latter so pleasurable. In his treatise about the passions, the French philosopher Jean-François Senault (*c*.1601–72) averred, 'the beauty of the Triumph depends upon the greatness of the Combat...so...nothing adds more to Pleasure than the Pain that hath gon before it'.[95] The use of military imagery here made sense, because recovery was conceived as a battle between Nature and the disease.[96] The most popular metaphor, however, was a sensory one. The medical writer William Folkingham wrote in his treatise on the key to a long life, published in 1628, '[he] who never felt the disgust of the bitter cup of *Sicknesse* cannot rightly relish the sweet tast[e] of *Sanitude*'. He continued:

> Contraries are best...distinguisht by their contraries; and he, that after...sharpe Torture of a grievous *Disease*, happily recovers...well knowes..., that...sanitude is a...most delicious condiment, and the best seasoning to relish the Nectar of...*Life*.[97]

Convalescents were thus in a unique position to appreciate health—the sweetness of ease could best be felt when juxtaposed with the bitterness of illness.[98] This was a common idea, frequently articulated by patients throughout the period,[99] and across a range of socio-economic levels. In a miracle account from 1691, Lydia Hills, a poor spinster lodging at Widow Elli's near Drury Lane, after years of 'extream and extraordinary Pains', found 'wonderful Ease', and 'had a Night of sweet Rest'.[100] Although this statement may have been edited by the scribe, the use of these words must have seemed credible in this context in order to make the miracle convincing.

Sweetness was thus at the heart of feeling better. No longer required to take bitter medicines, and able at last to detect the true tastes and smells of foods, convalescents probably came to associate recovery with this quality.[101] This word choice may also have stemmed from its positive nutritional and religious connotations: as Ken Albala has explained, the sweeter the food, the more nourishing it was thought to be to the body.[102] In Scripture, 'sweet' is used figuratively in reference to God's words and love; it refers both to the taste of honey, and to the smell of incense.[103] The reason sweetness was applicable to sleep as well as the abatement of pain and nausea, relates to moisture: sweet flavours were high in moisture, and sleep was thought to moisten the body: it irrigated the brain and organs with a '*mild and pleasant vapour*'.[104] This quality also denoted the pleasant dreams experienced by the recovering patient, which replaced the nightmares that had accompanied the sickness. The natural philosopher from the Isle of Wight, Robert Hooke (1635–1703),

---

[95] Senault, *The use of passions*, 468.   [96] See Chapter 1, pp. 39–40, 43, 51–2.
[97] Folkingham, *Panala medica*, to the reader.   [98] Harris, *Hezekiahs recovery*, 35.
[99] For example, Brilliana Harley, *Letters of the Lady Brilliana Harley*, ed. Thomas Taylor Lewis (1853), 49; John Buxton, *John Buxton, Norfolk Gentleman and Architect: Letters to his Son, 1719–1729*, ed. Alan Mackley, Norfolk Record Society, vol. 69 (Norwich, 2005), 45.
[100] *A relation of the miraculous cure of Mrs Lydia Hills of a lameness* (1695), 4–5.
[101] See pp. 101–3 in this chapter.   [102] Albala, *Eating Right*, 82.
[103] *DBI*, 832–4.   [104] Hart, *Klinike*, 332.

recorded that when he recovered from fever and giddiness in 1672, 'I slept pretty well and pleasantly', and dreamed of 'eating cream'.[105] Perhaps this sort of experience could be the origins of the expression, 'Sweet dreams'!

As well as referring to sweetness, patients described the pleasantness of abated suffering as 'soft'. John Kettlewell (1653–95), an ailing minister, longed to be 'allured by ease into…soft Slumbers'.[106] The word 'soft' derives from the Old English *softe*, meaning 'easeful, comfortable, calm'; it also means 'not stiff, not coarse, fine, smooth'.[107] Although associated particularly with the sense of touch, it could also be applied to hearing: quiet sounds were said to be 'soft'.[108] These various connotations rendered the word especially apposite for describing sleep: as shown earlier, disrupted sleep was described in opposite language—the bed seemed hard—but with recovery, the mattress once more felt soft and comfortable.[109] This was because the skin lost its heightened sensitivity once illness was over, and patients probably returned to their customary, feather beds after their temporary transference onto coarser, but more absorbent, mattresses. Improved sleep was also portrayed as 'quiet', a word which clearly relates to the sense of hearing: the rhythm of the patient's breathing was soft and gentle, in contrast to the earlier tossings and turnings of wakefulness. This vocabulary is almost onomatopoeic, since phonetically the repetition of 's' in the words 'slumber', 'sweet', and 'soft', resembles the *hiss* of the exhaled air during sleep.

Just as physical suffering produced powerful emotional reactions in patients, so too did the coming of bodily ease. The mitigation of mild to moderate discomfort occasioned cheerfulness. The physician and naturalist Sir Thomas Browne (1605–82) remarked that his grandson Tommy, who had been sick of fever, is now 'in a better temper and prettie chearly'.[110] Cheerfulness was understood to be a calm, tranquil form of happiness, which made the body's spirits expand, and move up to the mouth, 'from where laughter is formed'.[111] For this reason, laughter and joking were regarded as signs of the patient's growing ease and improved humoral balance. Perhaps this is why the phrase, 'sense of humour', has come to mean the appreciation of comedy.[112] John Yorke wrote in 1723 to his convalescing brother-in-law, James Clavering, 'It is further confirmation to me that you are eas'd of your pains, because you are dispos'd to show…wit and mirth [by making me]…the object of your merriment' in a previous letter.[113]

---

[105] Robert Hooke, *The Diary of Robert Hooke (1672–1680)*, ed. H. W. Robinson and W. Adams (1935), 27.

[106] John Kettlewell, *Death made comfortable* (1695), 212.

[107] See Online Etymology Dictionary, <http://www.etymonline.com/index.php?allowed_in_frame=0&search=soft> (accessed 15/4/16).

[108] See OED, 'soft' (adjective): 'Of a sound…low, quiet, subdued' (accessed 15/04/16).

[109] See pp. 104–5 in this chapter.

[110] Thomas Browne, *The Works of Sir Thomas Browne, vol. 6: Letters*, ed. Geoffrey Keynes (1931), 222. See also Chapter 2, p. 84.

[111] See Sandra Cavallo and Tessa Storey, *Healthy Living in Late Renaissance Italy* (Oxford, 2013), 184.

[112] On the links between comedy and the bodily humours, see Sullivan, *Beyond Melancholy*, 110–12.

[113] James Clavering, *The Correspondence of Sir James Clavering*, ed. Harry Thomas Dickinson, Surtees Society, vol. 178 (Gateshead, 1967), 149–50.

By contrast, the speedy mitigation of extreme suffering sparked stronger emotions: joy and amazement. A vivid example is provided in the testimony of a thirteen-year-old French girl called Mary Maillard, who was allegedly cured by miracle from a painful deformity of her legs in *c*.1693. At the time she was living in London, serving as a companion to an Englishwoman. Mary recalled, 'my Joy and Suprize was so great, that I could not sleep the whole Night, but was frequently shoving my Mistress', with whom she shared a bed, saying, ["]Madam, I feel no Pain, I am Easy, I am Well["] ... in this Surprize of Joy I spent the Night'.[114] Although the sudden mitigation of suffering was characteristic of miraculous healings, natural recoveries could also take place rapidly on occasions.[115] The Presbyterian Lancashire shopkeeper Roger Lowe (d. 1679) recorded in his diary that after a 'sad night ... in paine' in 1663, he awoke 'in health'; he praised God with the words, 'weepeing may endure for a night, but joy comes in the morneing', taken from Psalm 30:5.[116] Thus, the fast transformation from suffering to ease occasioned a correspondingly swift alteration in emotions—from grief to joy.

In short, the abatement of suffering produced a range of delightful sensations and feelings, including ease, comfort, pleasure, cheerfulness, and joy. What was the relationship between these various feelings? Nowadays, it would be usual to classify ease, comfort, and pleasure as bodily sensations, and cheerfulness and joy as emotions.[117] However, in the early modern period, the distinctions between sensations and emotions were less clear-cut: although ease and pleasure were associated primarily with the body, it was also possible for the soul to experience these sensations. Coeffeteau affirmed, '*pleasure ... is framed in our soules with a certain sweetnes which filles our senses with contentment and joy*'.[118] Pleasure was thus located in the soul, as well as in the body's senses. The same applied to the emotions: joy and cheerfulness, while usually classed as 'passions of the soul', could also be felt by the body. Drawing on Psalm 52:8, the Shropshire minister Edward Lawrence (d. 1695) wrote, 'now God hath given thee health, he hath caused *thy bones to rejoyce*, and *filled thy heart with food and gladness*'.[119] Here, the bones are capable of happiness, and the heart—the seat of the passions—is able to enjoy the sensation of eating. The reason

---

[114] *An exact relation of the wonderful cure of Mary Maillard* (1730, first publ. 1694), 7–8.

[115] David Gentilcore, *Healers and Healing in Early Modern Italy* (Manchester, 1998), 187–8.

[116] Roger Lowe, *The Diary of Roger Lowe of Ashton-in-Makerfield, Lancashire, 1663–1674*, ed. William Sachse (1938), 41.

[117] The OED defines 'pleasure' as the 'sensation induced by the experience or anticipation of what is felt to be good or desirable', and 'indulgence in physical ... sensual or sexual gratification'. The use of the words 'sensation' and 'sensual' implies that it is a bodily experience, since the latter means 'pertaining to the senses or physical sensation'. By contrast 'joy' is defined as a 'state of being highly pleased or delighted; exultation of spirit', and 'The expression of glad feeling', all of which indicate an emotion. Similarly, 'cheerful' means 'gladsome, blithe, lively and in good spirits', which again suggests an emotional rather than a sensual experience. These definitions are all in current usage (accessed 16/05/16).

[118] Coeffeteau, *A table*, 246–7.

[119] Lawrence, *Christ's power*, 262. This verse was also cited by patients—for example, Henry Newcome, *The Autobiography of Henry Newcome*, ed. Richard Parkinson, Chetham Society, vol. 26 (Manchester, 1852), 81. Other verses which refer to the soul's delight in food include Psalm 63:5 and Isaiah 55:2—my thanks to van Dijkhuizen for these references.

for this sharing of experiences was once again the close connection between the body and soul. Senault explained:

> [B]y a secret contagion...all their good...and bad estate is shared between them...For while [the soul] is in the body, she seems to renounce her Nobility; and...ceasing to be a pure spirit, she interesses her self in all the Delights, and all the Vexations of her Hoste: his health causeth contentment in her; and his sickness is grievous to her.[120]

Effectively, the soul—though the superior part—loved the body so much that it condescended to partake in all its states, including the coming of ease during recovery. In turn, the soul's joyful response to the mitigation of discomfort redoubled on the body, so that every organ rejoiced. The sharing of states could also be explained by reference to the structure of the soul: in Aristotelian philosophy, the five senses—the perceivers of bodily suffering and ease—were functions of the same part of the soul that produced the passions, the animal or sensitive soul.[121]

Thus, we have seen that the transition from feeling ill to feeling better was a double joy for patients, experiences usually described through sensory metaphors, especially those relating to touch and taste. It must be acknowledged, however, that a proportion of patients never reached a state of perfect health and ease, remaining chronically sick.[122] There were also occasions when the various symptoms might recede, giving the patient an impression of returning health, only to find moments later that their sufferings were back. A patient of William Walywn, 'upon a suddain seem'd to find himself so well' that he 'cal'd for his Diet'; but when supper arrived, 'alas', he 'could not endure the smell, nor swallow one bit', and 'hast[ens] to bed'.[123] Feeling better could thus be deceptive. Even those patients whose bodily sufferings *did* completely disappear might experience haunting 'remembrance[s] of those sore and dreadful' pains.[124] Perhaps the most frightening prospect for recovered patients, however, was relapse. John Donne observed that 'Man is most intimidated with those *paines* which...by a wofull' experience, he has endured 'in former afflictions'; therefore, after illness 'wee tremble at a *relapse*'. These fears far exceed those faced prior to the first bout of illness, on the grounds that 'wee can scarce fix a *feare*' on a disease that has not yet come, 'because wee know not what to feare; but the *feare* [of relapse] is the *busiest* and *irksomest affection*', since the illness is 'but newly gone, the *nearest object*' to memory.[125]

Another circumstance that could temper the patient's joy was spiritual anxiety. Due to the entrenched idea that suffering was sent by a loving God for their

---

[120] Senault, *The use of passions*, 478–82.

[121] Sullivan, *Beyond Melancholy*, 21. This idea came from Aristotle's *De Anima*, the most influential model of the soul in the early modern period: *Aristotle: De Anima in Focus*, ed. Michael Durrant (1993), 15.

[122] For example, Whitelocke, *The Diary*, which describes his chronic piles. Many other examples could be given.

[123] William Walwyn, *Physick for families* (1669), 75.

[124] Donne, *Devotions*, 597. On the spiritual advantages of remembering pain, see Chapter 4, pp. 138, 144–5, 155.

[125] Donne, *Devotions*, 596–612. On the spiritual advantages of contemplating relapse, see Chapter 4, pp. 145–6.

benefit, pious individuals occasionally cherished pain as a sign of divine care, and felt nostalgic upon its abatement. When eleven-year-old Margaret Muschamp from Northumberland recovered from diabolical possession in the 1640s, she reflected wistfully, 'My paynes were always with joy, never sorrowful...Now my torments are at an end'.[126] Given that suffering was thought to 'stop the torrent of sin', and wean the Christian 'from the world', both crucial in the Christian's attainment of salvation, perhaps we should not be so shocked by this response.[127] Even individuals noted for their 'scientific' outlook, like Robert Boyle, acknowledged the religious benefits of suffering: this man remarked that every symptom of disease had some useful purpose; for instance, the sleepless 'Silence of the Night' makes the patient begin to 'take some notice of his own [spiritual] Condition[,] and his Eyes, for want of outward Objects, are turn'd inwards'.[128] Such experiences complicate the historiographical notion that the religious valorization of suffering was on the decline in seventeenth-century Protestant cultures.[129]

FAMILY AND FRIENDS

Our attention can now shift from patients to their loved ones. In a nutshell, relatives and close friends usually shared the emotional transformation of the patient—from grief to joy. This is illustrated poignantly in an account of the recovery of eleven-year-old Martha Hatfield, by her uncle, the Sheffield minister James Fisher. Martha was diagnosed with 'Spleen-winde' in 1652, a disease which 'occasioned extream torments'. Fisher lamented that the girl's 'terrible crying' was:

> [V]ery grievous and afflictive to the spirits of all that heard her; and the whole Family [was] so continually under sadnesse, and their sleep so broken, that you might have seen *Every one with their hands upon their loines, as a woman in travel [labour], and all faces turned into palenese.*[130]

The depth of the family's distress is conveyed through its physical effects.[131] Nine months later, however, Martha's sufferings began to abate, and finally, one December evening, she 'laughed, and rejoyced, and said[:] Me is pretty well, I praise God...I am neither sick, nor have any pain'. Now, her relations expressed emotions of the opposite kind: they shed 'many tears of joy', and their 'hearts were mightily ravished'

---

[126] Mary Moore, *Wonderful news from the north. Or, a true relation of the sad...torments...on the...children of Mr George Muschamp* (1650), 19–20. See also Lambeth Palace Library, London, MS240, fol. 34r (Prose and verse meditations of Alathea Bethell, 1655–1708).

[127] Jeremy Taylor, *The rule and exercises of holy dying* (1651), 110. This treatise was one of the most popular of the century, reaching nineteen editions by 1695. On the value of suffering in Christian culture, see Newton, *The Sick Child*, 204–8; Jan Frans van Dijkhuizen, 'Partakers of Pain: Religious Meanings of Pain in Early Modern England', in Van Dijkhuizen and Enenkel (eds.), *The Sense of Suffering*, 189–220.

[128] Boyle, *Occasional reflections*, 212.

[129] Bourke, *The Story of Pain*, 91, 121–5. She does acknowledge that some people continue to find solace in religious interpretations of pain.

[130] Fisher, *The wise virgin*, 138. The italicized words are from Jeremiah 30:6.

[131] On the physical effects of grief, see Erin Sullivan, 'A Disease unto Death: Sadness in the Time of Shakespeare', in Carrera (ed.), *Emotions and Health*, 159–81.

at 'such a glorious end to this affliction', ease and health.[132] This dramatic alteration of feelings was reported throughout the period, and in a variety of sources.[133]

The tendency for relatives to share the experience of the patient was conceived in the early modern period as an instance of 'fellow-feeling'. This term meant 'to partake with him in all his occasions either of joy or sorrow'.[134] Other, closely related terms were sympathy, compassion, and pity, all of which denoted 'sorrow at the sight of another man's miserie'.[135] Since recovery was experienced as a transition from anguish to joy, the term 'fellow-feeling' is more suitable in this context, because it covers happy responses as well as distressing ones. While some work has been conducted on the history of compassion, fellow-feeling has rarely been explored, perhaps because the term is no longer widely used.[136] Throughout the period, this response was regarded as a 'Commendable Quality' in Christians, a sign of 'true humanity'—Romans 12:14 exhorts its readers to '*Rejoice with them that rejoice, weep with them that weep*'.[137] The exemplar of fellow-feeling is Christ, who came down from heaven to share in earthly sufferings, and was prepared to die on the Cross to spare humankind from eternal pain.[138]

Explanations for fellow-feeling centred on the emotion of love. Coeffeteau provides a detailed exposition of this theory in his treatise on the passions. He averred:

> A signe of true *Love*… [is that] friends rejoice & grieve for the same things;… a perfect friend should wish that he to whom he hath ingaged his affection, should have all things happy;… but… if it chance that hee fall into any infirmity, he must participate of his paine.[139]

As a result, the depth of fellow-feeling was thought to vary in accordance with the level of affection between the two parties. Those most prone to this response were people 'strictly tied unto us by… blood', like offspring, wrote Coeffeteau: their afflictions 'touch us so neere, we have a feeling more violent then… pitty: [we] are full of horror & amazement'.[140] Since 'a child is a part of the parent made up in

---

[132] Fisher, *The wise virgin*, 159–60.

[133] For example, Thomas Shepard, *God's Plot: The Paradoxes of Puritan Piety, Being the Autobiography and Journal of Thomas Shepard*, ed. Michael McCiffert (Amherst MA, 1972), 36–7; John Hervey, *Letter-Books of John Hervey, First Earl of Bristol, vol. 1, 1651–1715* (Wells, 1894), 300; *A narrative of the late extraordinary cure wrought in an instant upon Mrs Elizabeth Savage* (1694), 10–11; Walwyn, *Physick*, 97, 100.

[134] Richard Allestree, *The practice of Christian graces* (1658), 309–11.

[135] Thomas Bilson, *The survey of Christs sufferings* (1604), 27.

[136] A few exceptions include Katherine Ibbett, 'Fellow-Feeling', in Susan Broomhall (ed.), *Early Modern Emotions: An Introduction* (Abingdon, 2017), 61–4, and for an earlier period, Gillian Clark, 'Caritas: Augustine on Love and Fellow-Feeling', in Ruth Caston and Robert Kaster (eds.), *Hope, Joy and Affection in the Classical World* (Oxford, 2016), 209–25.

[137] Timothy Nourse, *A discourse upon the nature and faculties of man* (1686), 145–6; Richard Braithwaite, *Essaies upon the five senses* (1635, first publ. 1620), 124. This verse is quoted in Allestree, *The practice*, 311. Such a positive attitude to fellow-feeling was not universal, however—Lynda Payne has shown that Neostoics saw it as a weakness: *With Words and Knives*, 62–8.

[138] On God's compassion, see Psalm 86:15; Lamentations 3:22–3. On Christ's compassion, see John 11:25–33; Matthew 14:14; Mark 1:40–1; John 3:17.

[139] Coeffeteau, *A table*, 111–12, 117–19. See also Bilson, *The survey*, 27; Allestree, *The practice*, 309–11.

[140] Coeffeteau, *A table*, 369–70.

another skin', compassion for the plight of children was extreme.[141] Fellow-feeling was also deemed especially acute between lovers or married couples, who enjoy 'a Union of *Souls* as well as *Bodies*'.[142] Slightly lower in the hierarchy of fellow-feeling were close friends or 'soul mates', who were united by 'natural affinity'.[143] Next came acquaintances, and below them, strangers, whose circumstances were found to be much less moving, especially if they were 'remote from us', living far away.[144] Finally, at the bottom of the hierarchy were adversaries, whose afflictions and joys were assumed to elicit emotions of the opposite character: Coeffeteau lamented, 'wee know our miseries are a sweete and pleasing spectacle' to our foes, despite Christ's command to 'love your enemies'.[145] Since this study is concerned with the experiences of relatives and close friends, it may come as no surprise that the fellow-feeling uncovered in this study was intense.

Besides the relationship between the parties, the depth of fellow-feeling was thought to depend on whether or not the individual had personally experienced the patient's illness. '*Compassion* ... comes to no great *degree*', declared Donne, 'if wee have not *felt*, in some *proportion*, in ourselves, that which wee ... condole in another'.[146] In his treatise on afflictions, the ejected minister Thomas Case (*c*.1598–1682) echoed, in cases of '*Stone, Toothache, Gout,* ... and the like evils, ... experience doth melt the heart into tears of ... fellow-feelings, while strangers to such sufferings stand wondering'.[147] This was so for the friends of the Norfolk MP Robert Paston (1631–83): he received a letter from four friends in 1676, wishing him 'speedy freedome' from the gout; they wrote, 'some of us can experimentally sympathize ... having to purpose felt the tortures of the goutt'.[148] The same applied to relatives' happy responses upon the patient's recovery. The Herefordshire gentlewoman Brilliana Harley (*c*.1598–1643) told her son Edward in 1639, 'It is my joy that you are well' from 'your ... sore eyes', for 'by experience, I know it to be a greate paine; for I once had sore eyes ... [and] feele how tender the eye is'.[149] Other factors which influenced the level of fellow-feeling were gender and age. Olivia Weisser has shown that females were expected to effuse more pity than males: the abundance of moisture in women's hearts made them softer—or more 'tender-hearted'—than those of men, and more deeply affected by the miseries and joys of others.[150] The Anglican writer Richard Allestree (1619–81) declared that the 'highest human instance' of compassion could be found in 'the female sex', owing

---

[141] John Flavel, *A token for mourners* (1674), 3.

[142] Marcus Tullius Cicero, *Cicero's laelius a discourse of friendship* (1691), preface.

[143] Coeffeteau, *A table*, 369. See also George Berkeley, *Historical applications and occasional meditations* (1667), 115–16.

[144] Coeffeteau, *A table*, 371.

[145] Ibid., 493. See also Justus Lipsius, *A discourse of constancy*, trans. Nathaniel Wanley (1670, first publ. in Latin in 1584; first English edn. 1574), 48. On sadism, see Wilson-Yamamoto, *Pain, Pleasure and Perversity*, ch. 5. The Bible verse is Matthew 5:44.

[146] Donne, *Devotions*, 598–9.

[147] Thomas Case, *Correction instruction, or a treatise of afflictions* (1653), 10–11.

[148] Robert Paston, *The Whirlpool of Misadventures: Letters of Robert Paston, First Earl of Yarmouth 1663–1679*, ed. Jean Agnew, Norfolk Record Society, vol. 76 (2012), 263.

[149] Harley, *Letters*, 36.   [150] Weisser, *Ill Composed*, 94–8.

to their 'softer mold', which is 'more pliant and yielding to the impressions of pitty'.[151] Children's hearts were similarly moist.[152] Nonetheless, as we will see below, in practice even those with the driest hearts could share the sufferings and eventual relief of the patient: they simply had to have ears and eyes.

The main avenues to fellow-feeling were the senses of sight and hearing. The Bishop of Winchester, Thomas Bilson (1546/7–1616), confirmed that 'the eyes and eares, upon a thousand occasions, when the bodie is not touched [with illness], bring feare and griefe to the heart'.[153] Although the other senses were also affected by sickness—for instance, many diseases produced disgusting smells—it was chiefly the 'nobler senses' of sight and hearing that came to be associated with fellow-feeling. The likely reason is that this sentiment was judged to be morally superior to the more visceral responses elicited by stench, such as disgust.[154]

Before examining the sounds and sights of suffering and its abatement, I will briefly outline how sensation was thought to work. In early modern cognition theory, an amalgamation of Aristotelian and Galenic ideas, sound was defined as 'a quality issuing out of the Aire', caused by the 'sudden and forcible collision of hard and solid bodies'.[155] The disturbed air 'altereth that ayre that is next it, and so by succession' it enters the 'instrument of Hearing', the ear, where three 'little bones' hit the 'little skinne' (eardrum). The sound then makes its way through a 'winding...labyrinth', to 'the Auditory Nerve', and 'thence unto the common Sense', the faculty of the brain responsible for processing all sensory information.[156] The sense of sight operated slightly differently: all objects were thought to emit visual resemblances or replicas of themselves, called 'species', which travel to the eyes, where they are absorbed by a special 'crystalline humour'.[157] The 'opticke Nerves' at the back of the eye then 'convayes the sight to the common sense' in the brain. This faculty proceeded to compute all the data from the various senses, which it passed on to the 'imagination', the 'internal sense' responsible for creating a mental image of the external world, or in this instance, the sickchamber.[158] It was this mental picture—the 'mind's eye'—to which the soul responded with its passions.[159]

What noises could be heard in the sickchamber? Undoubtedly, the most distressing sounds of sickness were the cries and groans of the patient. Addressing the

---

[151] Richard Allestree, *The ladies calling* (1673), 48–9.

[152] Newton, *The Sick Child*, ch. 1. On children's inclination to compassion, see Bilson, *The survey*, 30.

[153] Bilson, *The survey*, 25.

[154] Richard Firth-Godbehere is undertaking a PhD on early modern disgust, 'Understanding the Opposites of Desire: The Prehistory of Disgust, c.1600–1760' (PhD in progress, Queen Mary, University of London).

[155] Helkiah Crooke, *Mikrokosmographia a description of the body of man* (1615), 609. This was a standard definition—for example, see Robert Burton, *The anatomy of melancholy* (1621), 34. On hearing, see Bruce Smith, *The Acoustic World of Early Modern England: Attending to the O-Factor* (1999). On the differences between Galenic and Aristotelian understandings of the senses, see François Quiviger, *The Sensory World of Italian Renaissance Art* (London, 2010), 15–17.

[156] Crooke, *Mikrokosmographia*, 531, 574, 583, 592, 603.

[157] Stuart Clark, *Vanities of the Eye: Vision in Early Modern European Culture* (Oxford, 2007), 2, 15–19. Clark complicates the ocular-centric model by showing that this period witnessed increasing scepticism about the reliability of vision.

[158] Burton, *The anatomy*, 33.   [159] Ibid., 531, 574, 583, 592, 603.

relations of the sick in 1691, Timothy Rogers lamented, 'your hearts...s[i]nk within you with the doleful and unintermitted accents of their Groans and Sighs'.[160] Religious writers taught that the very purpose of these sounds was to elicit this sorrowful response. The Arminian bishop Jeremy Taylor (*c.*1613–67) confirmed in his popular treatise on death, 'Sighes and groans' are the 'proper voice[s] of sicknesse', instigated by God to generate 'mercy and pity' in onlookers: by groaning, the patient's 'anguish of...spirit' is 'sent forth...into the...heart of the man that stood [by]'.[161] He seems to have been right: relatives frequently emphasized the emotional effects of these sad sounds. The newly married Mary Penington recorded that the groans of her sick husband 'were dreadful. I may call them roarings'. Forty years later, she still remembered his groans, and added another auditory memory: the sound of his convulsing limbs as they slammed against the bed in his convulsion fits. She wrote:

> [H]e snapped his legs and arms with such force, that the veins seemed to sound like the snapping of cat-gut strings, tightened upon an instrument of music. Oh! this was a dreadful...sound to me; my very heartstrings seemed ready to break, and let my heart fall from its wonted place.[162]

By applying the metaphor of breaking strings to both her own emotions and her husband's fits, Mary conveyed the depth of her fellow-feeling—her heart was mimicking his experience. The roaring mentioned in the above extract was usually reserved for male patients—women were more likely to be described as crying or shrieking; the former word carried connotations of masculine fierceness which were deemed incompatible with femininity.[163] Although women were thought to be more prone to pity than men, there is plenty of evidence to indicate that males were also grieved by hearing patients' cries. Bulstrode Whitelocke recorded in 1649 that when his wife was gravely sick, 'hearing [her] grones' brought him 'much more weeping than sleep'.[164] For both mothers and fathers, the cries of children were found to be agonizing.[165] Other sounds in the sickchamber, which provoked repugnance or vexation as well as grief, included the coughing up of phlegm, sniffing and sneezing, vomiting, and flatulence.[166] Perhaps polite diarists considered such sounds as inappropriate subjects for mention in their memoirs. Little change over time has been detected in the soundscape of the early modern sickchamber, despite the fact that the period witnessed advances in sound-proofing techniques, such as glazing and panelling, and a relocation of beds to upstairs chambers.[167]

---

[160] Rogers, *Practical discourses*, 19, 91.   [161] Taylor, *The rules*, 82–3.
[162] Penington, *Experiences*, 70–1, 93. The association between music and suffering dates back to Cassiodorus' biblical commentary, which reads the phrase 'Exsurge cithara' ('Arise, harp') in Psalm 57 as a metaphor for Christ's agonies on the cross; Cassiodorus imagines the stretched tendons of Jesus. My thanks to van Dijkhuizen for this observation.
[163] See Gina Bloom, *Voice in Motion: Staging Gender, Shaping Sound in Early Modern England* (Philadelphia PA, 2007), 9.
[164] Whitelocke, *The Diary*, 238.   [165] Newton, *The Sick Child*, 127.
[166] Reactions to these sounds will be examined in my new Wellcome Trust University Award project (2016–21: reference: 200326/Z/15/Z), 'Sensing Sickness in Early Modern England'.
[167] On sound-proofing, see Emily Cockayne, *Hubbub: Filth, Noise and Stench in England 1600–1770* (2007), 118–19; on bed location see Handley, *Sleep*, ch. 4.

This may have been because, as Emily Cockayne has suggested, 'quieter [homes]...led to a heightened sensitivity towards noise'.[168] In any case, these architectural developments would have done little to affect the experiences of poorer people, whose dwellings probably offered 'little resistance to noise intrusion', especially in subdivided houses of multiple occupancy.[169]

During recovery, the sounds of the sickchamber altered dramatically. The 'deep fetcht groanes' of the patient were replaced by 'the voice of Gladness'.[170] The London woodturner Nehemiah Wallington (1598–1658) recorded in his diary in 1631 that his 'sweete childe' Sarah:

> [B]eing very merrey all...day and pratteling to mee prettily...could not but make me call to mind Gods great love in preserving...it...I thought with in my selfe whereas now I am delighting to see my childe meray...I might have bine heavie and weeping over it: to heere the dolefull scrikes...of it.[171]

For this father, the contrast between his daughter's merry chatter, and the imagined sound of her sad cries, heightened his happiness at her health and ease. Cheerful conversations were accompanied by 'a loud, but inarticulate voice, which we call *Laughter*'.[172] The Suffolk MP and landowner John Hervey (1665–1751) informed his wife that their grandson 'is so wonderfully altered for the better...as is not to be imagined...and was in so good humour yesterday that he laughd near half an hour incessantly'.[173] The cause of laughter in medical theory was the repeated contractions and relaxations of the heart and lungs in moments of joy: this shaking movement 'sends forth much heat and Spirits...to the Face', which makes a *'sweet contraction of the Muscles of the face, and a pleasant agitation of the vocall organs'*.[174] Although theologians and medics warned that excessive laughter was spiritually and physically pernicious, they conceded that in moderation it was an innocent pleasure, beneficial both to those who emitted and heard it.[175] The Dutch physician Levinus Lemnius (1505–68) claimed that laughter purifies the blood 'from all grossenes', making 'the Spyrits...pure, bright and cleare shyninge', and in turn, this purity 'causeth the mynde to rejoyce, and amonge meery companions to laughe and delight'.[176] Thus, laughter was self-perpetuating:

---

[168] Cockayne, *Hubbub*, 118–19.   [169] Ibid.

[170] Rogers, *Practical discourses*, 269.

[171] Nehemiah Wallington, *The Notebooks of Nehemiah Wallington, 1618–1654: A Selection*, ed. David Booy (Aldershot, 2007), 434–5.

[172] Walter Charleton, *Natural history of the passions* (1674), 44. On the history of laughter, see Keith Thomas, 'The Place of Laughter in Tudor and Stuart England', *Times Literary Supplement* (2/01/77), 77–81; Albrecht Classen (ed.), *Laughter in the Middle Ages and Early Modern Times* (New York, 2010); Stephen Pender, 'The Moral Physiology of Laughter', in David Beck (ed.), *Knowing Nature in Early Modern Europe* (2015), 29–48.

[173] Hervey, *Letter-Books*, vol. 2, 190.

[174] Ambroise Paré, *The workes of that famous chirurgion Ambrose Parey*, trans. Thomas Johnson (1634), 39; B.A., *The sick-mans rare jewell* (1674), 29–30; Alexander Ross, *Arcana microcosmi, or, the hid secrets of man's body* (1652, first publ. 1651), 176; Charleton, *Natural history*, 144–5.

[175] On the dangers of excessive laughter see Colin Jones, *The Smile Revolution in Eighteenth Century Paris* (Oxford, 2014), 29–36. On the health benefits of laughter, see Pender, 'The Moral Physiology of Laughter'.

[176] Levinus Lemnius, *The touchstone of complexions*, trans. Thomas Newton (1576), 138.

it conditioned the spirits into a state conducive to further mirth. This use of visual metaphors—of brightness and shining—to describe an auditory experience is an example of what historians call 'intersensoriality', the interconnections between the various senses.[177]

Another sound that could be heard during recovery was the singing of 'chearful Praises' to God for His gift of healing.[178] This response is enshrined in the biblical command, 'Is any among you afflicted? let him pray. Is any merry? let him sing psalms'.[179] The Suffolk diarist Elizabeth Bury (1644–1720) recorded that when her husband was no longer in 'great Hazard of his Life', her 'Soul was filled with Praise': she and her friends enjoyed a 'sweet Day of Praise for Mercies...in the House', singing psalms.[180] Sweetness was primarily associated with taste, but here it is used to describe auditory perceptions, another example of intersensoriality.[181] This dual application may have been inspired by Scripture: in the Psalms, the sound of God's voice is described as 'sweeter than honey to my mouth!'[182] Contributing to the delight of song was the notion that God Himself possessed a sense of hearing, and enjoyed the music.[183] A Presbyterian minister from Norwich, Thomas Steward (1668/9–1753), observed in a sermon he preached upon his own recovery, 'The mutual, joynt, united praises of the Saints are sweet Musick,... delightful Melody in the Ears of the Almighty, and...our own Hearts [are] more warmed and enlarged...when we joyn in Consort to Sing'.[184] Ultimately, this 'mutual praising' of God was a 'resemblance of Heaven', the sound of which 'transport[s] us' imaginatively to this place.[185]

The above descriptions imply that the sounds that accompanied suffering and its abatement exerted a direct impact on the listener's heart, the 'seat and organ of all passions'.[186] The sharp, spiky accents of the patient's cries, followed at last by cheerful laughter and singing, were thought to penetrate loved ones' bodies, and hit this organ instantly. We might think that these descriptions are merely metaphorical, but this was not the case: sound was believed to make a real impact on the heart. Jennifer McDermott has shown that anatomists considered the recently discovered Eustachian tube as a direct link between the heart and ear.[187] The Danish physician Thomas Bartholin (1616–80) explained that the heart is encircled by 'a Vein' called the *coronaria*, which 'arises from the Cava...about whose Basis it Expatiates in a

---

[177] See note 19 in this chapter.
[178] Rogers, *Practical discourses*, 269. On the duty of praising God in song, see Chapter 4.
[179] James 5:13.
[180] Elizabeth Bury, *An account of the life and death of Elizabeth Bury* (Bristol, 1720), 153.
[181] On the pleasure of music, see Christopher Marsh, *Music and Society in Early Modern England* (Cambridge, 2010), 64–5. See also Chapter 4, pp. 160–1.
[182] Psalm 119:103.
[183] On God's senses, see Elizabeth Swann's forthcoming chapter, 'God's Nostrils: The Divine Senses in Early Modern England', in her edited volume, *Sensing the Sacred: Religion and the Senses in Medieval and Early Modern Culture* (Aldershot, 2017). See also Y. Avarhami, *The Senses of Scripture: Sensory Perception in the Hebrew Bible* (New York, 2012).
[184] Thomas Steward, *Sacrificium laudis, or a thank-offering* (1699), 19–20.
[185] Ibid., 20.   [186] Burton, *The anatomy*, 152–3.
[187] Jennifer Rae McDermott, '"The Melodie of Heaven": Sermonizing the Open Ear in Early Modern England', in Wietse De Boer and Christine Gottler (eds.), *Religion and the Senses in Early Modern Europe* (Leiden, 2012), 177–97. This tube was first described by the anatomist Bartolomeo Eustachi in 1562.

large tract from the...Eare[s]'.[188] A more prevalent explanation for the association between the heart and ears, however, was the perceived affinity between sound and the spirits. Penelope Gouk has argued that sounds, like the heart's spirits, were airy vapours that moved in a rhythmic manner, and tended to 'take on' the 'patterned movement' of the noise, which in turn provoked emotions of a similar nature.[189] This idea was articulated by the priest Thomas Wright (d. 1624) in his treatise on the passions: he explained that the 'shaking, crispling or tickling of the air' in the ear 'paseth thorow' the body 'unto the heart, and there beateth and tickleth it in such a sort, as it is moved with semblable passions', in this case, grief during illness, and joy upon recovery.[190] Owing to this link—between sounds and passions—the sense of hearing was sometimes regarded as the most emotionally moving of all the senses, despite the fact that, in general, sight was esteemed the 'noblest sense'.[191] It was the heart's sensitivity to vibrations that gave hearing the upper hand: this organ '[is] most delicate and sensitive, so it perceiveth the least motions and impressions as may be', wrote the famous English anatomist Helkiah Crooke (1576–1648).[192] It thus seems fitting that the words 'hear' and 'ear' are contained within 'heart'.[193] The Protestant privileging of hearing as the route to salvation may have contributed to this perception.[194]

Having explored how the sense of hearing acted as an avenue to fellow-feeling, we can turn to the sense of sight. During the illness of her husband, the puritan courtier from Durham, Mary Cowper (1685–1724), recorded in her diary, 'I am out of my Wits to see him suffer, which I declare is ten Times worse than Death to me'.[195] So great was the anguish of seeing her husband in pain, this woman thought it had tipped her into temporary insanity.[196] What exactly did she see that evoked such a response? The keenest cause of grief was the look in the patient's eyes, a tendency which reflects the popular belief that the eyes were the windows of the soul.[197] A poem composed by the Devonshire gentlewoman Mary Chudleigh (*c*.1656–1710), concerning her gravely ill daughter, Eliza Maria, encapsulates this experience poignantly:

> Rack'd by Convulsive Pains she meekly lies,
> And gazes on me with imploring Eyes,
> With Eyes which beg Relief, but all in vain,
> I see, but cannot, cannot ease her Pain.[198]

---

[188] Thomas Bartholin, *Bartholinus anatomy* (1668), 98. My thanks to my undergraduate dissertation student Matthew Norris for this reference.

[189] Penelope Gouk, 'Music and Spirit in Early Modern Thought', in Carrera (ed.), *Emotions and Health*, 221–39, at 227–8; Penelope Gouk, 'Some English Theories of Hearing in the Seventeenth Century', in Charles Burnett, Michael Fend, and Penelope Gouk (eds.), *The Second Sense: Studies in Hearing and Musical Judgement from Antiquity to the Seventeenth Century* (1991), 95–113.

[190] Thomas Wright, *The passions of the minde* (1630, first publ. 1601), 169–70.

[191] For example, Crooke, *Mikrokosmographia*, 308.   [192] Ibid., 169.

[193] Religious writers made puns with these words—see McDermott, '"The Melodie"', 180, 193–4.

[194] See Chapter 4, p. 160.

[195] Mary Cowper, *Diary of Mary, Countess Cowper*, ed. John Murray (1864), 76.

[196] On distraction caused by grief, see Sullivan, *Beyond Melancholy*, 59–66.

[197] Clark, *Vanities of the Eye*, 11.

[198] Mary Chudleigh, 'On the death of my dear daughter Eliza Maria Chudleigh', in her *Poems on several occasions* (1713), 95.

Adding to this woman's grief was her inability to alleviate her daughter's suffering. Relatives also commented on the sight of the patient's facial expression, which was typically contorted in pain, and wet with tears.[199] The physician Timothy Bright provides a vivid picture of the 'deformitie of the face in weeping' in his treatise on melancholy: 'The lip trembleth', the 'countenance is cast downe', and 'all the parts [are so] filled with…moisture…that not finding sufficient way [out] at the eyes, it passeth through the nose'.[200] This unhappy sight was so distressing to loved ones that it caused them to weep in return, a response which brought further dolour to the patient.[201] Ralph Thoresby (1658–1725), an antiquary from Leeds, recorded in his diary that his 'violent' chest pain 'drew tears from my dear wife, who sat weeping over me for two hours, which wounded me deeply'.[202] In certain contexts, tears were denigrated as unmanly, but moralists conceded that 'love puts a grace upon gestures otherwise undecent', which in this case was compassionate weeping.[203]

In addition to observing patients' sad faces, relatives bewailed the wasting of their bodies. As we saw earlier, acute illness often took away the patient's appetite; in more prolonged diseases, this faculty did not disappear completely, but digestion often became weak.[204] The emaciated appearance of the patient was a source of sorrow to relatives. In 1726, John Yorke lamented that 'every day appears more melancholly when I see poor Jem', his young nephew, 'in such piteous and languishing a condition. Nothing that he has taken [for sustenance] these 3 days stays with him'.[205] The sick also lost their natural beauty and colour. Rogers asked the families of the sick, 'Where is his former Comeliness and Beauty…his lovely Features? You can…have no mind to look upon that very person that…a while ago, was the Delight of your Heart'.[206] As this minister implies, these sights sometimes prompted relatives to look away, or to 'draw the Curtains about' the bed, 'that they may not contemplate his grim Visage'.[207] Such a reaction could turn into outright repugnance if the illness was accompanied by the 'detestable and loathsome Sight' or 'noysome smell' of disfiguring pustules or swellings.[208]

---

[199] On facial grimaces, but for a later period, see Bourke, *The Story of Pain*, ch. 6.

[200] Bright, *A treatise*, 153–4.

[201] For example, see Isaac Archer, 'The Diary of Isaac Archer 1641–1700', in Matthew Storey (ed.), *Two East Anglian Diaries 1641–1729*, Suffolk Record Society, vol. 36 (Woodbridge, 1994), 41–200, at 160.

[202] Ralph Thoresby, *The Diary of Ralph Thoresby*, 2 vols., ed. Joseph Hunter (1830), vol. 2, 391.

[203] William Houghton, *Preces & lachrymae: a sermon on Acts* (1650), 22. On attitudes to male weeping, see Bernard Capp, ' "Jesus Wept" But did the Englishman? Masculinity and the Display of Emotion in Early Modern England', *Past & Present*, 224 (2014), 75–108. Other scholars point out that crying was also deemed acceptable—even laudable—during prayer and repentance in Christians of both sex: Alec Ryrie, *Being Protestant in Reformation Britain* (Oxford, 2013), 187–94; Raymond Anselment, 'Mary Rich, Countess of Warwick, and the Gift of Tears', *The Seventeenth Century*, 22 (2007), 336–57.

[204] On the diet of the sick, see Chapter 2, pp. 78–9, 80, 82. On the different diets for chronic and acutely ill patients, see William Bullein, *The government of health* (1595, first publ. 1558), 28.

[205] Clavering, *The Correspondence*, 162.

[206] Rogers, *Practical discourses*, 228–9.

[207] Henry Atherton, *The Christian physician* (1686), 206–7.

[208] Robert Gould, *A poem most humbly offered to the memory of her late sacred majesty, Queen Mary* (1695), 13. For an example of relatives' reactions to nauseous smells, see Clavering, *The Correspondence*, 159. Michael Stolberg mentions the repugnance of onlookers to skin lesions/smells in *Experiencing Illness and the Sick Body in Early Modern Europe* (Basingstoke, 2011, first publ. in German in 2003),

Recovery often reversed these mournful sights: the patient's grimaced gaze melted into joyful smiles. When the aforementioned Martha Hatfield began to recover from 'Spleen-winde' in 1652, her uncle reported she could be seen 'lifting up her eye with smiling'.[209] Her relatives smiled back, a response which would come as no surprise to the historian Colin Jones, who has commented, 'It appears to be rather difficult to greet a smile without smiling in return'.[210] A lovely description of such expressions is provided in a late sixteenth-century treatise on laughter, by the Montpellier-trained physician Laurent Joubert (1529–82):

> Certainly there is nothing that gives more pleasure…than a laughing face, with its wide, shining, clear and serene forehead, eyes shining…and casting fire as do diamonds; cheeks vermillion …, mouth flush with the face, lips handsomely drawn back (from which are formed the small dimples…in the very middle of the cheeks).[211]

Thus, the smile affected the whole face—it lit up the eyes, and flushed the cheeks. Joubert's references to diamonds, light, and colour fit with contemporary theories of eyesight: the organ of sight was the sparkling 'crystalline humour' in the eye, its medium, 'the illumination of the aire', and its objects, 'colours & all shining bodies'.[212] The reason the lips curved up rather than down was that the passion joy caused the heart to propel the animal spirits—the instruments of animation— upwards and outwards.[213]

Another happy sight was the improved appearance of the patient.[214] Loved ones were relieved when the once lean frame of the sick person became 'plumpe and fatt', the 'colour return[ing] againe' to the hitherto 'white as marble' skin.[215] Preaching on a verse in Job relating to 'the sick mans recovery', the ejected clergyman Joseph Caryl (1602–73) reflected how, 'He shall be fresh-coloured, who before was pale and wan, he shall be full-fleshed, who before was fallen and leane'.[216] These sights were especially welcome to those relatives who had feared that the patient's recovery had been exaggerated. The Dorset doctor and musician Claver Morris (1659–1727) recorded in his diary that his dying wife was 'in great concernment' about her son Willey, who had been sick of smallpox in 1723. She was 'so affected with distrust' of her son's recovery,

> [T]hat to satisfie her Fear I was fain to make him…come to her [in the middle of the night]; And the sight of him seemd…to please her, & she looking upon him,…ordered

109, 119; see also Cockayne, *Hubbub*, 22, 31; Weisser, 'Boils, Pushes, Wheals', 327; on the sights/smells of smallpox, plague, and venereal disease, see Raymond Anselment, *The Realms of Apollo: Literature and Healing in Seventeenth-Century England* (1995), chs. 3, 4, 5. On the sights of skin diseases, and their legacies, see Wilson, *Surgery, Skin and Syphilis*, 61–2, 152–5. On the emotions evoked by seeing disfigured bodies, see Turner, *Disabilities*, 81–94.

[209] Fisher, *The wise virgin*, 144–5.   [210] Jones, *The Smile Revolution*, 7–8.

[211] Laurent Joubert, *Treatise on laughter*, ed. and trans. Gregory David de Rocher (Tuscaloosa AL, 1980; first publ. in French, 1579), unpaginated dedication at front of volume.

[212] Burton, *The anatomy*, 33; see Clark, *Vanities of the Eye*, 10.

[213] B.A., *The sick-mans rare jewell*, 29–30.

[214] For example, Josselin, *The Diary*, 487; Clavering, *The Correspondence*, 115.

[215] Josselin, *The Diary*, 635; Whitelocke, *The Diary*, 763, 768.

[216] Joseph Caryl, *An exposition…upon the thirty second, the thirty third, and the thirty fourth chapters of the booke of Job* (1661); this was in reference to Job 33:25 ('His flesh shall be fresher than a child's: he shall return to the days of his youth').

by me to turn himself... to the Light of her Candle [so] that she [could] perfectly see his Face,... [she] said she never saw him look better in her Life.[217]

It seems that it was the sight, rather than the sound, of this boy that convinced his mother of his full recovery. This finding fits with the philosophical notion that vision was pre-eminent when it came to the acquisition of knowledge, even if the sense of hearing was sometimes found to be the most moving of the two.[218]

Other sights that occasioned joy in relatives and friends included seeing the patient doing things that had been impossible during illness. In 1659, the Cheshire minister Henry Newcome (*c.*1627–95) sent his four-year-old daughter Betty who had rickets 'into the country' for a course of treatment; a month later, 'her mother and I went... to see her... and she met us on her feet, which was a great rejoicing to us'. That evening, their daughter was able to 'dance to the virginals', which amazed them when they considered that previously they had thought they 'should never have seen her go' (i.e. walk).[219] Poorer families as well as the affluent reacted in this way. An advertisement for a medicine, printed in 1717, describes the response of the London alehouse keepers Charles and Mary Pearce to the successful workings of the remedy: 'We... hereby affirm' that 'the Child got up upon his Feet to play, to our great Amazement, and has ever since so visibly recover'd and thriv'd'.[220] This testimony is reminiscent of miracle accounts, where typically the lame jump to their feet, and throw away their crutches.[221] For pious families, these wonderful sights were enjoyed on a spiritual as well as an emotional level: part of the happiness stemmed from the fact that they believed that God was the ultimate agent of recovery. This is evident in Martha Hatfield's biography: when she at last overcame her long illness in 1652, her family and friends gathered for a thanksgiving service. Her uncle reported that:

> [S]he was able to come forth into the Hall to meet and welcome us;... it was wonderful in our eyes, so that our hearts did rejoice with a kind of trembling at the glory of the Lord, which appeared in that Object, and it did the more affect [us], because [she had recovered] more then many... of us heard of before we came into the house.[222]

The visitors' joy was all the greater because they had not expected to find Martha so well, an experience which philosophers would have attributed to the fact that 'things... not expected, provoke most joy in our hearts'.[223] It was, however, the combination of sight and sound that sparked the greatest happiness. This is evident in an account of the recovery of eleven-year-old Margaret Muschamp from Northumberland, who had been diagnosed with diabolical possession in the 1640s. One day her mother, who had been out on an errand, returned home to see her daughter, 'whom she [had] left in so bad a condition', at the garden gate 'with her cloathes on, calling, ["]Mother, Mother, welcome home["]'. Writing in the

---

[217] Claver Morris, *The Diary of a West Country Physician, 1648–1726*, ed. Edmund Hobhouse (1935), 117.

[218] Stuart, *Vanities of the Eye*, ch. 1.   [219] Newcome, *The Autobiography*, vol. 1, 93.

[220] POB, Ref: a17170117-1 (accessed 12/05/16).

[221] See the Introduction, note 154 on the similarities between miracle accounts and advertisements.

[222] Fisher, *The wise virgin*, 159.   [223] Coeffeteau, *A table*, 302.

third person, her mother said, 'Now the Mother's joy may be imagined, but not expressed'.[224]

Thus, relatives shared the emotions of the patient in the transition from disease to ease, and the chief pathways to fellow-feeling were the senses of hearing and sight. It was not always possible to be present during a loved one's illness and recovery, however. How did fellow-feeling operate in these individuals? The answer is by correspondence. When relatives were awaiting news of the patient's condition, the experience of opening the letter was one of trepidation. A lawyer from Hackney, William Lawrence (1636/7–97), wrote that when he spied the envelope which he knew would contain information about the state of his brother Isaac, 'my heart trembled and for many hours I could not break the seals, but when I had hovered thus till night, full of anxiety...I at last opened the suspected paper, and read...the news of your escape'.[225] Emotional responses to the good news varied according to who had written the letter: when it was the patient him or herself, loved ones expressed great joy, since the ability to write was regarded as proof of recovery—it demonstrated that the patient had sufficient cognitive and physical strength to sit up and hold a pen.[226] John Hervey told his wife in 1711, 'The good news your letter brought me this evening of your pains being so abated...gives me joy inexpressible...for thy precious life is of so inestimable a value to me'.[227] Relatives often commented specifically on the handwriting. The poet and playwright John Dryden (1631–1700) told his recovering cousin, Elizabeth Steward, 'Your letter puts me out of doubt...because it was written with your own hand'.[228] However, if relatives found that the letter had been written in another hand, they instantly feared that the recovery had been overstated, since it suggested the patient was too weak to be able to sit up. This was the case for the Wiltshire gentlewoman Joan Thynne (1558–1612), who responded in 1577 to her husband's dictated letter with the following lines:

> I do not a little marvel that I hear from you but not by your own [hand], which surely giveth me occasion to think that you are not in good health. Wherefore sir, to put away such doubts [I] humbly desire you... [to] take so much pains as to write to me yourself.[229]

This man acquiesced to his wife's request, and Joan replied contentedly, 'I heartily thank you' for 'your letter I have received'.[230] Interestingly, recipients of such letters frequently referred to the senses of hearing and sight, even though they were not

[224] Moore, *Wonderful news*, 4.

[225] William Lawrence, *The Pyramid and the Urn: Life in Letters of a Restoration Squire: William Lawrence of Shurdington, 1636–1697*, ed. Iona Sinclair (Stroud, 1994), 55.

[226] On letter-writing as proof of recovery, see Chapter 6, pp. 211–12. For non-medical reasons why people preferred to receive letters that had been written in the correspondent's own hand, see James Daybell, *Women Letter-Writers in Tudor England* (Oxford, 2006), 110–13.

[227] Hervey, *Letter-Books*, vol. 1, 300.

[228] John Dryden, *The Letters of John Dryden*, ed. Charles Ward (Durham NC, 1942), 108–9.

[229] Alison Wall (ed.), *Two Elizabethan Women: Correspondence of Joan and Maria Thynne 1575–1611*, Wiltshire Record Society, vol. 38 (Devizes, 1983), 4.

[230] Ibid.

directly present in the patient's home. For example, they might say 'we...rejoiced to *see* a letter from you', or 'I...*hear* you are so fin[e]ly well' (my italics).[231] This tendency can be explained by the common practice of reading letters aloud, as well as seeing the printed word.[232] Gary Schneider offers another interpretation: he has noted that, 'Faith in the letter's representational capacities is often transmuted into a persuasive and determined fantasy of oral/aural intercourse and bodily presence'.[233]

In short, loved ones shared the patient's transition from grief to joy, and the main avenues to fellow-feeling were the ears and eyes, even for those not directly present. In what follows, it will be proposed that this empathy was physical as well as emotional: relatives and friends frequently implied that they were able to feel something akin to the physical suffering, and eventual ease, of the patient. In his widely published *Essays*, the French philosopher Michel de Montaigne (1533–92) wrote:

> The very sight of anothers Pain does materially work upon me, and I naturally usurp the Sense of a third Person to share with him in his Torment. A perpetual Cough in another tickles my Lungs and Throat...I take possession of the disease I am concerned at and lay it too much to heart.[234]

Englishmen reported similar experiences. In 1700, Richard Bentley wrote to his fiancée from his Cambridge college to express sorrow at the news of her toothache; he lamented, 'I am more sensibly touchd with any thing that befalls you, than if my self was the sufferer'.[235] By referring to the sense of touch, this man implies that he is practically feeling her pain. The notion that it is possible to vicariously experience another person's suffering or ease challenges the traditional view, associated with Elaine Scarry, that pain is unsharable. It also supports recent findings of the pain historians Jan Frans van Dijkhuizen and Joanna Bourke who have argued that compassion can 'take on the intensity of physical experience, and become a kind of pain itself'.[236] Incidentally, this idea has been partially endorsed by modern cognitive neuroscientists,[237] who have shown—from functional neuroimaging studies—that 'the perception of pain in others relies at least partly on the activation of...common neural systems'.[238]

---

[231] William Fitzwilliam, *The Correspondence of Lord Fitzwilliam of Milton and Francis Guybon, His Steward 1697–1709*, ed. D. R. Hainsworth and Cherry Walker, Northampton Record Society, vol. 36 (1990), 126; Buxton, *John Buxton*, 104.

[232] On reading aloud, see Andrew Cambers, *Godly Reading: Print, Manuscript and Puritanism in England, 1580–1720* (Cambridge, 2011), *passim*.

[233] Gary Schneider, *The Culture of Epistolarity: Vernacular Letters and Letter-Writing in Early Modern England, 1500–1700* (Newark NJ, 1984), 111, 113.

[234] Michel de Montaigne, *Essays of Michael, seigneur de Montaigne* (1685), 134.

[235] Trinity College Library, Cambridge, Additional MS a 331, letter 4 (Correspondence of Richard Bentley, 1662–1742). See also SHC, DD/WO 55/7/47-1 (Richard Carpenter to father-in-law, John Trevelyan, 24 March 1619, reporting on his wife's responses to his pains).

[236] Van Dijkhuizen, *Pain and Compassion*, 29, 234–7. Bourke's argument relates to a later period: *The Story of Pain*, ch. 8.

[237] Philip Jackson, Pierre Rainville, and Jean Decety, 'To What Extent Do We Share the Pain of Others? Insight from the Neural Bases of Pain Empathy', *Pain*, 125 (2006), 5–9, at 5.

[238] These scientists do not think sufferers' and witnesses' feelings were identical, however; see ibid., 6–8; T. Singer, B. Seymour, J. O'Doherty, H. Kaube, R. J. Dolan, and C. D. Frith, 'Empathy for Pain

There were various ways in which relatives and friends came close to sharing the patient's bodily suffering and relief. Most obviously, the use of the term 'bowels of compassion' to describe fellow-feeling—a phrase from 1 John 3:17—suggests that relatives could feel visceral movement when witnessing pain, just as the sick commonly experienced disturbance in their bowels and intestines.[239] This was the case for the Hertfordshire gentlewoman Sarah Cowper (1644–1720): she wrote in her diary in *c.*1713, 'this Day my Bowels Quake to see my dear son so Indispo'd with shaking fits' of ague.[240] Her handwriting mirrors her son's fits, as she herself acknowledges (see Figure 7). Secondly, family members, like patients, often suffered from insomnia during illness, and enjoyed peaceful sleep in recovery.[241] Ralph Josselin noted in his diary in 1650, 'my litle sonne' had 'rested very ill 3 nights' with sore eyes, but 'the 4th night god heard our prayer and refreshed his wearied mother'.[242] The cries of the patient, together with the demands of round-the-clock nursing, thus made sleep difficult for relatives, an experience recorded by men as well as women.[243] Other common bodily experiences included the tendency of loved ones to shed tears of sadness while witnessing the patient's suffering, and weep for joy upon their recovery. Thirteen-year-old Mary Maillard, who was miraculously cured from a deformity to her legs, described her father's tearful reaction: 'coming into the Shop, and seeing me go upright, he was so overcome with Surprize, as to burst out into excessive Weeping, which was so loud, as to be heard out into the Street'.[244] The fact this father shed tears in such a public way shows once again that males did not always feel constrained by the contemporary view that 'to weepe...is not so decent in a man'.[245]

The ultimate form of shared bodily suffering and ease was when relatives themselves fell ill or recovered in line with the patient. This was caused by their own emotional distress or joy, which was believed to be capable of procuring or curing disease.[246] The Essex minister Anthony Walker (*c.*1622–92) recorded that when he and his wife were both unwell:

> I recovered first, and when I could leave my Bed, and creep into her Chamber, the sight of me was like Life from the Dead. She hath oft told me,...what alteration it made in her, the joy so revived her Spirits, it helped to cure her.[247]

The spirits were the vehicles through which the body's healer, Nature, operated, and therefore their sudden expansion could speed up recovery.[248] Olivia Weisser

---

Involves the Affective but not the Sensory Components of Pain', *Science*, 303 (2004), 1157–61; Jean Decety and Claus Lamm, 'Human Empathy through the Lens of Social Neuroscience', *The Scientific World Journal*, 6 (2006), 1146–63, at 1150.

[239] On this phase, see Wilson-Yamamoto, *Pain, Pleasure and Perversity*, 134–5.
[240] Cowper, *Diary*, vol. 7, 271.   [241] Bury, *An account*, 152.
[242] Josselin, *The Diary*, 191–2.   [243] Hervey, *Letter-Books*, vol. 1, 275.
[244] *An exact relation*, 9.
[245] George Puttenham, *The arte of English poesie* (1589), 243. For a general history of crying, see Thomas Dixon, *Weeping Britannia: Portrait of a Nation in Tears* (Oxford, 2015); see also note 202 in this chapter.
[246] On fear as a cause of disease, see David Gentilcore, 'The Fear of Disease and the Disease of Fear', in William Naphy and Penny Roberts (eds.), *Fear in Early Modern Society* (Manchester, 1997), 184–208.
[247] Elizabeth Walker, *The vertuous wife*, ed. Anthony Walker (1694), 55–6.
[248] See Chapter 1 on Nature's role in recovery.

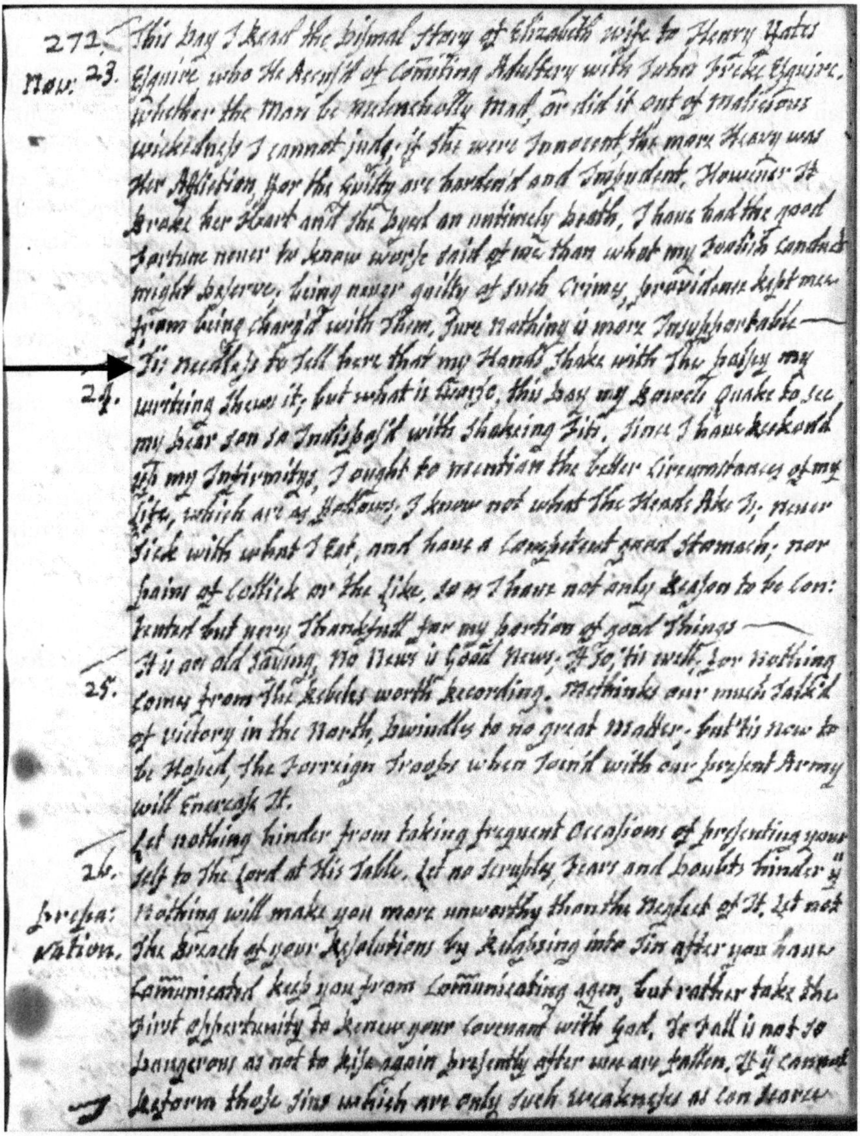

Figure 7. Shaky handwriting of Sarah Cowper during her son's 'shaking fits', 24 November 1715; 'Diary of Dame Sarah Cowper', vol. 7, p. 271, Hertfordshire Archives and Local Studies, MS D/EP/F35. This diary entry is material evidence of fellow-feeling: Cowper links her shaky handwriting to her son's shaking fits, as well as to her own illness, palsy (weakness with tremor). She writes, 'Tis needless to tell here that my Hands shake with the palsey my writing shews it; but what is worse, this Day my Bowels Quake to see my dear son so Indispo'd with shaking fits'. Thank you to the County Archivist, Chris Bennett, for granting permission for the use of this image.

has explored this phenomenon in her illuminating study of gender and illness: she shows that while women described the instant effects of emotion on their health, men highlighted the physiological steps involved, hoping that this would enable them to maintain 'manly virtues of reason, self-governance, and strength'.[249] There was one context, however, in which men *did* claim to suddenly sicken or recover, and that was courtship. A letter-writing manual from 1669 instructs suitors to address their ailing sweethearts with the following lines:

> I am so happy to sympathize with you in your want of Health [that]...you cannot be distempered...but I must be too...I have had an extream fit...Now I am somewhat amended...I do desire, that your condition is the same, otherwise, rather than you should want a Companion in your misery, I would choose to be ill again.[250]

We might expect this degree of male sensitivity to be expressed by the mid-eighteenth century, the era associated with the cultural movement of sensibility, but such expressions appear throughout the 1600s.[251] One explanation is that these responses were in fact rooted in the much older tradition of chivalry, which predated the cult of sensibility by a number of centuries.[252]

In short, families and friends usually shared the experiences of patients—illness was a double misery, and recovery, a double joy. I should add a caveat here, however: the sources in this study over-represent loving, 'functional' relationships, wherein fellow-feeling is likely to have been especially acute. Even so, occasional examples of less harmonious relationships indicate that fellow-feeling might still be experienced, albeit to a lesser degree. Sarah Cowper, who rarely had a good word to say about her husband, remarked that when her eye became infected in 1703, he no longer 'teaze[s] me with needless grievances as he was wont', because the sight of her afflictions 'moves so much compassion in him'.[253] Nonetheless, it is undeniable that some individuals experienced little empathy for their relations. In 1716, Dudley Ryder visited his sick aunt, Lomax; he recorded that as soon as she heard him knock at the door, 'she began to make a most hideous noise and crying, as if she was extremely sick, but it looked so much as if it had been done with design that I had not the least sentiments of pity'. As they conversed, 'she seemed to forget she was ill and talked as well and brisk as if not at all out of order'.[254] This man's suspicion that his aunt was feigning her suffering accounted for his uncompassionate attitude; it may also have been a sign of his lack of real affection for this relation.

---

[249] Weisser, *Ill Composed*, ch. 3, at 100.
[250] Charles Sackville, *The new academy of complements* (1669), 76.
[251] On sensibility and sympathy in the 1700s, see Bourke, *The Story of Pain*, ch. 8.
[252] On the vitality of chivalric codes in the seventeenth century, see Alex Davis, *Chivalry and Romance in the English Renaissance* (Woodbridge, 2003).
[253] Cowper, *Diary*, vol. 2, 53.
[254] Ryder, *The Diary*, 213. Another example is provided in the diary of Ralph Josselin, who remarked on how 'strange' it was that one Mrs Eldred 'never pittied' her husband when he was ill of the stone, 'nor spoke a good word of god in his recovery'. The fact that Josselin was shocked by this woman's response suggests that it was probably not very common: Josselin, *The Diary*, 517.

CONCLUSION

The transition from feeling ill to feeling better was often a 'double joy' for early modern patients, of their bodies and souls. During sickness, the soul, 'by its sympathy with its dear Companion', the body, felt 'anguish and vexation', but upon recovery this nobler part of the human being, together with every body part, rejoiced.[255] Recovery was also a double joy for family members and friends—they shared the distress, and subsequent relief, of the patient, an experience known as *fellow-feeling*. Van Dijkhuizen attributes these responses to the concept of pain, suggesting that one of its inherent properties was its tendency to elicit compassion in others.[256] I have suggested that fellow-feeling was also linked to the passion of love: the defining feature of this emotion was its 'uniting vertue', which enabled the sharing of states, good and bad, physical and emotional. This applied both to the love between the patient's body and soul, and to the affection between patients and their relatives. By exploring these experiences, the chapter has sought to demonstrate how apparently esoteric philosophical ideas exerted a powerful impact on the lived experience of illness and health. The discussions have also revealed just how much relatives and friends professed to love one another, especially parents and children, courting or married couples, and siblings. Given cultural attitudes to gender and emotion, we might have expected fellow-feeling to have been restricted in males—with drier hearts and more rational minds, tearful pity and joy could be regarded as effeminate at this time.[257] While it is true that husbands often emphasized their wives' tender hearts, this chapter has demonstrated that they too were capable of deep compassion.[258] This may have stemmed from codes of chivalry, an ideology that celebrated compassion in romantic heroes, together with the Christian veneration of the compassionate Christ. The idea that the sensitive 'man of feeling' only emerged in the later eighteenth century may thus require reconsideration.

Through investigating the experience of abated suffering, it has been possible to interrogate the meanings of the elusive, rarely defined terms, 'feeling ill' and 'feeling better'. Three of the most ubiquitous and unchanging facets of these experiences were the presence or decline of pain, nausea, and sleeplessness. While valuable studies have been conducted on the first of these components, the others have largely gone unnoticed. I think this is because pain has proved such a huge and challenging subject that it has absorbed all the attention, a trend evident in other disciplines too. The intention behind highlighting these additional aspects of illness is to reach a closer empathy for sick and recovering patients in the past, and perhaps also in the present, while encouraging further studies into other common symptoms of illness. We have seen that the experience of these forms of suffering and their subsequent disappearance was fundamentally sensory in nature, linking particularly to touch and taste. Pain was sharp and bitter, nausea made food seem sour and slimy, and the inability to sleep evoked sensations of

[255] Rogers, *Practical discourses*, 98–9.   [256] Van Dijkhuizen, *Pain and Compassion, passim*.
[257] Capp, '"Jesus Wept"', 76–7.
[258] For examples of the former, see Newton, *The Sick Child*, 103, 126, 142–3.

hardness; the mitigation of this suffering was experienced as sweet and soft ease, comfort, and pleasure. When the Lancashire minister and medical practitioner James Clegg (1679–1755) found himself 'much better in all respects' from a month-long ague, he exclaimed, 'O how sweet is rest and ease after Sickness and pain'.[259] While historians have long recognized the importance of metaphorical language in descriptions of pain, pleasurable sensations have been subjected to less analysis of this kind.

Whereas patients tended to refer to the senses of touch and taste in their accounts of suffering and its abatement, relatives and friends were more likely to mention sight and hearing, the 'nobler senses'. As I began to realize in my previous work on sick children, the agony of hearing and seeing a loved one suffer surpassed all other afflictions, even death. During the illness of his baby daughter Mary in 1669, Isaac Archer lamented, 'Oh what griefe was it to mee to heare it groane, to see it's sprightly eyes turne to mee for helpe in vaine!'[260] Upon recovery, these 'sad accents and lookes' turned into happy smiles and cheerful chatter, to the unspeakable joy of families and friends. So effective were the ears and eyes at communicating the feelings of another person, loved ones frequently claimed to *feel* something akin to the physical suffering and eventual relief of the patient. The fact that different senses were privileged by patients and their loved ones supports revisionist work on sensory hierarchies, showing that even within one context—the sickchamber— multiple rankings coexisted. Indeed, it is likely that the level of emphasis placed on each of the senses must have depended to a large extent on the disease in question: for instance, some illnesses gave rise to putrid smells, or directly affected the sensory powers of the sufferer. Further research on this subject is needed to fully explore these aspects of illness.[261]

A striking feature of the accounts of feeling better is the way patients and their families almost always mention God when describing their ease. While this ten- dency could be put down to the widespread belief that recovery was brought by the Lord, I think there was another, more intriguing reason.[262] The enjoyment of appetite, sound sleep, and sweet ease that accompanied recovery were of somewhat dubious moral status in Christian culture, since they were regarded as 'pleasures of the flesh'.[263] In order to render such things legitimate sources of celebration, pious patients and their relations emphasized their providential origins. Effectively, this turned sensual joys into spiritual ones, and in so doing, preserved, or even enhanced, individuals' pious identities.[264] This trend is visible across the early modern period, which reflects the endurance of Christian attitudes to bodily pleasures

---

[259] Clegg, *The Diary*, 114, 116. See also Josselin, *The Diary*, 120.

[260] Archer, 'The Diary', 120.

[261] I am undertaking a Wellcome Trust University Award on this subject, entitled 'Sensing Sickness in Early Modern England'.

[262] On the role of God in recovery, see Chapter 1, pp. 36–7, and Chapter 4.

[263] On the religious dangers of sensory pleasures, see Clark, *Vanities of the Eye*, 21–7; Corine Schleif and Richard Newhauser, *Pleasure and Danger in Perception: The Five Senses in the Middle Ages and the Renaissance*, Special Issue of *Senses & Society*, 5 (2010).

[264] Erin Sullivan has detected a similar trend in the context of sorrow: she has found that what could have been interpreted as 'profane' sadness, such as the excessive grief that followed the death of a loved one, was often transformed by sufferers into 'godly sorrow': *Beyond Melancholy*, ch. 4.

over time. Finally, it should be noted that not all patients reached a state of complete ease, nor did their families and friends necessarily find their senses entirely free from distressing stimuli, since many diseases left lasting 'footsteps', such as scars.[265] Worst of all, were the 'trembling feares' and 'hot Alarms' of the return of suffering— relapse—together with the occurrence of new symptoms and pains.[266] As the Hertfordshire gentlewoman Sarah Cowper put it in *c*.1701, after one illness had abated, 'I was seizd with an Exquisite pain in my shoulder which put me in mind not to be over solicitous to have any one Temporal Evil remov'd, because in a moment another, and perhaps a worse [one] may succeed'.[267]

[265] On smallpox scars, see Anselment, *The Realms of Apollo*, 187–212; Stolberg, *Experiencing Illness*, 51–2. Michelle Webb's PhD explores this subject, ' "As Fowle a Ladie as the Smale Pox could Make her": Facial Disfigurement in Sixteenth and Seventeenth-Century England' (University of Exeter, in progress).
[266] Boyle, *Occasional reflections*, 235–7.   [267] Cowper, *Diary*, vol. 1, 79.

4

'A Double Delight':
Thanking God

Behold thou art made whole. Sin no more, lest a worst thing come unto thee.[1]

Offer unto God thanksgiving; and pay thy vows unto the most High. Call upon me in the day of trouble: I will deliver thee, and thou shalt glorify me.[2]

I will extol thee, O Lord, for thou hast lifted me up.[3]

I have not hid thy righteousness within my heart; I have declared thy faithfulness and thy salvation.[4]

Sing unto the LORD, O ye saints of his, and give thanks at the remembrance of his holiness.[5]

Recovery from disease was an event of profound religious significance in early modern England, because it was thought to be ordained by God. This chapter investigates the perceived impact of bodily recovery on spiritual well-being, and asks how patients and their loved ones reacted to the belief that ultimately it was the Lord who had raised them from the sickbed. While scholars have explored providential interpretations and responses to illness, little attention has been paid to religious reactions to divine healing.[6] I show that across the Protestant spectrum, the spiritual experience of recovery was shaped by what can be called 'the art of recovery', a set of moral duties and devotional practices derived from Scripture, which were supposed to be performed in the wake of illness. Reminiscent of the 'art of death' with which historians are familiar, it was possible to make a good or

---

[1] John 5:14.   [2] Psalm 50:14–15.   [3] Psalm 30:1.
[4] Psalm 40:10.   [5] Psalm 130:4.
[6] For example, Andrew Wear, 'Puritan Perceptions of Illness in Seventeenth Century England', in Roy Porter (ed.), *Patients and Practitioners: Lay Perceptions of Medicine in Pre-Industrial Society* (Cambridge, 2002, first publ. 1985), 55–99; Andrew Wear, 'Religious Belief and Medicine in Early Modern England' in Hilary Marland and Margaret Pelling (eds.), *The Task of Healing: Medicine, Religion and Gender in England and the Netherlands, 1450–1800* (Rotterdam, 1996), 145–69; Raymond Anselment, *The Realms of Apollo: Literature and Healing in Seventeenth-Century England* (1995), 24–9; David Harley, 'The Theology of Affliction and the Experience of Sickness in the Godly Family, 1650–1714: The Henrys and the Newcomes', in Ole Peter Grell and Andrew Cunningham (eds.), *Religio Medici: Medicine and Religion in Seventeenth-Century England* (Aldershot, 1996), 273–92; Jan Frans van Dijkhuizen, 'Partakers of Pain: Religious Meanings of Pain in Early Modern England', in Jan Frans van Dijkhuizen and Karl Enenkel (eds.), *The Sense of Suffering: Constructions of Physical Pain in Early Modern Culture*, Yearbook for Early Modern Studies, vol. 12 (Leiden, 2008), 189–220; Jenny Mayhew, 'Godly Beds of Pain: Pain in English Protestant Manuals (ca. 1550–1650)', in van Dijkhuizen and Enenkel (eds.), *The Sense of Suffering*, 299–322.

bad recovery depending upon one's ability to cultivate certain holy emotions and life changes.[7] When patients were able to meet the requirements, recovery was a 'double delight'—their souls as well as their bodies were better. But, on those occasions when they failed to live up to the expectations, the joy of recovery was significantly undermined. The stakes were high: ultimately, the healing of the soul signified the individual's likely salvation, whilst relapse into sin was tantamount to impending damnation. These ideas were rooted in the Christian concept of predestination, a doctrine of great influence amongst second-generation Protestants; it held that everyone's eternal destinies had been decided from the beginning of time, and that people should seek out assurance of their election by examining the states of their souls.[8] Significantly, recovery itself was not evidence of salvation, since 'wicked men, as well as godly men' were raised from sickness; rather, it was patients' subjective sense of spiritual well-being following illness, together with their behavioural responses to deliverance, that counted.[9] Through these arguments, the chapter reveals the close relationship between bodily and spiritual health, and medicine and religion more broadly in early modern culture. It also illuminates a variety of wider themes within the historiography of lived religion, including the hazy relationship between private and public devotion, attitudes to psalm-singing and music, and the use of bodily gestures in acts of devotion.[10]

Religious historians have tended to focus on the gloomy effects of Protestant doctrine. Jean Delumeau's book *Sin and Fear* (1990) traces the emergence of a 'western guilt culture', sparked by puritans' emphasis on human depravity.[11] John Stachniewski asserted that the Calvinist belief in predestination produced 'incalculable' volumes of despair in Christians.[12] Others have focused on Hell, and the 'intense and unremitting fear of death' it evoked.[13] By examining responses to God's mercies rather than his judgements, this chapter showcases the happier side of Protestantism. It reveals that divine deliverance was often found to elicit exquisite emotions called 'holy affections', feelings kindled by the presence of the Holy

[7] On the art of death, see Nancy Lee Beaty, *The Craft of Dying: A Study in the Literary Tradition of the Ars Moriendi in England* (1970); Lucinda Beier, 'The Good Death in Seventeenth-Century England', in Ralph Houlbrooke (ed.), *Death, Ritual and Bereavement* (1989), 43–61; Ralph Houlbrooke, *Death, Religion and the Family in England, 1480–1750* (Oxford, 1998), 183–219.

[8] On this doctrine, see Leif Dixon, *Practical Predestinarians in England, c.1590–1640* (Abingdon, 2014); Matthew Reynolds, 'Predestination and Parochial Dispute in the 1630s: The Case of the Norwich Lectureships', *The Journal of Ecclesiastical History*, 59 (2008), 407–25; Arnold Hunt, *The Art of Hearing: English Preachers and their Audiences, 1590–1640* (Cambridge, 2010), ch. 7.

[9] Nicholas Byfield, *A commentary: or, sermons upon the second chapter of the first epistle of Saint Peter* (1623), 284.

[10] On these themes, see Alec Ryrie, *Being Protestant in Reformation Britain* (Oxford, 2013); Hunt, *The Art of Hearing*; Jessica Martin and Alec Ryrie (eds.), *Private and Domestic Devotion in Early Modern Britain* (Farnham, 2012).

[11] Jean Delumeau, *Sin and Fear: The Emergence of a Western Guilt Culture, 13th–18th Centuries* (New York, 1990).

[12] John Stachniewski, *The Persecutory Imagination: English Puritanism and the Literature of Religious Despair* (Oxford, 1991). This negative assessment of the doctrine of predestination has been challenged by Dixon in his book, *Practical Predestinarians*, and Hunt, *The Art of Hearing*, ch. 7.

[13] David Stannard, *The Puritan Way of Death: A Study in Religion, Culture, and Social Change* (Oxford, 1977), 79.

Spirit in the soul, such as praise and love for God. These findings support recent historiographical assertions that intense emotion was central to the daily lives of early modern Protestants, in contrast to earlier depictions of reformed Protestantism as an inherently intellectual, rather than an affective, faith.[14]

An entrenched assumption in the history of early modern medicine is that England was undergoing a secularizing process in the late seventeenth century. Ian Mortimer avers that from 1690, 'the English turned from praying... to paying for medicines when struggling with grave illness'.[15] Focusing on the doctrine of providence, Andrew Wear has suggested that after 1660, 'God the healer... receded into the background', and that 'it was generally only Nonconformists... who seemed to view the occurrences of life in... providential terms'.[16] Other scholars have suggested that the 'tenor' of spirituality was changing: in the wake of the Civil Wars, there was widespread aversion to what was called 'enthusiasm', the puritan emphasis on intense spiritual emotions.[17] This chapter adds to revisionist work which casts doubt on these various teleologies: it reveals that deliverance from disease continued to be interpreted as a divine mercy into the eighteenth century amongst conformists and nonconformists alike.[18] Whilst enthusiasm may have evoked censure in some contexts, it seems that deliverance from disease was regarded as a legitimate occasion for hyperbolic spiritual rapture, even by Anglicans. This interpretation fits with Alec Ryrie's assertion that 'the division between

---

[14] Hunt, *The Art of Hearing*; Ryrie, *Being Protestant*; Alexandra Walsham, 'Deciphering Divine Wrath and Displaying Godly Sorrow: Providentialism and Emotion in Early Modern England', in Jennifer Spinks and Charles Zika (eds.), *Disaster, Death and the Emotions in the Shadow of the Apocalypse, 1400–1700* (Basingstoke, 2016), 21–43. Other influential studies on the emotion and religion, but for different places or periods, include Susan Karant-Nunn, *The Reformation of Feeling: Shaping the Religious Emotions in Early Modern Germany* (Oxford, 2010); Phyllis Mack, *Heart Religion in the British Enlightenment: Gender and Emotion in Early Methodism* (Cambridge, 2008).

[15] Ian Mortimer, *The Dying and The Doctors: The Medical Revolution in Seventeenth-Century England* (Woodbridge, 2009), 2. Similar views are put forward by Michael Macdonald, 'The Medicalization of Suicide in England: Laymen, Physicians and Cultural Change, 1500–1870', *Milbank Quarterly*, 67 (1989), 69–91; Charles Webster, 'Paracelsus Confronts the Saints: Miracles, Healing and the Secularization of Magic', *SHM*, 8 (1995), 403–21; John Sommerville, *The Secularization of Early Modern England: From Religious Culture to Religious Faith* (Oxford, 1992).

[16] Wear, 'Puritan Perceptions', 75–6. See also Keith Thomas, *Religion and the Decline of Magic: Studies in Popular Beliefs in Sixteenth- and Seventeenth-Century England* (1991, first publ. 1971), 126–7.

[17] Hunt, *The Art of Hearing*, 89, 93; Ryrie, *Being Protestant*, 90; Thomas Dixon, 'Enthusiasm Delineated: Weeping as a Religious Activity in Eighteenth-Century Britain', *Litteraria Pragensia: Studies in Literature and Culture*, 22 (2012), 59–81; Michael Heyd, 'The Reaction to Enthusiasm in the Seventeenth Century: Towards an Integrative Approach', *Journal of Modern History*, 53 (1981), 258–80; Michael Heyd, *Be Sober and Reasonable: The Critique of Enthusiasm in the Seventeenth and Early Eighteenth Centuries* (Leiden, 1995).

[18] Revisionists include Sophie Mann, 'A Dose of Physic: Confessional Identity and Medical Practice within the Family', in John Doran and Charlotte Methuen (eds.), *Studies in Church History: Religion and the Household*, 50 (Woodbridge, 2014), 284–95; Jane Shaw, *Miracles in Enlightenment England* (2006); Blair Worden, 'The Question of Secularization', in Alan Houston and Steve Pincus (eds.), *A Nation Transformed: England after the Restoration* (Cambridge, 2001), 20–40. Walsham believes that there was some sort of change happening, but it was not as rapid as has been previously assumed, 'Deciphering Divine Wrath', 34–5.

puritan and conformist Protestants...almost fades from view when examined through the lens of devotion and lived experience'.[19]

One of the difficulties presented by the task in hand is assessing how far the primary sources convey the 'real' experiences of the authors. Alexandra Walsham has observed, 'it is difficult to gauge the depth of the pious rhetoric...and to disentangle sincere conviction from conventional formulae'.[20] Pious authors may have presented the ideal religious response to recovery in order to create a powerful didactic message for readers. Sermons and conduct books about recovery—termed here the 'art of recovery literature'—provide templates for how to behave, even supplying patients with statements to utter. 'Now you feel yourselves Well, say... *This is the Lords doing!*', instructed the author of *A perfect recovery* (1714).[21] It is conceivable that patients replicated such phrases in their personal documents without fully endorsing them.[22] Nevertheless, the unique advantage of spiritual meditations from this period is their authors' apparent honesty about discrepancies between what they called 'inward' and 'outward' affections. Reformation scholars have shown that devout Protestants were terrified of hypocrisy, and deeply wary of expressing false feelings.[23] Consequently, they were willing to admit when they found it difficult to muster up the required holy responses. The other major challenge encountered in this chapter is the over-representation of the Protestant godly—and especially ministers—in the sources; this issue has been discussed at length in the Introduction, and so will not be repeated here.[24]

The first section investigates the perceived impact of bodily recovery on spiritual health; the rest of the chapter is structured around the key components of the art of recovery: repudiate sin, cultivate 'holy affections', and join together in collective thanksgiving.

BODY AND SOUL

In early modern England, the human being was conceived as 'a double substance', the body and soul. The former was 'terrestriall, composed of the elements', while the latter was 'more sublime and celestiall...neither composed of any elementary substance...and therefore...immortal'.[25] Theologians on both sides of the confessional spectrum taught that the states of these two spheres were usually analogous. John Harris (d. 1719), an Anglican minister from Sussex, declared in 1676,

---

[19] Ryrie, *Being Protestant*, 6. On inter-confessional relations in the context of medicine, see Alexandra Walsham, 'In Sickness and in Health: Medicine and Inter-Confessional Relations in Post-Reformation England', in C. Dixon, Freist Dagmar, and Mark Greengrass (eds.), *Living with Religious Diversity in Early Modern Europe* (Aldershot, 2009), 161–82; Mann, 'A Dose of Physic'.

[20] Alexandra Walsham, *The Reformation of the Landscape: Religion, Identity, and Memory in Early Modern Britain and Ireland* (Oxford, 2011), 436.

[21] Cotton Mather, *A perfect recovery. The voice of the glorious God, unto persons, whom his mercy has recovered from sickness* (Boston, 1714), 20–1.

[22] Timothy Rogers, *Practical discourses on sickness and recovery* (1691), 177–8.

[23] Ryrie, *Being Protestant*, 4, 15, 70.   [24] See the Introduction, pp. 26–8.

[25] James Hart, *Klinike, or the diet of the diseased* (1633), 341–2.

[T]here is an agreement... between the Affections of the Soul, and the Temperature of the Body[:] ... experience... demonstrate[s] their joint influence... in the production either of Health or Diseases.[26]

The body and soul were depicted as close friends or bound servants, who shared in one another's prosperities and afflictions. 'The chains that bind them together, are so straight, that all their good and bad estate is shared between them', explained the French Catholic philosopher Jean-François Senault (c.1601–72).[27] In view of this close connection, the illness of the body was commonly regarded as a sign of spiritual illness—sin. Since God sent disease to punish human transgressions, or to provide opportunities for reformation, the implication was that the soul must also be sick.[28] The popular conformist preacher Nathaniel Hardy (1619–70) confirmed in a sermon published in 1653, 'Mans *soule* was first *sick of sinne*, and so the *body* becommeth infected with *sicknesse for sinne*'.[29] Sin was the spiritual equivalent to bad humours, and it was described in similarly evocative language—it was 'peccant', 'stinking', 'hideous', 'odious', and 'putrefying'.

The double sickness of the body and soul was a distressing experience: patients often felt overpowered by guilt, and some worried that they might be destined for Hell. The late sixteenth-century puritan minister Richard Kilby described his feelings of a 'loaden conscience' whilst suffering from kidney stones in his published autobiography: he lamented, 'Woe is me! my soule is wholly over-runne with a most foule filthy leprosie'.[30] These experiences were not confined to puritan clergymen. The apprentice clothier Joseph Lister (1627–1709), aged about eighteen, confessed that when he fell sick from 'a death-threatening distemper', he suffered 'sharp and piercing' fears and 'soul-trouble', in which 'agony I lay some weeks oppressed under the burden of guilt'.[31] The use of metaphors of weights and loads is common in descriptions of guilt, a choice which fitted with medical understandings of this emotion: it was associated with the humour melancholy, a dense, heavy liquid.[32] The guilty conscience was also likened to the 'nauseous... sower recoilings of our stomack' in acute illnesses, a symptom only too familiar to many of the patients in this study.[33] This emotion was experienced by patients' close relatives

[26] John Harris, *The divine physician, prescribing rules for the prevention, and cure of most diseases, as well of the body, as the soul* (1676), 'To the reader'.

[27] Jean-François Senault, *The use of passions*, trans. Henry Earl of Monmouth (1671, first publ. 1649), 479.

[28] Historians tend to assume illness was always a punishment, but as Jan Frans van Dijkhuizen has pointed out, it could also be a test of faith, or a benevolent prompt from God to repent. My thanks to Jan Frans for sharing with me his forthcoming article, '"Never Better": Affliction, Consolation and the Culture of Protestantism in Early Modern England', *Past & Present*.

[29] Nathaniel Hardy, *Two mites, or, a gratefull acknowledgement of God's singular goodnesse... occasioned by his late unexpected recovery of a desperate sickness* (1653), 5.

[30] Richard Kilby, *Halleluiah: praise yee the Lord, for the unburthening of a loaded conscience* (Cambridge, 1635), 112.

[31] Joseph Lister, *The Autobiography of Joseph Lister of Bradford, 1627–1709*, ed. Thomas Wright (Bradford, 1842), 29.

[32] Olivia Weisser discusses the physical sensations of guilt in *Ill Composed: Sickness, Gender, and Belief in Early Modern England* (2015), 68.

[33] John Collinges, *Several discourses concerning the actual Providence of God* (1678), 355. On nausea, see Chapter 3, pp. 101–3.

and friends, as well as by the sick themselves, because God was believed to use the
sickness of a loved one to correct or punish the sins of others.[34] Although guilt was
unpleasant, it must be remembered that it was regarded as a rational, commendable response to sin in the early modern period. As Erin Sullivan has shown, guilt
for sin was called 'godly sorrow' in this era, on the grounds that it was a virtuous
emotion: it was indicative of a diligent conscience, and necessary for inspiring
repentance.[35] This positive attitude may have made guilt more bearable, and in
some cases, joyful.[36]

Recovery from illness had the potential to dramatically alter the above perceptions: the departure of bodily disease was often interpreted as a sign of spiritual
healing and forgiveness. John Harris explained, 'sin, being taken away, the effect
which is bodily sickness ... must needs cease and be removed'.[37] The mechanism
through which sin was removed was the spiritual equivalent to the expulsion of
bad humours that took place during bodily recovery: repentance, the discharging
and forsaking of sin.[38] Robert Harris (*c.*1581–1658), a moderate nonconformist
Oxfordshire rector, instructed his parishioners:

> Come forth of affliction ... purged from your drosse: let sicknesse draine the soule as well
> as the bodie, and leave your humours, your pride; self-love, worldlinesse, hyporisie, &c.
> weaker than it found them.[39]

Since earnest repentance usually involved the shedding of tears, this analogy was
literal as well as metaphorical—something was actually leaving the body.[40] Of
course, repentance alone could not cure the soul: to imply that this was so would
be to suggest that humans could coerce God. Just as the efficacy of physic depended
on the Lord's blessing, the effects of repentance hinged on His forgiveness of sin.
Forgiveness was defined as release 'from the *Guiltiness*, wherein we are bound over,
to undergo his Infinite Wrath ... and we now *Stand as without Fault before the
Throne of God!*'[41] It was synonymous with the recovery of the soul, as is confirmed
in contemporary collections of scriptural metaphors.[42] The Bible provides precedents
for forgiveness upon recovery: James 5:14–15 states: 'Is any sick among you? let

---

[34] For parents' guilt, see Hannah Newton, *The Sick Child in Early Modern England, 1580–1720*
(Oxford, 2012), 131–3.

[35] Erin Sullivan, *Beyond Melancholy: Sadness and Selfhood in Renaissance England* (Oxford, 2016),
16, 30–4, 126–62, esp. 146–55. See also Ryrie, *Being Protestant*, 49, 54; Raymond Anselment, 'May
Rich, Countess of Warwick, and the Gift of Tears', *The Seventeenth Century*, 22 (2007), 336–57, at
343, 345–51.

[36] See note 35. Harris, for instance, stated that the 'acrimony' of 'godly sorrow' is 'corrected by the
sweet inward ingredient of inward Consolation': Harris, *The divine physician*, 62.

[37] Harris, *The divine physician*, 139; John Andrews, *Andrewes repentance, sounding alarm to return
from his sins* (1631), image 10; *An earnest exhortation to a true Minivitish repentance* (1642), 1.

[38] On the expulsion of humours, see Chapter 1, pp. 48–56.

[39] Robert Harris, *Hezekiahs recovery. Or, a sermon, shewing what use Hezekiah did, and all should
make of their deliverance from sicknesse* (1626), 37.

[40] On tears in repentance, see Ryrie, *Being Protestant*, 187–94; Dixon, 'Enthusiasm Delineated';
Walsham, 'Deciphering Divine Wrath'; Anselment, 'Mary Rich'.

[41] Cotton Mather, *Mens sana in corpore sano: a discourse upon recovery from sickness* (Boston, 1698),
12, 14.

[42] Thomas De Laune, *Tropologia, or a key to open Scripture metaphors* (1681), 165–6.

him call for the elders of the church; and let them pray over him... And the prayer of faith shall save the sick, and the Lord shall raise him up; and if he have committed sins, he will be forgiven'.[43]

How did patients experience this dual healing of body and soul? Phrases such as 'double delight' and 'double joy' were common.[44] When the Essex clergyman Ralph Josselin (1617–83) found his sore mouth was 'much abated' in 1655, he noted 'my mind was also very peaceable to Godward which is a doubling of mercies on mee'.[45] In fact, the joy could be more than doubled, on the grounds that the soul—as the immortal part of man—was far superior to the body. Richard Baxter (1615–91), an Anglican minister from Shropshire, averred, 'if... the cure' of 'a mans Sickness [and] Pain... brings ease and joy; How much more ease and joy may it bring, to be cured from all the grievous Maladies of reigning sin?'[46] Nonconformists agreed.[47] Patients used metaphors of lifted weights, and the washing away of dirt, to capture the wonderful relief that came with spiritual healing.[48] A poem by Henry Wotton (1568–1639), a diplomat from Kent, compared the sickbed to a bath, which has 'cleanse[d] my sordid *soul*... of Sin'.[49] Patients also likened their relief to the sensation of 'euphoria' which followed the expulsion of bad humours from the body.[50] Robert Cawdrey's *A treasurie or store-house of similies* (1600) states, 'As they which have... store of ill humours, are eased if they vomit them up: So if sinners... doo Confesse their sinnes to God, they shal finde ease in their soules and consciences'.[51] In short, the healing 'of the whole man', body and soul, was 'the Crown of all Mercies', spelling eternal life.[52]

However, recovery from bodily disease did not always have a positive impact on the patient's spiritual well-being. It was possible to recover from physical illness, but to remain spiritually distempered. '*Wo, wo, wo* to them, who being recovered from *sickness*, are not yet recovered from *Sin*', warned the puritan New England preacher Cotton Mather (1663–1728); 'Let us not count our *Sickness* well gone, Except our *Sin* be gone too'.[53] Vivid similes were used to describe this paradox. Rogers declared, 'to be diseased in our Souls whilst our Bodies thrive, is as if the House in which one lives, were very well... adorned to all advantage, [but] the Man that dwells in so fair an Habitation were forced to go in raggs'. He concluded, the patient 'is composed of Contradictions,... he is... well as to his Body, but his Soul is dead in... Sins'.[54] Rogers hoped this metaphor would make what otherwise might seem a rather abstract idea understandable to his parishioners. Laypeople

[43] Cited in Thomas Steward, *Sacrificium laudis, or a thank-offering* (1699), 11.

[44] James Burdwood, a minister from Devon, wrote that in the 'healing [of] Souls and Bodies together... we enjoy a double sweetness': *Helps for faith and patience in times of affliction* (1693), 235, 237.

[45] Ralph Josselin, *The Diary of Ralph Josselin 1616–1683*, ed. Alan Macfarlane (Oxford, 1991), 343.

[46] Richard Baxter, *Compassionate counsel to all young-men* (1681), 56.

[47] Rogers, *Practical discourses*, 118, 212–13.

[48] Kilby, *Halleluiah*, 57–8; Adam Littleton, *Hezekiah's return of praise for his recovery* (1668), 30.

[49] Henry Wotton, 'A hymn to my God in a night of my late sickness', in Izaak Walton, *Reliquiae Wottonianae, or, a collection of lives, letters, poems with characters of sundry personages* (1651), 361–2.

[50] See Chapter 1, p. 53, and Chapter 3, pp. 96, 107, on euphoria.

[51] Robert Cawdrey, *A treasurie or storehouse of similies* (1600), 125.

[52] Littleton, *Hezekiah's return*, 5–6.   [53] Mather, *A perfect recovery*, 42; Mather, *Mens sana*, 30.

[54] Rogers, *Practical discourses*, 214–15.

also recognized the possible coexistence of spiritual illness and bodily health. In the 1650s, the London woodturner Nehemiah Wallington (1598–1658) awoke at four in the morning to examine his soul: 'upon serch' he found 'I have a fatt body, but a lean soule[,]...an helthfull body but a...sickly soul[,] A body without sores and blains but a soule with...sinns and corruptions...that break out daily'.[55]

The reason this contradictory situation could arise, was that the sick and their families did not always fully repent of their sins during illness. This was not necessarily their fault—true repentance was 'onely the work of the holy spirit', not falling 'within the compasse of mans abilitie'.[56] Under these circumstances, God might relinquish His corrective efforts, and remove the disease, yet know that the person would eventually die and go to Hell.[57] The doctrine of predestination was relevant here—some individuals had been chosen for damnation just as others had been called for election, irrespective of the states of their bodies.[58] One might expect that this thinking would have lessened the individual's sense of personal culpability for failing to repent, but it did not. Contemporaries assumed that God had foreseen their inadequate repentance, and built it into His grand plan.

SIN NO MORE

Thus, in ideal circumstances, the recovery of the patient's body was accompanied by the recovery of the soul. But this is only the beginning of the story: the cornerstone to the art of recovery was proving and preserving one's newfound spiritual health. There were three main components, around which the rest of this chapter is structured. The first was to sin no more, a command taken from John 5:14: after Jesus had healed a cripple, He told him, 'Behold, thou art made whole: go away and sin no more, lest a worse thing do come unto thee'. Patients sought to achieve this goal by cultivating a new disgust for sin. The wake of illness was an ideal time for doing this, because the painful effects of sin were still fresh in the mind. Recalling his own illness in the 1690s, Timothy Rogers wrote in his sermon on recovery:

> In whatsoever disguise [sin] may come to us hereafter...when it wraps it self in... alluring colours, let us remember what an hideous and frightful Look it had when Sickness took the mask away.[59]

Rogers anticipated that this memorable image of masked deformity would help his readers, and himself, to retain their impression of the true horror of sin.[60] Patients also used metaphors of taste in this context: 'I have found by Experience the bitter

---

[55] Nehemiah Wallington, *The Notebooks of Nehemiah Wallington, 1618–1654: A Selection*, ed. David Booy (Aldershot and Burlington VT, 2007), 329–30.

[56] *An earnest exhortation*, 1; see also Daniel Dyke, *Two treatises. The one, of repentance* (1616), 6–7.

[57] Harris, *The divine physician*, 10.

[58] For example, Eusabius Pagit, *A verie fruitful sermon...concerning Gods everlasting predestination* (1583), A5r–A7v.

[59] Rogers, *Practical discourses*, 202, 206–7.   [60] Hunt, *The Art of Hearing*, 87, 112.

wayes of sin, and the sweet wayes of believing and walking with God', wrote the Oxford-educated clergyman James Allen (1632–1710).[61] Taste was a powerful analogy in the early modern period, perhaps more so than it is today: in nutrition theory, bitterness indicated a divergence between the quality of the body and the ingested food, while sweetness signified that it would be wholesome.[62] Taste was also spiritually significant: in Scripture the word 'bitter' is used to describe anything shameful, painful, or sinful.[63] Given that patients had probably tasted bitter medicines during illness, it is unsurprising that they made this linguistic choice when describing their feelings about sin.[64]

As well as cultivating a hatred for sin in general, patients were advised to repudiate their 'special sins' and to keep their 'sickbed promises'.[65] Special sins were the particular vices that had provoked God to send the illness in the first place; sickbed promises were solemn resolutions made to the Lord during sickness: patients vowed to reform their lives, and abstain from habitual sins, in exchange for recovery. In the early part of the Reformation, the tradition of covenant-making was rejected by Protestants on the grounds that sin was unavoidable, and to promise to abstain meant placing undue faith in one's own willpower. By the late sixteenth century, however, the practice was creeping back, and by the 1630s it was 'almost within the pale of Protestant acceptability'.[66] Sickbed promises were rife amongst all shades of Protestants. The royalist high churchman John Kettlewell (1653–95) endorsed the words of the biblical character David: 'I will pay thee my Vows, *O! God*, which my Lips have uttered, and my Mouth hath spoken when I was in trouble'.[67] At the other end of the spectrum, the dissenting Presbyterian medical practitioner and preacher James Clegg (1679–1755) recorded that he 'promisd if God would spare my son I would…make it my care and business in the world henceforward to advance the honour of God'.[68]

How successful were patients and their loved ones at keeping their sickbed vows, and sinning no more? Some individuals claimed that they did achieve their resolutions. Upon recovery from toothache and 'rhewme' in 1678, the moderate puritan clergyman from Suffolk, Isaac Archer (1641–1700), stated in his diary, 'I am wonderfully weaned from that wherin I had offended…in conquering the inward corruption'.[69] Children might also report these experiences. Before the age of eleven, Robert Blair (b. 1593?), had shown 'unruliness toward my two sisters'; God sent a 'sudden and short sickness' as punishment, which 'madest me to detest

[61] James Allen, *Serious advice to delivered ones from sickness* (Boston, 1679), 22.
[62] Ken Albala, *Eating Right in the Renaissance* (2002), 66.   [63] *DBI*, 315.
[64] See Chapter 3, pp. 99–101, for the use of 'bitter' in descriptions of pain.
[65] Samuel Cradock, *Knowledge and practice: or a plain discourse…[on] salvation* (1673, first publ. 1659), 109.
[66] Ryrie, *Being Protestant*, 132–3, 139.
[67] Psalm 66:13–14, cited in John Kettlewell, *Death made comfortable* (1695), 126.
[68] James Clegg, *The Diary of James Clegg of Chapel-en-Frith 1708–1755*, vol. 1 (1708–36), ed. Vanessa Doe, Derbyshire Record Society, vol. 5 (Matlock, 1978), 98.
[69] Isaac Archer, 'The Diary of Isaac Archer 1641–1700', in Matthew Storey (ed.), *Two East Anglian Diaries 1641–1729*, Suffolk Record Society, vol. 36 (Woodbridge, 1994), 41–200, at 157.

all strife' with his siblings for evermore.[70] Since the daily and lifelong goal of conscientious Christians was to improve the states of their souls, it is hard to overestimate the satisfaction that such an achievement occasioned. Ultimately, the happiness sprung from the notion that the ability to keep one's sickbed promises was itself an 'infallible token' of election to Heaven. The Anglican clergyman Richard Greenham (1540s–94) confirmed, 'An acknowledging of our offences with our whole heart, whiles we are sicke, and a verie dooing of it indeed, when we be recovered', is a 'sure signe' of election.[71]

Even more dramatic victories over sin were reported by those who had, prior to their illness, not been very interested in religion. Before her sickness at the age of eighteen, Mary Carey (*c*.1609–80), an aristocrat from Northumberland, 'knew not God'; she preferred 'worldly contentments' and 'delighting myself... in cards, dice, dancing,... going to plays... and the like'. Upon falling ill, she 'made a wish, *O that God would spare my life... I would ever quit all my vain company, leave my most beloved pleasures,... and give myself up to his service*'. When her desire was granted, she recorded that the mercy 'did so win upon my heart, that I found my resolutions, in the time of my sickness, much strengthened'.[72] Similar experiences were reported lower down the social scale, though the evidence is not from patients' own mouths. David Wright, a 'sinful and grossly ignorant' shepherd from Hertfordshire, was miraculously cured of scrofula at the age of 28; he immediately relinquished his 'vile and ignorant' ways, and began to 'shine in Grace'.[73] Sickbed vows could thus amount to a complete redirecting of one's life. These forms of religious awakenings—known as conversions—usually occurred in adolescence or early adulthood, occupying an important place in spiritual autobiographies.[74]

It was not easy to keep sickbed promises, however. The term used to describe the situation when patients broke their vows, or returned to their special sins, was 'spiritual relapse'. The equivalent to bodily relapse, it was caused by the re-admission of sin into the soul, and was usually more severe than the original distemper.[75] Succumbing to this 'feareful danger' was the defining feature of a bad recovery—it was a 'heartbreaking expression' of ingratitude, 'the greatest of all evils'.[76] Going by clergymen's accounts, spiritual relapse was common. John Beadle (1595–1667), a moderate nonconformist from Shropshire, remarked, 'How many are there that on

---

[70] Robert Blair, *The Life of Mr Robert Blair, Minister of St Andrews, Containing his Autobiography from 1593 to 1636*, ed. Robert McCrie, Wodrow Society (Edinburgh, 1848), 6–7. Parents tended to take the blame for their children's illnesses, but this did not always stop their offspring from feeling guilty—see Newton, *The Sick Child*, 131–4, 203–4.

[71] Richard Greenham, *A most sweete and assured comfort of all those that are afflicted in consicience* (1595), image 96.

[72] Mary Carey, *Meditations from the Note Book of Mary Carey, 1649–1657*, ed. Francis Meynell (Westminster, 1918), 16–18. See also Mary Rich, *Autobiography of Mary Countess of Warwick*, ed. T. Crofton Croker (1848), 10.

[73] *A true copy of a letter of the miraculous cure of David Wright, a sheppard* (1694), 1–2.

[74] Bruce Hindmarsh, *The Evangelical Conversion Narrative: Spiritual Autobiography in Early Modern England* (Oxford, 2005); Ryrie, *Being Protestant*, 436–41.

[75] On bodily relapse, see Chapter 2, pp. 67–8, 70, 74–5, 79, 83, 85, 87–9; Chapter 3, p. 111; Chapter 6, p. 206, 207, 217.

[76] Allen, *Serious advice*, 16.

their sick dayes make new promises, but being recovered, forget God, and follow their old lusts?'[77] Rogers provided an answer: 'scarce fifty' of a thousand patients 'perform their Vows, when they are recovered'.[78] Although clergymen were notoriously pessimistic in their judgements of the piety of the 'vulgar masses', evidence from other sources, such as popular literature and legal depositions, suggests that it was a familiar concept.[79]

Several reasons were given for spiritual relapse. Besides the 'proneness that is in mans nature to return again to sin', it was believed that everyone was 'addicted' to a particular sin.[80] Elizabeth Deleval (née Livingston, 1649–1717), an Anglican aristocrat from Lincolnshire, admitted that her 'beloved crime' was 'I yeeld to eate that for my tooth when my stomacke doth not requier it'.[81] She had committed this sin so many times that it had become 'an infirmity', the equivalent to a chronic bodily complaint. Language of affection was used to describe these sins—they were 'darlings', like beloved children, of whom parents would say, 'I love them all so well that I know not which I love best'.[82] Another reason for spiritual relapse was the abatement of bodily suffering during recovery, which served to erase the association between pain and sin. Rogers mused, 'Those good Purposes which they had were the Products of their Fears, and when those are over, their intended Goodness does also vanish'.[83] Put another way, sickbed promises were triggered 'not because sin is sinful, but because it is painful'; as such, the disappearance of pain takes away the abhorrence of sin.[84] Once again, colourful metaphors were used to make sense of this tendency—the strength of the patient's resistance to vice was compared to an iron that had been removed from the fire, and 'quickly returns to its old coldness', or to the morning dew, that 'can no longer resist the powerfull beames of the sun'.[85] Patients were also likened to sailors during storms, a profession notorious for forgetting promises upon reaching safety. 'Trust not a passionate resolution[:] it is raised in a storm, and will die in a calm', declared the ejected minister Thomas Watson (d. 1686).[86] This analogy was so familiar that it was used as a literary trope.[87]

Intriguingly, men were thought to be more vulnerable to spiritual relapse than women. This is evident in the many cautionary tales published on this theme, the majority of which involve males. John Bunyan (1628–88), a popular religious

---

[77] John Beadle, *The journal or diary of a thankful Christian* (1656), 2.

[78] Rogers, *Practical discourses*, 254.

[79] For example, Thomas Gills, *Thomas Gills of St. Edmund's Bury in Suffolk, upon the recovery of his sight* (1710), 3–4; Daniel Defoe, *Robinson Crusoe* (2012, first publ. 1719), 5–7; POB, Ref: OA16950712 (accessed 16/01/17).

[80] Allen, *Serious advice*, 16.

[81] Ibid.; Elizabeth Delaval, *The Meditations of Lady Elizabeth Delaval, Written Between 1662 and 1671*, ed. D. G. Greene, Surtees Society, vol. 190 (1978), fol. 17r.

[82] Henry Newcome, *The Autobiography of Henry Newcome*, ed. Richard Parkinson, Chetham Society, vol. 26 (Manchester, 1852), 49. See also Rogers, *Practical discourses*, 185–6. The terms 'bosom' or 'beloved sins' were common too—see Richard Sibbs, *A consolatory letter to the afflicted conscience* (1641), dedicatory epistle.

[83] Rogers, *Practical discourses*, 254.   [84] Thomas Watson, *The doctrine of repentance* (1668), 10.

[85] Matthew Hale, *A letter from Sr Matthew Hale... to one of his sons, after his recovery from the smallpox* (1684), 5; Delaval, *The Meditations*, 103.

[86] Watson, *The doctrine*, 10.   [87] Defoe, *Robinson Crusoe*, 5–7.

writer from Bedfordshire, described the archetypal scenario in his book, *The life and death of Mr Badman*. The caricature of immorality, Mr Badman, had promised that 'if God would but let him recover this once, what a new...penitent man he would be[come]'. But upon his recovery, 'the contrary showed itself': no sooner had 'his trouble began to goe', he 'never minded Religion more, but betook...again to the world, his lusts and wicked companions'.[88] Whether or not the story was true—Bunyan claimed that it was—it must have been credible enough for it to be deemed an effective moral tale. Indeed, there are anecdotal reports of real people like Mr Badman. The nonconformist Halifax minister Oliver Heywood (*c*.1630–1702) mentioned one Mr Longley in his diary: when this man was 'judged near death', he made 'resolutions of reformation', but during his recovery, he was 'wonderful stupid', and showed no wish to 'speak of spiritual things'.[89] It was not just notorious sinners, however, who succumbed to spiritual relapse. Some of the pious diarists and letter-writers confessed to breaking sickbed promises, including Heywood himself.[90]

The main reason for men's heightened vulnerability to spiritual relapse was that they were more likely than women to attend wild social events to celebrate recovery. The sixteenth-century Dutch physician Levinus Lemnius complained:

> [W]hen *men* recover of their diseases, many witty...companions come to see them, and they invite them to rejoyce, and make merry...Hence they eat, and drink healths... and commonly...sing bawdy songs...To this[,] I add the...voluptuous meats, which the humours being augmented by, do stimulate...the obscene parts...and cause erection. Hence...they return to...gluttony, and profuse lusts.[91]

Thus, the feasting and drinking that took place after recovery provided opportunities for sinful behaviour. Although women were not excluded from these celebrations, alehouse culture carried connotations of male sociability.[92] The physiological workings of men's genitalia provided a further reason. Doctors taught that when males overcome disease they are 'very prone to venery' because the penis is 'the first organ to recover' after illness: directly connected to the liver, 'the nutriments are first carried' to the 'secret parts'.[93]

What was it like forgetting a sickbed promise? Four short case studies of patients from various religious and social backgrounds provide insights into this experience: firstly, a royalist soldier called John Hutchins, tried for murder at the Old Bailey in 1684. Originally born into a 'plentiful Estate' in Somerset, he had, through 'Profuse' spending, 'wasted most or all of it'. The Ordinary's account reports that as a youth this man had fallen into 'a great fit of Sickness', which had inspired him to promise God that if he recovered he 'would Reform his Loose

---

[88] John Bunyan, *The life and death of Mr. Badman* (1680), 275–81.

[89] Oliver Heywood, *The Rev. Oliver Heywood, B.A: His Autobiography, Diaries, Anecdote and Event Books*, ed. Horsfall Turner, 4 vols. (1883), vol. 1, 345–6.

[90] Ibid., 177–8.

[91] Levinus Lemnius, *The secret miracles of nature* (1658, first publ. 1559), 135.

[92] See Chapter 6, notes 153, 154, for the historiography on gender and alehouses.

[93] Lemnius, *The secret miracles*, 185.

Conversation'. Yet 'contrary to his Resolution, he continued very Vain'. He confessed that this failure 'lay as a heavy burthen on his Conscience, by calling to mind that Counsel' of Christ, who had told the man at Bethsaida, 'Behold thou art made Whole, Sin no more'. He believed that God eventually punished him 'for sinning against…his Conscience' by letting him 'run into further Wickedness', which ultimately led him to commit murder. As he awaited his execution, Hutchins lay 'under [the] horrid Imprecation' that he would go straight to Hell. This incident was not connected directly to the murder, so it is fair to say that it is unlikely to have been invented by the Ordinary.[94]

The second example concerns an Anglican wigmaker of lower-middling status, Edmund Harrold, aged 34. Following a series of drink-induced distempers in 1712, Edmund and his wife made a bargain: 'Shes to refrain washing cloth[e]s and I'm to refrain drinking to excess…and we have shaked hands and kissed as a ratification'. His wife had been taking in neighbours' laundry to make ends meet, and hoped to be able to stop this work once Edmund gave up his expensive alcohol habit. Harrold then set himself a 'tryal'—he visited a local tavern, the 'Coatch and Horses', and vowed to 'drink little'. To his great satisfaction, he succeeded, spending a modest five pence on alcohol. Some time later, however, he made 'a foul slip': being sent to an inn to run an errand, he bumped into some friends, and was persuaded to have a drink—which soon turned into several, until at last 'I acted all tempers', he admitted. Harrold was 'heartily sorrey' and deeply frustrated with himself. He pleaded, 'O my soul, wilt thou lose eternall pleasures for momentary ones'. With hindsight, he blamed the deaths of '2 dear wives and 5 sweet infants' on his repeated failings, and anticipated that 'I for my part am likly to be next'.[95] Thus, the satisfaction of achieving a reformation was crushed, and replaced with self-loathing and a fear of further divine retribution.

Our third case study comes from the upper-middling classes, an Oxford-educated puritan minister from Kent, Richard Kilby, who suffered from kidney stones all his life. During a severe fit in 1613, he 'prayed earnestly' that God would 'ease me of…that paine, with [the] condition that if I did not presently enter into a very reformed course of life, the disease should return upon mee and kill me'. The pain abated, but the next morning he 'performed not' his promise. His 'breast quaked as [a] leafe shaken with the winde', for fear of 'the wrath of my Lord'. In response to this initial failure, Kilby devised a new set of rules, far more elaborate than the original ones, taking up twenty-seven pages in his autobiography; they included 'striv[ing] to have a more hungry…desire of the grace of God', praying three times a day, and 'conscionably detest[ing] and resist[ing] my sinnes'. Unfortunately, Kilby could not keep to his rules: he lamented, 'Woe is mee!… I cannot stedfastly continue in the purpose of resisting my sins…Oh mine heart is so divellishly bent to sine, that no vowes, no oathes, nothing can turne it'. Eventually, he prayed that God would allow him to 'shut up' his former vows, and

[94] POB, Ref: OA16841217 (accessed 16/01/16).
[95] Edmund Harrold, *The Diary of Edmund Harrold, Wigmaker of Manchester 1712–15*, ed. Craig Horner (Aldershot, 2009), 32, 76, 84, 90.

replace them with the following single resolution: 'I either reforme my selfe from this day forward, or for default thereof, leave the Ministery'.[96] Kilby died shortly afterwards.

The final example comes from the top echelons of society, the 18-year-old royalist aristocrat Elizabeth Delaval. In her memoirs, she recorded numerous unsuccessful attempts to curb her habit of overindulging in sweet foods, a sin which she believed drew the providential punishment of stomach-ache. She recorded, 'Wo is me that though I have lived yet but few yeares, I have broke[n] more vows that I can number… Tho[ugh] upon serious consideration I make strict resolutions against my sins, yet am I still inclined to evill'. The love of sweet things was a sin associated especially with women: in medical treatises, females were described as 'sweet toothed': sweet foods were high in moisture, and since the bodies of females abounded in moist humours, they naturally craved these substances.[97] Delaval's experience in some ways mirrored those of the others—all were exasperated with themselves. But there are subtle differences: Delaval was not unduly frightened by the consequences of her broken promises—indeed, the purpose of her meditations was to 'stir up' fear, so that she would cease sinning. 'O let the feare of thy judgements make me dread to offend thee any more', she urged her soul.[98]

There are some clear similarities and differences between the experiences of the four individuals. All expressed a desire to keep their vows, and felt remorse when they failed. Clearly, they accepted full responsibility for their broken promises: the doctrine of predestination did little to negate human agency on this front.[99] But there is a slight difference in tone: Kilby's expressions are more hyperbolic, with frustration verging on self-hatred. At first glance, it is tempting to interpret these distinctions as effects of the writers' different religious affiliations—Kilby exhibited the archetypal puritan 'enthusiasm' identified by historians, in contrast to the Anglicans, Hutchins, Delaval, and Harrold. However, perhaps a more convincing explanation relates to the different nature of Kilby's disease: whereas the other three suffered from transient conditions, Kilby's illness was agonizing and chronic, and attached to no single sin. This was why his vows were more elaborate than those of the other diarists, and his frustrations and desires, more acute. Kilby's autobiography was also intended for publication, so he may have wished to make it more engaging by emphasizing the highs and lows of his life story. Together, the examples reveal the flipside to the art of recovery: when the expectations were not met, the result was severe distress, an experience shared by patients across the socio-economic and Protestant spectrum.

Fortunately, the art of recovery literature offered practical strategies for preventing spiritual relapse. The main one was for patients to 'call to mind' and 'keep alive' the '*sad discourses* and *reasonings*, their *fears* and *tremblings*,…they had in *time* of

---

[96] Kilby, *Halleluiah*, 56–92, 132–3.
[97] Children were also thought to crave sweet foods: see Newton, *The Sick Child*, 54, 85–6.
[98] Delaval, *The Meditations*, 100–3.
[99] This issue is discussed by Alexandra Walsham in reference to collective repentance: *Providence*, 153–4.

their *distress*.[100] Through its sheer unpleasantness, the memory of pain would prolong the abhorrence of sin, and help the patient to resist it. Diaries were ideal forums for these recollections: patients could set down in detail their recent sufferings for future re-reading. Oliver Heywood used his diary to 'study to regain the thoughts and impressions my soul had...in the day of my Affliction:...Remembering...my misery'.[101] Relatives and friends might also write accounts of this sort on behalf of the patient. The Anglican judge and author Matthew Hale (1609–76) composed a 'little Volume' for his convalescing son, 'touching [his] late sickness', smallpox. He wrote, 'sick-bed promises are forgot, when sickness is over', and,

> [T]herefore I shall give you an account of your sickness, and your recovery: And let them never be forgotten by you, as often as those Spots...in your Face are reflected to your view from the Glass.[102]

The use of scars as a spur to extemporary spiritual meditation was common, and could be applied to any of the 'footsteps of disease', as they were known.[103] This positive function of disfigurement helps balance the deeply negative interpretation of smallpox scarring that dominates the historiography.[104]

Other ways to keep alive the associations between disease and sin were to visit the sick, and attend 'lively sermons' about illness. On entering the sickroom, visitors were instructed to observe the patient's misery, to 'heare it, view it[,] see how it racks and tortures the poore man, and reflect upon thy selfe'.[105] The best sermons were those inspired by the clergyman's own sickness, which contained vivid accounts of what it was like to be ill. Arnold Hunt has shown that Protestant preaching was 'designed not merely to impart doctrinal information but to elicit an affective response', to which end ministers employed various rhetorical devices, including metaphor and gesture.[106] Possibly the most striking metaphor in recovery sermons likened spiritual relapse to an unsavoury habit of dogs: 'take heed you doe not lick up those vomits you have vomitted out in time of distress'.[107] Vomiting, along with all other evacuations, was regarded as Nature's method for expelling superfluous or corrupt humours from the body; as such, to 'lick up' one's vomits was a sure way to bring relapse.[108] By drawing on well-known medical theory, this metaphor turned an abstract notion into something more comprehensible, and quite simply, disgusting.[109]

If the above techniques proved unforthcoming, patients could strengthen their resolve to keep their sickbed promises by dwelling on the threat embedded in the aforementioned Bible verse, 'Sin no more, lest a worst thing come unto

---

[100] Cradock, *Knowledge and practice*, 109.
[101] Heywood, *The Rev. Oliver Heywood*, vol. 3, 258–9.   [102] Hale, *A letter*, 5.
[103] See Chapter 2, pp. 65, 69–71, on the footsteps of disease. On extemporary meditation, see Ryrie, *Being Protestant*, 115–17.
[104] For this historiography, see Chapter 3, note 265.
[105] Harris, *Hezekiahs recovery*, 37.   [106] Hunt, *The Art of Hearing*, 11, 84, 86–7, 90, 112.
[107] Allen, *Serious advice*, 12–13; Mather, *A perfect recovery*, 37. This saying is derived from Proverbs 26:11.
[108] On the role of vomiting and other evacuations in recovery, see Chapter 1, pp. 51–6.
[109] On medical metaphors, see David Harley, 'Medical Metaphors in English Moral Theology, 1560–1660', *Journal of the History of Medicine*, 48 (1993), 396–435, at 397.

thee'—God would punish the offender harshly.[110] To quantify the severity of the retaliation, preachers referred to Leviticus 23–4: '*If ye will not be Reformed...then I will Punish you yet seven Times for your Sins*'.[111] The potential penalties encompassed all earthly and spiritual afflictions, from bodily relapse to damnation. Cotton Mather thundered in a sermon published in 1714, 'Oh! Hear with a trembling Soul...they who go on in their Sins after a *Recovery from Sickness*', may 'Rationally expect nothing but a *Banishment from God*, into the *Place of Torments*'.[112] Ironically, the fear of relapse thus became the solution to the fear of relapse.

HOLY AFFECTIONS

The second component of the art of recovery was to praise God for His gift of healing, and to foster a new love and trust in Him. These responses were known collectively as 'holy affections'—they were a set of special spiritual emotions in Christian culture, developed in the writings of the medieval theologians St Augustine of Hippo and St Thomas Aquinas.[113] The very purpose of human existence was to express these feelings: Isaiah 43:21 states, 'This people have I formed for myself; they shall shew forth my praise'. The holy affections were therefore morally superior to all other emotions, a status confirmed by their location in the soul: these feelings emanated from the rational soul in Classical Christian philosophy, as opposed to the middle section, the animal or sensitive soul, which was responsible for all the other passions.[114] Walter Charleton (1620–1707), a physician and natural philosopher from Somerset, explained in his treatise on the passions, 'our love of God, and all other real goods...belong only to the *Reasonable* Soul, which...[is] seated in a higher sphere...looking down...upon all tumults, commotions and disorders hapning in the inferior part of man', the sensitive soul.[115] It was within this 'higher sphere' that the Christian's relationship with God was conducted: the holy affections were the soul's chief communications with the Lord, and in turn He made His presence known through the spiritual feelings, sending in the Holy Spirit. Alec Ryrie's ground-breaking study, *Being Protestant*, reveals the vital importance of these emotions in the spiritual lives of Protestants: they were taken as signs of divine grace, and ultimately, of election to Heaven.[116] As shall become apparent, this belief rendered the holy affections highly desirable, and turned them into

---

[110] John 5:14.   [111] Mather, *A perfect recovery*, 39.   [112] Ibid., 45, 39.

[113] St Augustine, *The city of God*, Books IX and XIV, trans. P. Levine (1966); Thomas Aquinas, *Summa Theologiae*, trans. The Dominican Fathers (1964–81), especially Ia.75–83, on 'Man', and Ia.2ae.22–48 on 'The Emotions', 'Pleasure', and 'Fear and Anger'. The holy affections were also known as '*devout* and *religious Affections*': Walter Charleton, *A natural history of the passions* (1674), 77. My thanks to Thomas Dixon for recommending this treatise.

[114] Thomas Dixon, *From Passions to Emotions: The Creation of a Secular Psychological Category* (Cambridge, 2003), 54; Sullivan, *Beyond Melancholy*, 68–9.

[115] Charleton, *A natural history*, 55–6.

[116] Ryrie, *Being Protestant*, section 1. See also Charles Lloyd Cohen, *God's Caress: The Psychology of Puritan Religious Experience* (Oxford, 1986), 5–7, 11; Sullivan, *Beyond Melancholy*, 148–50.

'double joys'. Although the affections were inspired by the Holy Spirit, it was thought that they could—and should—also be actively 'stirred' through conscious effort.[117] The art of recovery literature taught that deliverance from disease was an ideal context for doing this.

The first step in the cultivation of holy affections was to acknowledge God's role in recovery. This obligation was rooted in John 5:14, 'Behold thou art made whole', a statement uttered by Jesus after healing a cripple. Expounding on this passage, James Allen wrote, 'That which Christ herein calls' us to do, is make 'a diligent observance of the mercy God had bestowed'.[118] The personal documents of patients and their relatives show that this duty was taken seriously. In 1728, the poet and courtier from Wiltshire, Frances Seymour (1699–1754), penned the following statement upon her recovery from fever:

> In the name of God Almighty…I, the Right Honorable Frances Countess of Hertford, do make this grateful acknowledgement of his special mercy vouchsafed unto me… I do entirely attribute my recovery to the blessings of God…And I do think myself bound to give this solemn testimony on the mercies of the Almighty in raising me… from the jaws of the grave.[119]

The formal style of this statement reveals the importance of the duty. Diaries and autobiographies were the obvious locations for such acknowledgements, since one of their main functions was to record God's interventions.[120] In the case of recovery from especially dangerous distempers, patients and their relations remembered God's role on multiple occasions, often annually. Lady Anne Clifford (1590–1676), a noblewoman from Westmorland, recalled the recovery of her two-year-old daughter Margaret from ague almost every year during her old age.[121] Even individuals who were not renowned for their piety made these sorts of regular acknowledgements—the naval officer and famous diarist, Samuel Pepys (1633–1703), for instance, observed the anniversary of the successful extraction of his bladder stone most years in his diary.[122]

After recognizing God's role, patients and their loved ones expressed, in writing and speech, the holy affections of praise and thankfulness. 'The lords name bee praised', exclaimed Ralph Josselin in his diary, for 'bringing health' to his infected navel in 1651.[123] To praise meant 'to proclaim or commend the excellence of'.[124]

---

[117] Sullivan agrees that the emotions were 'more voluntary, willful, and indeed empowering' than historians have hitherto assumed: *Beyond Melancholy*, 67.

[118] Allen, *Serious advice*, 2.

[119] Frances Seymour, *The Gentle Hertford: Her Life and Letters*, ed. Helen Hughes (New York, 1940), 91.

[120] For example, see Alice Thornton, *The Autobiography of Mrs Alice Thornton*, ed. Charles Jackson, Surtees Society, vol. 62 (1875), 259, 150.

[121] Anne Clifford, *The Diaries of Lady Anne Clifford*, ed. D. D. H. Clifford (Stroud, 1990); the illness occurred in 1617.

[122] The operation was on 26 March 1658. A typical example of commemoration, from 1661, reads, 'This is my great day, that three years ago I was cut of the stone—and blessed be God, I do yet find myself very free from pain'. He only omitted mentioning the operation in 1666 and 1668; cited in Weisser, *Ill Composed*, 131.

[123] Josselin, *The Diary*, 235.   [124] OED, verb 1 (accessed 19/05/17).

It was used interchangeably with 'bless', 'extol', 'magnify', 'glorify', and 'worship', all of which implied elevated praise.[125] Thanking God was to 'express gratitude' for a kindness received.[126] Such feelings were considered to be natural, logical reactions to divine deliverance, stemming from a sense of common courtesy. The Presbyterian Suffolk minister Thomas Steward (1668/9–1753) commented, 'Reason it self tells us, that we should be thankful to our Benefactors…we cannot but praise, and admire…the God of our Mercies…[;] why should it not excite and stir us [to praise]?'[127] Nonetheless, thankfulness was not just a matter of polite etiquette: it was a 'commanded Duty'.[128] Two Bible verses were cited to prove that this was so—the song of David upon his recovery from illness: 'I will extol thee, O Lord, for thou hast lifted me up', together with Asaph's psalm, 'Call upon me in the day of trouble: I will deliver thee, and thou shalt glorify me'.[129] The duty was described in financial or legal terms—the Lord was owed praise in return for His deliverance, and His assistance was a binding contract, which brought certain duties.

The art of recovery literature taught that the volume and intensity of thankfulness should correspond to the 'greatness of the mercy'. Various tips were given for how to cultivate appropriate levels of praise. Timothy Rogers suggested:

> This excitation of our selves [to praise] is not acquirable by a few cold and transient Thoughts…but [by]…arguing and pleading the Case with our Souls, till the Fire of our…Thankfulness begin to burn…We should think of the Mercies of God till our Hearts, under the sense of his Goodness, begin to melt…Then will the Holy Spirit cherish our Endeavours.[130]

Praising God was thus an active process, which might require sustained effort—only then would the Holy Spirit assist human attempts. This understanding is also evident in lay documents: patients and their families entreated themselves to 'enlarge' their praises. When her husband recovered from ague in 1658, the puritan aristocrat Lady Anne Harcourt (d. 1661) addressed her soul: 'O my soul, Labour for inlardgment in praysing God; be not content to do it in an ordinary maner'.[131]

Another way to enhance one's praise was to identify, and meditate upon, the most amazing features of the recovery. Top of the list were those cases where God had intervened directly. John Maillard, a French sword-cutler living in Westminster, gave his 'most humble Thanks to God' for the recovery of his daughter Mary from lameness, which he declared he and his wife 'cannot look upon but as miraculous'.[132] Patients and their relations also emphasized the rarity of the recovery, or more particularly, those instances of survival from a disease that had killed many others. Matthew Hale told his son in 1684 that 'The Disease' smallpox,

[125] OED, verb 4: states that to 'bless God' means, 'To call holy; to extol, praise, or adore (God) as holy, worthy of reverence' (accessed 19/05/17).
[126] OED, verb 4 (accessed 19/05/17).   [127] Steward, *Sacrificium laudis*, 15–16.
[128] Ibid., 14.   [129] Psalm 30:1, 50:15.   [130] Rogers, *Practical discourses*, 175–6.
[131] Anne Harcourt, *The Harcourt Papers in 14 volumes*, vol. 1, ed. E. W. Harcourt (1880), 183.
[132] James Welwood, *A true relation of the wonderful cure of Mary Maillard* (1694), 36–7.

[I]s now become ordinarily very Mortal...Look upon even the last yea[r']s General
Bill of Mortality, [and] you will find near Two Thousand dead...you might have been
one of that number![133]

He hoped this realization would 'engage us to make suitable returns to that God
who has spared us when he hath taken them away'.[134] At this time, it was thought
that the number of humans who would go to Heaven would be minuscule—some
estimated as few was one in a thousand.[135] Any divine mercy that distinguished
one individual from another was therefore cherished as possible evidence of election; these interventions were called 'singular' or 'special mercies'.

What was it like to feel the holy affections of praise and thankfulness? Philosophers
of both Protestant and Catholic faith taught that the holy affections were exquisite
to experience, far more delightful than ordinary emotions or sensual pleasures. The
philosopher Jean-François Senault stated, 'man cannot be [truly] satisfied, unless
the noblest part', the rational soul, 'be happy'. The 'pleasures of the Senses are
limited' because the body 'finds no contentment which gives satisfaction to all its
senses'. By contrast, the 'pleasures of the soul', the holy affections, 'have no bounds':
they 'present themselves all at once' to the soul, enlightening the understanding,
will, and memory simultaneously, so that 'her joy is universal'. He concluded, 'the
soul is wholly filled' with the holy affections, and they 'penetrate her [very]
Essence'.[136] Indeed, as well as saturating the soul, these feelings could be felt in the
body. Mary Carey addressed her soul in 1649, 'Let thee and I, my dear Body, all
thy members, all my faculties, even the whole man, give up ourselves unto our
God...Let us labour together to glorify God'.[137] This striking image—of the
entire body and soul engaged in praise—fitted with physiological theories of
the emotions: strong feelings were thought to have a real physical impact, especially on the heart.[138] For instance, Oliver Heywood recorded that when he found
his 'dear brother...wonderfully recovered' of a dangerous disease, 'oh what
endeared meltings of heart did god stirre up in me'.[139] Olivia Weisser has argued
that these experiences were gendered: the 'warm, broken frame' implicit in the
descriptions of holy affections 'resonated with seventeenth-century feminine virtues of docility, passivity, and humility', but 'could threaten manly markers of
bodily control and self-mastery'. Consequently, most men, with the notable exception of ministers, avoided references to their bodies in accounts of their spiritual
experiences.[140] Perhaps owing to the great piety of many of the men featured in my
study, little obvious distinction between female and male experiences has emerged.

One reason for highlighting the physical impact of the affections on the heart
was that internal sensations were regarded as evidence of the sincerity of emotions:

---

[133] Hale, *A letter*, 6.   [134] Rogers, *Practical discourses*, 253.
[135] Dixon, *Practical Predestinarians*, 41–3.
[136] Senault, *The use of the passions*, 451–2. See also Edward Reynolds, *A treatise of the passions and
faculties of the soule of man* (1640), 217–18.
[137] Carey, *Meditations*, 35–6.
[138] Gail Kern Paster, *Humoring the Body: Emotions and the Shakespearean Stage* (Chicago IL, 2004),
12–13; Ryrie, *Being Protestant*, 20–1, 25–6.
[139] Heywood, *The Rev. Oliver Heywood*, vol. 4, 104.   [140] Weisser, *Ill Composed*, 71.

the word 'heartfelt' meant quite literally that the affection could be felt in the heart.[141] In turn, sincere feelings were the surest signs of election, and the best protection against 'false assurance' (or 'security'), the ill-grounded confidence in one's election.[142] These concerns also explain another feature of spiritual praise: bodily gesture. Outward movements of the body were evidence of inward feelings, as explained by the theologian and cartographer John Norden (1548–c.1625): 'any outward action or gesture of the body...may argue the inward heart wel prepared, and that hee wanteth not the spirit of God'.[143] Holy affections were thought to begin in the heart, before quickly 'diffusing...through the whole man, and commanding...the knees [to] bend, the eyes and hands [to] lift up, and the whole body [to] testifie the inward veneration'.[144] Fruitful work has been conducted on Protestant gestures during prayer, such as kneeling, weeping, and the positioning of the hands, but less attention has been paid to those made in praise.[145] The gestures most frequently mentioned by patients and relatives were falling onto the knees, springing up to the feet, and the lifting up of arms and eyes. In 1652, eleven-year-old Martha Hatfield from Yorkshire, recovering from 'Spleen-winde', was observed 'holding up her hands, and lifting up her eye with smiling'.[146] About fifty years later, David Wright, a shepherd from Hertfordshire, was seen 'leaping and praising God as he...came home[,] adoring the love & grace of God' after his miraculous cure from scrofula.[147] Similar gestures were mentioned in imaginative literature, which indicates their prevalence in early modern culture.[148] Two reasons were given for the upwards direction of these gestures. Firstly, Christians tended to picture God in the heavens, beyond the clouds, even though they knew that He was omnipresent.[149] The soul had an instinctive yearning to be with God, and since the eyes were the 'windows of the soul', it made sense that they would also turn upwards during spiritual rapture.[150] The other reason was physiological: holy affections caused the outward diffusion of the body's 'spirits', the special vapours that carried out all mental and physical functions, from the heart to the 'extreme parts'.[151] Edward Reynolds (1599–1676), a minister in Northamptonshire, believed that of all the passions, spiritual joy had the most visible impact on the limbs: 'it exerciseth a kind of welcome violence...upon a man, as we see in' the

---

[141] The OED defines 'heartfelt' (adjective) as 'deeply or acutely felt; intense. Of words, actions, etc.: spoken or proceeding from the heart; genuine, sincere' (accessed 19/05/17).

[142] Dixon, *Practical Predestinarians*, 301, 305.

[143] John Norden, *A pathway to patience in all manner of crosses* (1626), 86.

[144] Joseph Hall, *The remedy of prophanenesse* (1637), 111–12.

[145] Ryrie, *Being Protestant*, 144, 170–1, 173, 177, 179–94. On the use of eyes/hands, see John Craig, 'Bodies at Prayer in Early Modern England', in Natalie Mears and Alec Ryrie (eds.), *Worship and the Parish Church in Early Modern Britain* (Farnham, 2013), 173–96. On groaning, see John Craig, 'Psalms, Groans and Dogwhippers: The Soundscape of Worship in the English Parish Church, 1547–1642', in Will Coster and Andrew Spicer (eds.), *Sacred Space in Early Modern Europe* (Cambridge, 2005), 104–23, at 109–13.

[146] James Fisher, *The wise virgin, or, a wonderful narration of the various dispensations towards a childe of eleven years of age* (1653), 145–6.

[147] *A true copy of a letter*, 1–2.   [148] Defoe, *Robinson Crusoe*, 92–3.

[149] Ryrie, *Being Protestant*, 184.   [150] This proverb probably comes from Matthew 6:22.

[151] See Chapter 1, p. 38 for a definition of the spirits.

Bible story of 'the lame Mans...leaping, and praising God, after hee had been cured of his lameness'.[152] Although these gestures were associated especially with puritans—satires of 'the godly' depicted them 'turning up the white of the eye'—it seems that in the context of recovery, Anglicans also used them.[153] Recovery was an event of such significance that any reservations about enthusiastic postures seem to have been temporarily forgotten.

Praise and thankfulness were not the only holy affections sparked by the conviction that God had brought recovery. Another widespread response was renewed love for the Lord. The greatest commandment in the Bible is 'to love the Lord thy God with all thy heart, and with all thy soul, and with all thy mind'.[154] Unfortunately, this commandment was not always easy to obey, especially during illness: despite recognizing that affliction was sent by a loving God for their spiritual benefit, patients found that the sense of the Lord's anger made it hard to love Him, or to imagine that He loved them. An anonymous relative of Oliver Cromwell confided in her diary in 1701, 'I was under a sevear Fit of the Ston[e], which is a sad Provedence in a double Respect' by reason of the 'great Feare in me, lest the Lord should be angry with me'.[155] The sick pictured the furious countenance of God.[156] However, with recovery, people's perceptions of God's feelings towards them radically altered, and the result was that it was much easier to love Him in return. During the illness of his daughter Ann in 1654, Ralph Josselin had felt a 'strangeness fallen in between god and mee, not having had any signal evidence of his taking notice of mee'; he interpreted her recovery as 'a token of love' from God, 'a pledge of his kindness to mee'.[157] Patients consciously meditated upon God's manifestation of love for them as a way to rouse their feelings of affection for Him. Addressing her soul in 1649, Mary Carey pleaded, 'Let the consideration of God's free, full, singular, continual, constant, eternal, best love to me, stir up and increase abundantly my love to him...Ah, love him, love him, my Soul'.[158]

An examination of the metaphors that were used to describe holy love provides further insights into the experience of this emotion, and confirms that human beings were regarded both as passive receptacles, and as active producers, of the holy affections. The first metaphor relates to sweetness. Isaac Archer described the recovery of his two daughters in 1678 as a 'token of God's love'; he declared, 'how should I love him who delivers from death!...he doth by sweetnes as well as severity draw mee after him'.[159] This metaphor implies that the individual played no part in generating the holy affections—God simply delivered the sugary morsel into their mouths, as a bird would her chicks. As mentioned earlier, sweetness was

[152] Reynolds, *A treatise of the passions*, 218.   [153] Cited in Craig, 'Bodies at Prayer', 185.
[154] The most widely cited wording is Matthew 22:37. For slightly different wording, see Deuteronomy 6:5; Mark 12:30; Luke 10:27.
[155] BL, Additional MS 5858, fol. 220v (Religious diary of a female cousin of Oliver Cromwell, 1687/90–1702). See also Lambeth Palace Library, London, MS 2240, fol. 25r (Prose and verse meditations of Alathea Bethell).
[156] Heywood, *The Rev. Oliver Heywood*, vol. 1, 168.   [157] Josselin, *The Diary*, 328–9.
[158] Carey, *Meditations*, 36.
[159] Archer, 'The Diary', 156. See also BL, Additional MS 5858, fols. 215v–216r (Cromwell relative); BL, Additional MS 42849, fol. 19r (Letters of the Henry family).

highly prized in early modern culture, so it is not surprising that this word was deemed an apt choice when describing love: in nutrition theory, the sweeter the food the more wholesome it would be to the body, and in the Bible over one hundred references to this quality can be found.[160] The second metaphor refers to fire. When Elizabeth Delaval was preserved from plague, she prayed that God would 'grant me thy grace so to blow every sparke of holy fier that it may be kindle'd into a pure flame of love to thee'.[161] This metaphor ascribes more agency to the human in the production of holy affections than the previous one: God sent a spark of love into the heart, but it had to be 'kindled' by human efforts for it to blaze. Although this metaphor might seem incongruous—fire was associated with Hell, a place utterly devoid of divine affection—it also held positive connotations of burnt offerings and sacrifices. Rogers commanded recovered patients to make God's 'Altar smoak with burning Frankinscence: we must cover it with our chearful Praise, and a flaming Love'.[162] Thirdly, God's love was described using metaphors of ravishment. The Northampton attorney Robert Woodford (1606–54) noted that when the Lord did 'heale & Cure' his baby boy in 1637, he experienced 'great & Ravishinge comforts'.[163] The verb 'ravish' meant to 'carry away by force', some-times implying subsequent rape; it also denoted to 'fill with ecstasy, [or] intense delight'.[164] These definitions suggest that God's love was experienced as a violent, but exquisite pleasure. Like the sweetness simile, it implies that the human was entirely passive, playing no part in the provocation of holy affections—such a notion was consistent with the belief that grace was 'irresistible' to the soul.

Together the three metaphors show that the holy affections were delightful feel-ings that filled the person's entire being—senses, body, heart, and soul.[165] What made these emotions all the more joyful was the belief that they were 'badges of election'. Thomas Tuke (1580/1–1657), a London conformist minister, confirmed in his treatise on election: 'he that [loves God] may assure himselfe of Gods love, and that hee is...in the *ranke* and *roll* of Gods elect; these being infallible tokens, and undoubted effects of Election, and fore-runners of eternall life'.[166] Patients and their relatives agreed on this point. When Ralph Josselin heard that his son Thomas was better from fever in 1670, he exclaimed, 'oh how sweet is it to be persaded [that] I am of gods mercy in the merits of christ for my salvacion'.[167]

---

[160] Albala, *Eating Right*, 82. On the biblical use of 'sweet', see Ryrie, *Being Protestant*, 89. Peter Marshall also notes the ubiquity of this word, but in the earlier period of the 1500s, in the context of evangelical conversion: *Religious Identities in Henry VIII's England* (Abingdon, 2006), 31–3. Eamon Duffy has shown that this term was used in Catholic religious discourse too: *The Stripping of the Altars: Traditional Religion in England 1400–1580* (1992), *passim*.
[161] Delaval, *The Meditations*, 86.   [162] Rogers, *Practical discourses*, 175–7.
[163] Robert Woodford, *The Diary of Robert Woodford, 1637–1641*, ed. John Fielding, Camden Society, vol. 42 (2012), 190.
[164] OED, verbs 1 and 4 (accessed 19/05/17).
[165] Elizabeth Isham, *Diary and Confessions: Constructing Elizabeth Isham, 1609–1654*, Warwick University Online Editions, ed. Elizabeth Clarke, Nigel Smith, Jill Millman, and Alice Eardley, <http://web.warwick.ac.uk/english/perdita/Isham/index_bor.htm> (accessed 15/05/17), fol. 17r.
[166] Thomas Tuke, *The high-way to heaven: or, the doctrine of election* (1609), 48. See also Byfield, *A commentary*, 288.
[167] Josselin, *The Diary*, 557.

The final holy affection to discuss is trust in the power of prayer.[168] Prayer was defined as 'an earnest talk with God, proceeding from a very inward, deep, or fervent affection of the heart, craving somewhat at the hand of God'.[169] During illness, patients and their loved ones prayed for the restoration of health, and interpreted their subsequent recoveries as answers to their petitions. This was often found to be the most moving spiritual experience in a person's life. James Clegg recorded that when his wife was 'in extreme danger' of death in 1721, he 'pour[ed] out prayers to God for her with great earnest and bitterness of soul'. By nightfall, 'God gave her rest', and she recovered. He wrote, 'This is one of the most evident and remarkable answers to prayer that I have ever experienced. This was plainly God's work, blessed be his name forever and ever'.[170] When the patient's revival coincided exactly with the moment at which relatives had been engaged in prayer, the experience was all the more special. The royalist gentlewoman from Yorkshire, Alice Thornton (1626–1707), recorded in 1665 that the 'very night, about that houer when we weare at praiers' for her husband in his *dangerous fitt of the palsie*, he 'wakened out of sleepe when Dr [Wittie] expected his departure;…and changed so fast in a way of recovery that it was admirable to all'.[171] Her husband's proximity to death, and his rapid recovery, served to enhance his wife's awe at God's power.

Once more, the trope of 'double joy' was used to describe the experience of this holy affection. As a sign of election, an answered prayer greatly enhanced the overall happiness of recovery. In the 1690s, Heywood recorded, 'my dear Lord fetcht me back again from the grave: it was…a double mercy…that it came as a return of prayer'. This man went on to imply that the prayers made on his behalf had been so potent that they had practically forced God into cooperating: 'the people of god would not let me dye:…many prayd with me and took hold of gods strength and stayd his hand from falling on me'.[172] At first glance, this description seems at odds with predestinarian theology: it hints that God was amenable to persuasion, and might even be cajoled into changing His mind by saving someone whom He had previously intended to let die. Contemporary ministers interpreted such impressions as 'mere feints or bluffs' on the part of God, designed 'specifically to…redouble our prayers'.[173] Alexandra Walsham believes that, for pastoral purposes, ministers felt bound to suggest to their parishioners that 'the Lord could be…browbeaten [and] brought round' to their desires, even though this could never be the case. If pressed, ministers resolved the contradiction by explaining that God's answers to

---

[168] On prayer by literary scholars, see Kate Narveson, 'Publishing the Sole-Talk of the Soule: Genre in Early Stuart Piety', in Daniel Doersken and Christopher Hodgkins (eds.), *Centred on the Word* (Newark NJ, 2004), 110–26. For historians' work on prayer, see Virginia Reinburg, 'Hearing Lay People's Prayer', in Barbara Diefendorf and Carla Hesse (eds.), *Culture and Identity in Early Modern Europe* (Ann Arbor MI, 1993), 19–39; Ryrie, *Being Protestant*, 97–256; Martin and Ryrie (eds.), *Private and Domestic Devotion*, and their sister-volume, *Worship and the Parish Church in Early Modern Britain* (Farnham, 2013).

[169] Thomas Becon, *The Catechism of Thomas Becon*, ed. John Ayre (Cambridge, 1844), 125.

[170] Clegg, *The Diary*, 14–15.   [171] Thornton, *The Autobiography*, 150.

[172] Heywood, *The Rev. Oliver Heywood*, vol. 3, 256.   [173] Ryrie, *Being Protestant*, 250.

prayers, however spontaneous they might appear to be, were choices 'foreseen from eternity and inbuilt into the original scheme'.[174]

The art of recovery literature advised patients and their loved ones to deploy their recent experiences of answered prayer to dissipate any former doubts they might have harboured about its efficacy. Rogers admonished:

> We have greatly dishonoured [God] in our former straits by our own unbelief: Let us in all future occasions…never…dispute his Power…Having tasted *how good the Lord is*…let us meet every new…danger with a greater Courage, and never admit the least doubt of Gods Ability.[175]

By imparting this advice, Rogers implies that there were substantial numbers of people who doubted the power of prayer, and needed success stories to bolster their faith. It is clear that these experiences *did* help in future afflictions. During the illness of his infant son John in 1637, Robert Woodford wrote in his diary, 'my Child…is grievously infested with a cold…in his head & lungs[;] oh Lord I pray thee heale & Cure him…thou hast restored him to us from former illnesses when we have prayed unto thee, Lord heare our poore prayers againe'.[176] Woodford was reminding God, as well as himself, of previous answered prayers, hoping that this memory might inspire the Lord to repeat the mercy. One of the reasons that Christians were so keen to strengthen their faith in the power of prayer was that it was necessary to believe a prayer would work in order for it to work. This idea is rooted in the Gospels: after healing the sick, Jesus tells patients, 'thy faith hath made thee whole'.[177]

In short, divine delivery inspired a host of delightful holy affections in patients and their loved ones, including praise and thankfulness, love for God, and faith in the power of prayer. However, it should be noted that these responses were not universal. Harris lamented, 'when we are delivered, we return like those Lepers in the Gospell, scarce one in ten, in twentie, in a hundred' to thank God.[178] He is referring to the story in Luke 17 of the ten lepers healed by Christ, of whom only one 'turned backe' to glorify and thank God.[179] Another common complaint was that recovered patients expressed 'empty praises', uttering words of gratitude without fully feeling the sentiments they were expressing. Rogers declared, 'there ought to be a Correspondence between our outward Expressions and the more undiscernable Motions of our Hearts', but 'There is nothing indeed more common than for People…to say, ["]I thank God for this or that["]; but the manner in which they speak it, plainly discovers that the sense which they have of the Divine Goodness is but light and superficial'. He called these false expressions 'toilsom Pomps of a ceremonious Gratitude, and outward Ostentations'.[180]

Evidence from diaries and letters reveals that the concerns voiced by religious authors were not entirely unfounded. Patients and relatives sometimes worried about the sincerity of their holy affections, and admitted when they struggled to

---

174 Walsham, *Providence*, 153.   175 Rogers, *Practical discourses*, 196.
176 Woodford, *The Diary*, 189.   177 For example, Luke 17:19; Matthew 9:22; Mark 5:34.
178 Harris, *Hezekiahs recovery*, 6.   179 Luke 17:11–19.
180 Rogers, *Practical discourses*, 177–8.

achieve the required pitch of emotional fervour. Lady Joan Barrington (1558–1641) from Essex received a letter from a friend in 1630, saying: 'now God hath graciously... mittigated his hand... Oh that I hade such a hart as to be *actually* thankfull to such a good God' (my italics).[181] About thirty years later, the clergyman Isaac Archer wrote, 'it pleased God to remove his hand, and I was very thankfull, outwardly at least'.[182] By referring to his 'outward' feelings, Archer hints that his gratitude might not have been internal. Metaphors of theatre plays were used to describe these outward 'shows' of emotion: spiritual affections entered the heart 'only in dress and imagery', passing away 'as scenes do when the show is done'.[183] Patients also referred to the physical state of their hearts, calling them 'cold luke warm', 'dead and listles', and 'darke'.[184] Since the holy affections were thought to enliven, melt, and ignite the heart, it made sense to use opposite terms when describing the absence of such feelings.

The art of recovery literature provided solutions to the challenges of cultivating sincere praise. For a start, it was possible for patients to avoid accusations of 'empty words' by choosing their words carefully: rather than stating that they were feeling the particular emotion, they could say they 'desired' to feel that emotion. Speaking of his love for God in 1708, James Clegg mused, 'I cannot say I am sure that I am sincere but I desire to be if my heart deceive me not'.[185] Alec Ryrie has shown that the 'desire' to feel a holy affection was a positive sign of grace, almost as good as actually feeling the emotion.[186] Another practical response was prayer: patients and their loved ones beseeched God to 'give us an heart answerable to [the] mercy'.[187] Since the affections were the work of the Holy Spirit, it was perfectly acceptable to request these feelings from the Lord. This did not mean that people could rest on their laurels, however: patients were advised to 'stir' their holy affections actively by comparing 'thy miserie past' with their present ease. Harris commanded his readers to 'lay both estates' of sickness and health 'together... and provoke thy selfe to thankfulnesse' by the dramatic contrast.[188] By 'setting our Sorrows and our Mercies together[,] our Praise may be the more harmonious', echoed Rogers.[189] The combination of prayer and meditation attests once more to the paradoxical nature of the holy affections—they were a gift from God, but also a product of human effort.

PUBLIC PRAISES

Thus far, we have concentrated on the deeply personal, inner spiritual experiences of patients and their loved ones. The final component to a good recovery was ostensibly a public one: the patient and family were enjoined to perform collective

[181] Arthur Searle (ed.), *Barrington Family Letters, 1628–1632* (1983), 172.
[182] Archer, 'The Diary', 77.   [183] Delaval, *The Meditations*, 106.
[184] Ibid., 99; Josselin, *The Diary*, 312. On 'stony hearts', see Ryrie, *Being Protestant*, 14–15. Olivia Weisser has also highlighted the use of this language in *Ill Composed*, 72.
[185] Clegg, *The Diary*, 1.   [186] Ryrie, *Being Protestant*, 64–5.
[187] Josselin, *The Diary*, 283.   [188] Harris, *Hezekiahs recovery*, 36–7.
[189] Rogers, *Practical discourses*, 157.

praise to God in the form of a thanksgiving service. The term 'public' is used here in the knowledge that it is a problematic concept, which sets up a stark, and possibly anachronistic, dichotomy between the domestic or private sphere, and the wider public or communal domain.[190] The use of this vocabulary, however, provides opportunities for its interrogation. In line with recent historiography, we will see that while contemporaries did make distinctions between private and public thanksgiving, they also recognized points of overlap.[191]

Considerable attention has been paid to the thanksgiving ceremony that was held for newly delivered mothers—a ritual called 'churching'—but very little scholarship has been conducted on the equivalent tradition for recovered patients.[192] This is probably because churching generated far greater controversy at the time: as David Cressy has shown, the ritual was criticized by nonconformists as a superstitious adherence to Mosaical and Levitical law. Puritans objected not to the thanksgiving function of churching, but to the lingering notion that it served a purification purpose.[193] Since thanksgiving for recovery from illness carried no such connotations, it did not generate the same debate. The lack of controversy, however, should not obscure its importance: although there are no statistical data from which the incidence of thanksgiving for recovery can be estimated, impressionistic evidence suggests that it was very common. Some clergymen mention it their diaries almost as frequently as they record funerals.[194]

Public thanksgiving was necessary for several reasons. Firstly, it was a milestone on the 'road to health': the duration of illness was measured in missed Sabbath services, and recovery was confirmed by the first trip to church. Anne Halkett (1623–99), an Anglican gentlewoman from London, recorded in 1649, 'The first Sunday that my health...would permitt...I went to the chapel...to offer up thanksgiving to my God who had raised mee from the gates of death'.[195] A more pressing reason for communal praise, however, was that it was a biblical command: Psalm 130:4 states, 'Sing unto the LORD, O ye saints of his, and give thanks at the remembrance of his holiness'. Steward explained that through this verse, '*David*...does...exhort others to join with him in this Work of blessing and

[190] For a discussion of this issue, see Erica Longfellow, 'Public, Private, and the Household in Early Seventeenth-Century England', *Journal of British Studies*, 45 (2006), 313–34.

[191] This relationship is explored in the sister volumes, Mears and Ryrie (eds.), *Worship and the Parish Church*, and *Private and Domestic Devotion*.

[192] For example, David Cressy, *Birth, Marriage, and Death: Ritual, Religion and the Life Cycle in Tudor and Stuart England* (Oxford, 1997), ch. 9; Adrian Wilson, *Ritual and Conflict: The Social Relations of Childbirth in Early Modern England* (Farnham, 2013), 175–8, 201–8; Kathryn McPherson, 'Dramatizing Deliverance and Devotion: Churching in Early Modern England', in Kathryn Moncrief and Kathryn McPherson (eds.), *Performing Maternity in Early Modern England* (Aldershot, 2007), 131–42; Gail McMurray Gibson, 'Blessings from the Sun and Moon: Churching as Women's Theater', in Barbara Hanawalt and David Wallace (eds.), *Bodies and Disciplines: Intersections of Literature and History in Fifteenth Century England* (Minneapolis MN, 1996), 139–54.

[193] Cressy, *Birth, Marriage, and Death*, 205–13.

[194] For example, Heywood, *The Rev. Oliver Heywood*. It is easier to generate statistics for the prevalence of churching, because one of the questions posed by bishops in their visitations related to this ceremony—see Wilson, *Ritual and Conflict*, 201.

[195] Anne Halkett, *The Autobiography of Anne Lady Halkett*, ed. John Gough Nichols, Camden Society New Series, vol. 13 (1875–6), 35. See also Newcome, *The Autobiography*, 120.

pra[i]sing God...[he] calls to the People...of God to help...him in the Celebration of the Divine Goodness'.[196] A third reason for collective thanksgiving was that it was thought to offer God more honour than private praise. Rogers stated, 'It is not enough that we have an inward and a silent Gratitude, *we must publish with the voice of thanksgiving, and tell of all his wondrous Works*'.[197] Steward echoed, 'My single Praises are not sufficient...we should not be content with [only] our...own private Praises...to God, but we should call upon others to joyn us'.[198] The clear message in these exhortations is that glory comes in numbers—the greater the congregation, the more powerful the praises. Metaphors of sunrays and streams were used to explain this idea: 'Beams of the Sun...united,...give a stronger Light', and 'many small Rivers united run with a swifter Course...to the Sea'.[199] It may seem strange that public praises were elevated above private thanksgiving: the value of 'secret' worship was that it avoided allegations of 'ostentation and hypocrisie'.[200] Matthew 6:5 warns, 'thou shalt not be as the hypocrites *are*: for they love to pray standing in the synagogues and in the corners of the streets, that they may be seen of men'.[201] However, private devotion also encountered a degree of criticism—it was tainted by associations of melancholy and popish monasticism.[202] In view of these ambivalent attitudes, it is not surprising that contemporaries advocated a mixture of private and public praise, and cautioned against ostentation in either context.

Public thanksgiving also performed an important evangelical function. The recovered patient was a 'living monument of the Power and Prevalency, the force and efficacy of fervent Prayer'.[203] It was hoped that the sight of the recovered patient in church would strengthen the faith of the congregation, and assure parishioners that 'he [who] hath delivered me, can also deliver you when you come to Straits'.[204] Preachers were right: the emotional and spiritual impact of seeing a friend or neighbour appear in public for the first time after an acute or prolonged illness could be extraordinary. James Fisher described the reactions of his friends to the sight of his newly recovered niece, eleven-year-old Martha Hatfield, when she appeared at her thanksgiving day: 'she was able to come forth...to meet and welcome us...[:] it was wonderfull in our eyes, so that our hearts did rejoyce with a kind of trembling at the glory of the Lord, which appeared in that Object'.[205] Clearly, the sight of the patient exerted a more powerful impact on onlookers than learning of a person's recovery second-hand.[206]

The practical arrangements of thanksgiving services varied. For Anglicans, the ceremony was usually held in the local church, at the request of the patient or the family. If the patient was a particularly esteemed member of the congregation,

---

[196] Steward, *Sacrificium laudis*, 6–7.   [197] Rogers, *Practical discourses*, 255.

[198] Steward, *Sacrificium laudis*, 7.   [199] Rogers, *Practical discourses*, 256.

[200] Cited by Ryrie, *Being Protestant*, 155–6.   [201] Matthew 6:5.

[202] Erica Longfellow, '"My now Solitary Prayers": *Eikon Basilike* and Changing Attitudes towards Religious Solicitude', in Martin and Ryrie (eds.), *Private and Domestic Devotion*, 53–72.

[203] Steward, *Sacrificium laudis*, 1–2.   [204] Rogers, *Practical discourses*, 268.

[205] Fisher, *The wise virgin*, 162.

[206] On attitudes to sight, see Stuart Clark, *Vanities of the Eye: Vision in Early Modern European Culture* (Oxford, 2007).

the service might be dedicated entirely to the occasion of thanksgiving.[207] Families that had their own chapels tended to delegate the organizing of the service to their curate.[208] Lower down the social scale, the ceremony was more likely to be incorporated within the normal Sunday service, without explicit mention of the particular patient. Religious affiliation also made a difference—nonconformists often preferred to hold the service in their homes rather than in the church, because it afforded them greater freedom: participants did not have to adhere to the thanksgiving liturgy in the Book of Common Prayer, and could choose their own Bible readings.[209] The length of the service could also be extended from the customary one or two hours, to half, or even a full, day, with refreshments served at various points.[210] In view of the domestic setting of nonconformists' thanksgiving services, it is tempting to re-classify them as forms of private worship. Such a categorization is problematic, however, because the attendees were often numerous and diverse, and included members of the wider community as well as relatives. The nonconformist minister Oliver Heywood recalled that his thanksgiving day was attended by '50 person and upwards'.[211] The Conventicle Act of 1664, a statute which forbade religious assemblies of more than five people from different families, indicates that from an official Anglican perspective, household thanksgiving services would have been classed as public.[212] Thus, it is perhaps best to see these events as semi-public.[213]

What happened at a typical thanksgiving service? The centrepiece was a sermon. A brief look at a printed thanksgiving sermon provides clues into what might have been preached, though we must heed Arnold Hunt's warning that printed and preached sermons were by no means identical.[214] Thomas Steward's sermon, which he gave at his own thanksgiving service in 1699, opens with a Bible passage relating to divine deliverance, Psalm 30:3–4; Steward then highlights several 'observations' on the chosen passage, such as 'God is the Author of our Deliverances'.

---

[207] The royalist clergyman from Northamptonshire, Thomas Fuller (1608–61), published a sermon upon the recovery of Sir John Danvers, 'a Person honourably extracted'; the sermon is about divine healing, and it refers explicitly to Danvers' own experience: *Life out of death: a sermon preached at Chelsey, on the recovery of an honourable person* (1655), 27.

[208] For example, a thanksgiving service was organized by John Gough (d. 1684), the rector of Robert Paston's Norfolk estate, Oxnead: Robert Paston, *The Whirlpool of Misadventures: Letters of Robert Paston, First Earl of Yarmouth 1663–1679*, ed. Jean Agnew, Norfolk Record Society, vol. 76 (2012), 167–8.

[209] Although the Book of Common Prayer does not provide a special service dedicated to thanksgiving for deliverance from disease, it does contain a chapter on 'Prayers and thanksgivings for several occasions', including 'For Deliverance from the Plague, or other common Sickness'; this prayer may have been used by conformists in their thanksgiving for recovery. Letters from John Gough, the curate who organized Robert Paston's thanksgiving service in 1675, show that while Anglicans did insist on the use of official church liturgy, they were prepared to customize the form to suit the occasion: Paston, *The Whirlpool of Misadventures*, 166, 168.

[210] For example, Newcome's thanksgiving lasted until 2 p.m., and was followed by a 'great dinner': *The Diary of Rev. Henry Newcome*, ed. Thomas Heywood, Chetham Society, vol. 18 (1849), 27.

[211] Heywood, *The Rev. Oliver Heywood*, vol. 4, 141.   [212] Longfellow, 'Public, Private', 319–21.

[213] This is how Ian Green classifies these sorts of gatherings, in 'Varieties of Domestic Devotion in Early Modern English Protestantism', in Martin and Ryrie (eds.), *Private and Domestic Devotion*, 9–31, at 10.

[214] Hunt, *The Art of Hearing*, 148–9, 153, 156.

Next, he expounds upon a number of applications for these observations, which include 'God [should] be praised for our Deliverances'.[215] The sermon concludes with a summary of the main duties of the recovered patient. If read verbatim, it would probably have lasted just over an hour.[216] While preachers drew on a range of scriptural passages, this basic structure and message is espoused in most of the thanksgiving sermons across the period. The other major component of the service was the singing of psalms, a form of worship embraced by most shades of Protestants, bar some Quakers and Baptists.[217] The version of the psalms that was most likely to have been sung in early modern England was known as the 'Sternhold and Hopkins', reputedly written by Thomas Sternhold and John Hopkins, and first published in 1548/9. Ian Green estimates that a staggering 482 editions came out between 1562 and 1640, and concludes that it was probably published more often than any other work in the early modern period.[218] Sung unaccompanied in unison, psalms were ideal for thanksgiving gatherings in the home as well in churches, as there was no need for an organ.[219]

The legitimacy of psalm-singing was rooted in the Psalms themselves—the prophet David says, 'O LORD, thou hast brought up my soul from the grave . . . Sing unto the LORD, O ye saints of his, and give thanks'.[220] Contemporaries held the Book of Psalms in high regard, viewing it as an epitome of the Bible; its vast range of themes made it suitable for every occasion, from funerals to weddings. Of all functions, however, the psalms were deemed especially apt for thanksgiving: their poetic, songlike quality was ideal for expressing joyous praise.[221] The reason the psalms were sung rather than read, relates to beliefs about the effects of music on the soul. Jonathan Willis and Penelope Gouk have shown that melodious sound was thought to be 'capable of lifting the soul to otherwise inaccessible states of holy contemplation'.[222] As one theologian put it, '*David* in penning Psalmes . . . taught us, . . . the vertue of musicke to stirre men up to devotion': rhythmic melodies 'beateth and tickleth' the heart to produce holy affections.[223] It was also hoped that the sound of everyone singing together would enhance the intensity of each individual's praises. Thomas Steward confirmed: 'Our own Hearts [are] more warmed and enlarged, and our Affections are raised and elevated, when we joyn in Consort

[215] Steward, *Sacrificium laudis*, 14.

[216] Estimates of sermon lengths are given by Ryrie, *Being Protestant*, 317–18.

[217] Ian Green, *Print and Protestantism in Early Modern England* (Oxford, 2000), 530–3; Jonathan Willis, *Church Music and Protestantism in Post-Reformation England: Discourses, Sites and Identities* (Farnham, 2010), 69, 76–7.

[218] Green, *Print and Protestantism*, 503.   [219] Ibid., 551.

[220] Psalm 3:3–4. See also Psalm 150; Colossians 3:16.

[221] Rivkah Zim, *English Metrical Psalms: Poetry as Praise and Prayer, 1553–1601* (Cambridge, 1987), ix.

[222] Jonathan Willis, 'Protestant Worship and the Discourse of Music in Reformation England', in Mears and Ryrie (eds.), *Worship and the Parish Church*, 131–50, at 147–8; Penelope Gouk, 'Music and Spirit in Early Modern Thought', in Elena Carrera (ed.), *Emotions and Health, 1200–1700* (Leiden, 2013), 221–39. See also Jonathan Willis, '"By These Means the Sacred Discourses Sink More Deeply into the Minds of Men": Music and Education in Elizabethan England', *History*, 94 (2009), 294–309; Willis, *Church Music*, 32, 41–2, 48.

[223] Thomas Wright, *The passions of the minde* (1630, first publ. 1601), 159–71, at 164.

to Sing'.[224] This preference for singing reflects Protestant privileging of the sense of hearing—faith comes through hearing God's word, a precept conveyed in Romans 10:17.[225] Of all the senses, 'God never commeth so neere a mans soule as when he entreth in by the doore of the eare', averred the sixteenth-century Protestant theologian Robert Wilkinson.[226]

How was the singing of psalms experienced? It was often regarded as the most enjoyable of all forms of religious devotion.[227] Diarists frequently noted the delight they took on these occasions. Oliver Heywood described the 'endeared meltings of heart [that] god [did] stirre up in me' at the thanksgiving service of his brother-in-law Joseph Dawson in 1684.[228] What made the praise all the more delightful was the sense that everyone was feeling the same emotions at once, a phenomenon known as fellow-feeling.[229] Jonathan Willis has confirmed that 'Coming together in song created a bond of unity through musical concord'.[230] At his own thanksgiving sermon, Rogers declared, 'let us joyn our thoughts, our voices and our hearts to give him with delight a common Song of Praise'.[231] Anglicans recorded similar experiences: Edmund Wharton (d. 1717), a clergyman at Sir Robert Paston's thanksgiving service in 1675, recorded, 'It did mee good methought to behold so fervent, so unanimous a devotion', in which the congregation 'were…in spirit and in affection…heartily joined'.[232] This communal experience once more exemplifies the crossover between public and private devotion: the spiritual joy of each individual was interior and personal, and yet it could also be shared by the whole church.

Adding to the pleasure of singing was the belief that God would enjoy the music too.[233] Steward confirmed, 'The mutual, joynt, united praises of the Saints are sweet Musick, pleasant and delightful Melody in the Ears of the Almighty'.[234] Ultimately, communal thanksgiving was regarded as the closest thing to Heaven on earth: humans were 'beginning that blessed Work which we hope to be employed in forever', singing God's praises like the angels in paradise.[235] Music and spiritual praise so inflamed the person's spirits, that they soared upwards, beyond

---

[224] Steward, *Sacrificium laudis*, 20. See also Rogers, *Practical discourses*, 256. On the functions of psalm-singing, see Beth Quitslund, 'Singing the Psalms for Fun and Profit', in Martin and Alec Ryrie (eds.), *Private and Domestic Devotion*, 237–58.

[225] On Protestant privileging of hearing, see Bryan Crockett, '"Holy Cozenage" and the Religious Cult of the Ear', *The Sixteenth Century Journal*, 24 (1993), 47–65; Hunt, *The Art of Hearing*. For a critique of this view, see Kathrin Scheuchzer, '"Eat Not, Taste Not, Touch Not": The Five Senses in John Foxe's *Actes and Monuments*', in Annette Kern-Stahler, Beatrix Busse, and Wietse de Boer (eds.), *The Five Senses in Medieval and Early Modern England* (Leiden, 2016), 219–36.

[226] Robert Wilkinson, *A jewell for the eare* (1602), images 6, 8. On the link between the ear and heart, see Gina Bloom, *Voice in Motion: Staging Gender, Shaping Sound in Early Modern England* (Philadelphia PA, 2007), ch. 3.

[227] Quitslund, 'Singing the Psalms'.

[228] Heywood, *The Rev. Oliver Heywood*, vol. 4, 104. See also Elizabeth Walker, *The vertuous wife*, ed. Anthony Walker (1694), 56.

[229] See the second part of Chapter 3 (sub-titled 'Family and Friends'), for a discussion of fellow-feeling.

[230] Willis, *Church Music*, 215.   [231] Rogers, *Practical discourses*, 272.

[232] Paston, *The Whirlpool of Misadventures*, 170.

[233] On the tendency to anthropomorphize God, see Walsham, 'Deciphering Divine Wrath'.

[234] Steward, *Sacrificium laudis*, 19–20.

[235] Rogers, *Practical discourses*, 266. On the links between Heaven and music, see Willis, *Church Music*, 19–21.

the confines of the human body to the skies, teetering on the cusp of the heavens, where they would experience something akin to the ecstasies of paradise.[236] These positive reports of psalm-singing contribute to recent efforts by historians to contradict the older notion that church 'must have been excessively dull' in the early modern period.[237]

Nonetheless, the joyfulness of public thanksgiving should not be overstated. The same individuals who at times experienced 'heart melting' praises, on other occasions found thanksgiving disappointing. Heywood admitted in 1667 that when he 'observed a solemn day of thanksgiving for the recovery' of his eleven-year-old son John, 'my heart was not so affected as sometimes it hath been in those dutys'.[238] Perhaps this could have been due to the poor quality of the singing: one churchgoer complained in 1619, 'some roar, some whine, some creak like wheels of carts'.[239] A more pressing concern, however, was that people did not always turn up to the thanksgiving service. Preachers compared the size of the congregations at thanksgiving services unfavourably with those at funerals, and attributed this tendency to mankind's natural proclivity to dwell more on sorrows than joys. 'Alass!', exclaimed Rogers: 'so many desire *Funeral Sermons* to be preached for their departed Friends, and few[er] desire any *Sermons* for their own *Recovery* from Sickness and Death'.[240] Ministers also grumbled that 'Some indeed when they recover... the first Visit they make' is not to church, 'but to their old *Good-fellows*'—the pub![241] Continuing this theme, James Allen's sermon on the healing of the man at Bethsaida in James 5, reminds its readers:

> The place where Christ found him [after his recovery] was... the Temple, where he was offering his Thank-offering... then observe... this healed mans Example also, there Christ finds him: he finds him not in a Tavern,... but in Gods house.[242]

Once again, this seems to have been a problem associated especially with males. Historians have observed that women made up the majority of church congregations, so this may come as no surprise.[243] Females may have been more accustomed to attending thanksgiving services than men, due to the churching ritual.

CONCLUSION

The previous chapter was about the bodily dimensions of recovery. This chapter has shown that getting better was also a deeply spiritual experience in early modern

[236] On the capacity of the spirits to leave the body and travel to the heavens, see Richard Allestree, *The art of patience and balm of Gilead* (1694, first publ. 1684), 13.
[237] Horton Davies, *Worship and Theology in England: From Andrewes to Baxter and Fox, 1603–1690* (Princeton NJ, 1975), 213–14; Christopher Haigh, 'The Church of England, the Catholics and the People', in Christopher Haigh (ed.), *The Reign of Elizabeth I* (Basingstoke, 1984), 179.
[238] Heywood, *The Rev. Oliver Heywood*, vol. 1, 246
[239] Cited in Green, *Print and Protestantism*, 504–5. Sarah Cowper gave a similarly critical view of the singing in her church, describing it as 'Bleating, Howling, Grunting, Squeeling, and what not': Cowper, *Diary*, vol. 2, 276.
[240] Rogers, *Practical discourses*, 265.   [241] Ibid., 210.   [242] Allen, *Serious advice*, 2.
[243] Patricia Crawford, *Women and Religion in England, 1500–1720* (1993), 78; Kenneth Charlton, *Women, Religion and Education in Early Modern England* (1999), 154.

England. The reason was that human beings were believed to be composed of a 'double substance'—the body and soul. Depicted as close friends or relations, these 'Twinns' usually shared one another's estates of sickness and health.[244] God sent bodily disease to punish or correct spiritual illness—sin—and He cured disease when He saw that the soul was better. As such, recovery from bodily illness could be experienced as a 'double delight', as both parts of the human were restored together. However, as soon as the immediate memory of sickness faded, it was feared that patients would return 'like dogs to vomit' to former vices, with the disastrous result of double relapse. This was where the 'art of recovery' came in: patients and their loved ones sought to preserve and enhance their newfound spiritual health by following the guidelines laid out in Scripture: sin no more, extol and love the Lord, and join together in praise. This forgotten art was the spiritual equivalent to analeptics, the branch of medicine discussed in Chapter 2, which was designed to restore bodily strength after illness, and prevent relapse into disease. Doctors and clergy regularly drew parallels between these two forms of post-illness care.[245] When patients succeeded in fulfilling the components of the art of recovery, the overall joy of getting better was greatly multiplied, on the grounds that the capacity to reform one's life and express heartfelt spiritual emotions was itself a 'token and signe' of election to Heaven.[246] On the other hand, a failure to meet the expectations served to undermine the happiness of recovery, or in the words of James Allen, 'disappoint[s] you of the good of your deliverance, [and] eat[s] out the good and sweet of it'.[247] For conscientious patients, the pressure to perform the duties could cause considerable stress, even if they eventually succeeded. Martha Hatfield, whose recovery inspired the subject of this book, told her mother, 'with a sigh, ["]Oh when the Lord is pleased to do great things for us, he expects…great things from us; even as the Husbandman that sowes a great deal of seed…looks for a great crop"'.[248] The fact that patients were keen to seize the spiritual opportunities brought by recovery shows that the doctrine of predestination did not usually produce a fatalistic attitude in Christians. It is hard to tell, however, whether patients believed their actions would actually alter God's plan for their eternal destiny, since they could argue that their behaviour had been foreseen and incorporated by the Almighty into His original scheme.

The spiritual experiences of patients and their loved ones were remarkably similar: gratitude to God and a determination to reform were expressed as much by relatives as by patients themselves. This shared experience—'fellow-feeling'—was put down to love: 'friendship…make[s] such a perfect union, that one cannot suffer but the other must have some share of it', wrote the Hackney lawyer William Lawrence (1636/7–97) to his younger brother in 1678.[249] Whereas in Chapter 3, I argued that fellow-feeling was most acute amongst the close relations and friends of the patient, here we have seen that in the context of the thanksgiving service, it

[244] Norden, *A pathway*, 8.   [245] Harris, *Hezekiahs recovery*, 38; Allen, *Serious advice*, 9, 20.
[246] Ryrie, *Being Protestant*, section 1.   [247] Allen, *Serious advice*, 19.
[248] Fisher, *The wise virgin*, 150–1.
[249] William Lawrence, *The Pyramid and the Urn: Life in Letters of a Restoration Squire: William Lawrence of Shurdington, 1636–1697*, ed. Iona Sinclair (Stroud, 1994), 54.

was imagined to extend to everyone in the congregation, owing to the combined efforts of the Holy Spirit and music.

The art of recovery was widespread, familiar to people from various socio-economic and occupational backgrounds. Even individuals known for their 'scientific' outlooks, like the naturalist Robert Boyle (1627–91), noted that it was vital to obey Christ's command *'Behold, thou art made whole, Sin no more'*. After his ague, he told his sister Katherine:

> [W]e should be more watchfull against falling back into the Sins, than into the Sicknesses…unless we would think that…[our] Nobler part deserv'd less of our care.[250]

The experiences of puritans and Anglicans were also alike: staunch royalists like Elizabeth Delaval expressed a similar repugnance of sin, and effusive thankfulness to God, as puritans like Oliver Heywood. Any discrepancies that did emerge probably owed more to the nature of the disease, or to the personality of the individual, than to religious affiliation. For instance, chronic illnesses like kidney stones tended to generate a greater sense of frustration for failed reform than acute illnesses, because the effect of sin—pain—was still being felt. One difference has emerged, however: namely, the tendency for nonconformists to hold thanksgiving in private homes rather than parish churches, for various religious and practical purposes. Even so, the content of the ceremonies was similar, comprising a sermon and singing. The reason for these limited differences was that recovery from life-threatening or painful illness was such a profound event that any pre-existing suspicions about enthusiastic devotional responses could be temporarily brushed aside.

Through revealing the vital importance of spiritual emotions in recovery, this chapter has built on Alec Ryrie's findings on the role of emotion in the daily lives of Protestants: this faith was characterized by intense feeling. The emotions experienced upon deliverance from disease were diverse, ranging from joyful praise and love, to sorrow for sin and fear of divine retribution. While the happier emotions help counter the rather depressing picture that has dominated the historiography of early modern religion, it is important to remember that contemporaries may have welcomed the sorrowful passions as well as the happy ones. Emotions such as guilt for sin, however unpleasant, were signs of the presence of the Holy Spirit in the soul. Ironically, the only emotional condition that would have been regarded negatively from a religious viewpoint was a lack of emotion—a state labelled 'stony-heartedness' by devout Protestants. Thus, perhaps we need to resist the intuitive urge to distinguish between pleasant and unpleasant feelings, since such a categorization does not reflect how they were viewed by past societies: the pious were more likely to judge emotions according to what they revealed about the state of the soul.

Several themes have emerged in this chapter. One is the impact of gender on spiritual experiences of recovery: it has been suggested that although the key religious duties incumbent on recovered patients were the same for both sexes, men were more closely associated with the stereotype of the 'bad recoverer' than

---

[250] Robert Boyle, *Occasional reflections upon several subjects* (1665), 235–7.

women—the allure of the alehouse tempted young men in particular to return to sin after illness. Whether or not this evaluation rings true is hard to tell, but the perception was unequivocal. Another theme has been the blurred boundary between private and public devotion: the spiritual emotions elicited upon recovery were interior, private experiences, the soteriological implications of which were only discernible to the individual. On the other hand, the call to join together in praise invited patients and their communities to unite their hearts and minds in shared adoration for God, a form of devotion that supports Andrew Cambers' assertion that Protestantism was more sociable than is often assumed.[251] The mixed location of services—in the church or in the household—further complicates the classification of this form of worship. The third theme concerns metaphor: we have seen that this rhetorical device was ubiquitous in the art of recovery literature, a technique which served to transform something intangible—the health of the immaterial soul—into something concrete. The fact that some of the most metaphor-rich sermons were those that were published in the last decade of the seventeenth century challenges the notion that this sort of language fell out of favour after the Civil Wars, owing to its associations with sectarian violence and 'enthusiasm'.[252] Ministers were acutely aware that printed sermons were not as 'affecting' as those which were delivered orally; using striking metaphors therefore helped to compensate for this deficiency. There also appears to have been a notable continuity in the spiritual experiences of recovery more broadly: the same basic obligations and affections required of the patient after illness were reiterated throughout the period, and deliverance continued to be interpreted providentially in the 1700s. In fact, until as late as the early nineteenth century, clergymen were publishing sermons which warned of the spiritual dangers associated with recovery, such as 'a fearful risk of thanklessness' and the likelihood of returning to one's 'special besetting sin'.[253]

---

[251] Andrew Cambers, *Godly Reading: Print, Manuscript and Puritanism in England, 1580–1720* (Cambridge, 2011), *passim*.

[252] Hunt, *The Art of Hearing*, 396–7. See also Worden, 'The Question of Secularization', 33.

[253] Robert Milman, *Convalescence, thoughts for those who are recovering from sickness* (1836), 62, 68.

5

'Pluck't from the Pit':
Escaping Death

In 1690, the ailing London minister Timothy Rogers (1658–1728) nearly died. Upon his recovery, he preached and published a sermon about his near-death experience. Addressing his congregation, he declared:

> Never was any[one], I believe, nearer to Death [than I], never was any compass'd with a greater Danger; never any had less hope of an Escape than I, and yet the Mercy of a God that is Omnipotent, has relieved me.

Rogers thought that his unusual proximity to death granted him special authority to preach on the subject; as he put it, 'the Words of one that has dwelt so long as in the very Grave, and in the nearest Confines of Eternity, ought to carry more than ordinary weight'. He implied that his experience had furnished him with unrivalled insights into what it might be like to die, a question of keen interest to all mortal beings, and yet one which was for the most part unfathomable, owing to the fact that 'none of the Millions of Souls that have past into th[at] invisible World have come again to tell us how it is'.[1]

Rogers was not as unique as he thought, however! Accounts of close shaves with death are ubiquitous in early modern sources. This chapter asks how patients like Rogers responded emotionally to the realization that they would not die, but live. While valuable work has been conducted on people's reactions to the prospect of dying, little has been said about responses to survival.[2] By examining mortality from this new angle, I seek to enrich our understanding of attitudes both to life *and* death, showing that these states were viewed ambivalently. The discussions also enable us to revisit and revise an entrenched teleology in the historiography of early modern religion: namely, that belief in the reality of a Christian afterlife was beginning

---

[1] Timothy Rogers, *Practical discourses on sickness & recovery* (1691), 156, 6.
[2] For example, David Stannard, *The Puritan Way of Death: A Study in Religion, Culture, and Social Change* (Oxford, 1977); Philippe Ariès, *The Hour of Our Death*, trans. Helen Weaver (1981); Lucinda Becker, *Death and the Early Modern Englishwoman* (Aldershot, 2003); Claire Gittings, *Death, Burial and the Individual in Early Modern England* (1984); Ralph Houlbrooke, *Death, Religion and the Family in England, 1480–1750* (Oxford, 1998); Hannah Newton, *The Sick Child in Early Modern England* (Oxford, 2012), ch. 6; Alec Ryrie, *Being Protestant in Reformation Britain* (Oxford, 2013), 460–68. On accidental/violent death, see Craig Spence, *Accidents and Violent Death in Early Modern London, 1650–1750* (Woodbridge, 2016).

to fade by the late seventeenth century.[3] As shall become apparent, even in the early 1700s, ideas about Heaven and Hell exerted a significant influence on people's responses to not dying.

Besides exploring patients' own responses to survival, the chapter examines the reactions of their families and friends. Considerable research has been undertaken on experiences of bereavement in early modern England, a body of literature which has successfully overturned the older view that grief was rare in this period.[4] But emotional responses to survival have received little attention.[5] Nor has much work been conducted on the reactions of individuals outside the 'nuclear family', such as friends and work colleagues, and wider kin like grandparents and cousins. By revealing the emotional responses of an array of individuals, the discussions showcase the diversity and depth of relationships enjoyed by early modern people. In so doing, it adds to the 'neo-revisionist' interpretation of family and social networks, which challenges the more established view that ties between members of the extended family were weak.[6] Nonetheless, in some cases, it is possible to discern a hierarchy of affection, with the most profuse emotions being professed by the patient's 'nearest and dearest'.[7] The chapter also contributes to the history of early modern emotion, unravelling the rarely examined interrelationships between different passions.[8]

It is worth briefly considering why so many people experienced recovery as an escape from death. The simplest explanation is that while mortality rates varied over time and place, acute disease was ever present, and usually ended either in death or recovery.[9] Doctors encouraged patients to see any illness, however apparently trivial, as potentially fatal, on the grounds that the bad humours could easily pass from the 'ignoble organs'—the regions of lesser physiological importance—to the 'noble' ones, the heart, brain, and liver.[10] This message was reinforced by the Protestant Church, which advised its flock to view every sickness as a dress rehearsal

---

[3] Daniel Pickering Walker, *The Decline of Hell: Seventeenth-Century Discussions of Eternal Torment* (1964); Ralph Houlbrooke offers a more tentative interpretation in, *Death, Religion and the Family*, 50–6, as does Keith Thomas, *The Ends of Life: Roads to Fulfilment in Early Modern England* (Oxford, 2009), 232–7.

[4] For example, Anne Laurence, 'Godly Grief: Individual Responses to Death in Seventeenth-Century Britain', in Ralph Houlbrooke (ed.), *Death, Ritual, and Bereavement* (1989), 66–71; Jennifer Vaught (ed.), *Grief and Gender, 700–1700* (Basingstoke, 2003); Raymond Anselment, *The Realms of Apollo: Literature and Healing in Seventeenth-Century England* (1995), ch. 2; Houlbrooke, *Death, Religion and the Family*, ch. 8; Newton, *The Sick Child*, ch. 4. The most famous exponent of the older view is Lawrence Stone, *The Family, Sex and Marriage in England 1500–1800* (1990, first publ. 1977).

[5] One exception is Olivia Weisser, who addresses the health-giving effects of news of a loved one's survival in *Ill Composed: Sickness, Gender, and Belief in Early Modern England* (2015), 99, 260, 264. I also touch on this subject in *The Sick Child*, 154–5.

[6] For a summary of this literature, see the Introduction, pp. 18–19.

[7] The term 'neo-revisionist' was coined by Naomi Tadmor in 'Early Modern English Kinship in the Long Run: Reflections on Continuity and Change', *Continuity and Change*, 25 (2010), 15–48, at 16–20.

[8] For an introduction to this literature, see Susan Broomhall (ed.), *Early Modern Emotions: An Introduction* (Abingdon, 2017).

[9] On regional variations, see Mary Dobson, *Contours of Death and Disease in Early Modern England* (Cambridge, 1996), *passim*. On the high incidence of acute illnesses, see James Riley, *Sickness, Recovery and Death: A History and Forecast of Ill Health* (Basingstoke, 1989), xi.

[10] See Chapter 1, pp. 43–4 on the humoral cause of disease.

for the deathbed.[11] Reflection on one's closeness to death helped patients to cultivate a sense of thankfulness to God for His deliverance, a vital religious duty at this time.[12] There were also social reasons behind this tendency, which may even have tempted some patients to exaggerate the severity of their illnesses. As Rogers implied, survival brought attention and respect: it was a sign of God's special favour.

One of the challenges faced when attempting to explore emotional responses to the escape from death is the possible gap between real feelings and cultural etiquette. Patients and their loved ones may have voiced emotions which they knew were appropriate in the circumstances, rather than expressing their 'true' feelings. Ministers taught that 'life prolonged' was 'a *choice* mercy indeed', to be joyfully received; those who failed to react in this way were deemed ungrateful.[13] In his epistolary handbook, William Fulwood (d. 1593), a member of the Merchant Taylors' Company, taught readers 'how to write Letters rejoycing for our frendes health': first they should say, 'we were so affrayde of his sickenesse', and second, 'declare the joy that we have had of his mending'.[14] Fulwood's model letters are virtually indistinguishable from real ones.[15] The etiquette described in these documents constitutes what Barbara Rosenwein would call an 'emotional community', a set of social rules governing emotional expression.[16] Although it is likely that patients and their loved ones were influenced by these conventions, to dismiss their professed feelings as artificial would be unwise. William Reddy believes that the expression of an emotion—in words or gestures—helps to bring it to fruition.[17] From this stance, we can be more confident about glimpsing something of the 'real' feelings of individuals. In any case, there were occasions when people admitted that they could not stir up the required feelings, or felt emotions contrary to expectations.[18] The first part of the chapter discusses the responses of patients, and the second half turns to their relatives and friends.

PATIENTS

A 'Hymn of Thanksgiving for Recovery', by the Yorkshire Anglican minister John Kettlewell (1653–95) sums up what it was like to escape death for many patients: quoting Psalm 30:11, he tells God, 'thou hast turned for me my mourning into dancing[,] thou hast putt off my Sack-cloth, and girded me with gladness'.[19] Appearing frequently in accounts of survival, this verse conveys the extraordinary

---

[11] Houlbrooke, *Death, Religion and the Family*, 69–70.

[12] See Chapter 4, pp. 146–51 on this duty.

[13] Nathaniel Hardy, *Two mites, or, a gratefull acknowledgement of God's singular goodnesse... occasioned by his late unexpected recovery of a desperate sickness* (1653), 27.

[14] William Fulwood, *The enimie of idlenesse teaching the maner and stile how to... compose... letters* (1568), 52.

[15] See the Introduction, p. 29.

[16] See the Introduction, note 173 for references to Rosenwein.

[17] See the Introduction, note 175 for references to Reddy.

[18] See pp. 189–90 in this chapter.

[19] John Kettlewell, *Death made comfortable* (1695), 125; this text was inspired by his own illness.

transformation of patients' feelings—from fear to joy. The sackcloth, a coarse, scratchy fabric made of goats' hair, and worn in biblical times as penitential or mourning garb, contrasts with the silky and soft texture of dresses more likely to have been worn by dancers.[20] Fear was defined as, 'A griefe and distresse of the soule, troubled by ... some approaching Evill wherewith man is threatned', which in this case was death.[21] It made the body 'growe pale and trembling' by driving the person's spirits and humours—the instruments of nutrition, animation, and life—from the outer parts of the body to the heart.[22] The passion of joy could not have been more different: it was 'the *rest* and contentment to the soule, which enjoyeth some good wherof she tastes the sweetness', wrote the French philosopher Nicolas Coeffeteau (1574–1623). In this passion, the heart was imagined as an opening flower, that propels the body's spirits and humours upwards and outwards, leading to the brightening of the eyes and cheeks, and the turning up of the mouth in smiles.[23]

Why did patients undergo this emotional transformation? There seem to have been three main reasons, the first of which can be labelled natural: mankind's innate fear of mortality and love of life. 'Who doth not dread ... the face of Death?', asked the popular religious writer Richard Baxter (1615–91): 'Death is an *Enemy* to *Nature[:]* ... it maketh a *Man* to become *No man*'.[24] Such instincts were thought to arise from the intimate connection between the body and soul: these two parts of the human being were personified as close relatives, who cared deeply for one another, and were 'loth to part'—death was defined as the separation of these constituents.[25] During an illness at the age of forty, the Wiltshire poet Hester Pulter (*c.*1595/6–1678) mused:

> Ah mee! how sore & how sad is my poor heart,
> How loath my Soule is from my flesh to part:
> Hath forty years acquaintance caus'd such love.[26]

The sick imagined the internal dialogue between their own bodies and souls, frequently implying that they would be conscious of their own disintegration.[27] In some cases, the interactions between these two parts bear an uncanny resemblance to the responses of parents or married couples to the prospect of the death of a child or spouse. This is evident in Rogers' account:

> [W]hen the day is come that the two Friends who have been so long acquainted and so dear to one another must part ... when [the soul] consider[s] ... what it is to have this Body, which we have tended with so long a Care, ... maintain'd at so vast a Charge

---

[20] OED, noun: 'sackcloth' (accessed 19/05/17).
[21] Nicolas Coeffeteau, *A table of humane passions*, trans. Edward Grimestone (1621), 430–1.
[22] Ibid., 17. See also Stephen Bradwell, *Physicke for the sicknesse, commonly called the plague* (1636), 37.
[23] Coeffeteau, *A table*, 254–5, 297–8.
[24] Richard Baxter, *A treatise of death* (1660), 4–5.
[25] Thomas Steward, *Sacrificium laudis, or a thank-offering* (1699), 5–6. See also Rachel Russell, *Letters of Rachel, Lady Russell*, ed. Thomas Selwood, 2 vols. (1853, first publ. 1773), vol. 2, 38.
[26] Brotherton Library, Leeds, MS. Lt q 32, fol. 48r–v (Hester Pulter's 'Poems Breathed forth By The Nobel Hadassas).
[27] Mary Carey, *Meditations from the Note Book of Mary Carey, 1649–1657*, ed. Sir Francis Meynell (Westminster, 1918), 13–15.

of Meat and Drink and Time... laid into the cold Grave, and there in a loathsome manner to putrifie... it cannot but occasion very great Commotions... [even in] the boldest and stoutest Man.[28]

At this time, the word 'friend' denoted family members as well as unrelated individuals; here, Rogers seems to be referring to close, cohabiting relatives, as can be inferred from his reference to the long-term provision of sustenance.[29] By suggesting that fear of death is universal, experienced by the strongest of men, Rogers may have been trying to reassure those male patients who were concerned that such a reaction was unmanly. The only individuals who seemed exempt from these urges were little children, whose bodies and souls had not yet attained the same degree of friendship as those of adults.[30]

In view of the love between the body and soul, it followed that the escape from death was experienced as the joyful embracing of these two parts of the human being, as they realized they would no longer have to part. Baxter confirmed, 'The Soul hath naturally a Love and Inclination to its Body: and therefore it feareth a separation before, and desireth a Restauration afterward[s]'.[31] The recent contemplation of parting was found to fill one's body and soul with a 'fresh kind of pleasure and delight' in life itself, as well as for each other.[32] A common analogy invoked in this context referred to sailors' responses to survival from shipwrecks. The French philosopher Jean-François Senault (c.1601–72) wrote:

> Mariners never taste the sweetness of life more than when they have escaped Shipwrack; and they are never more sensible of contentment, than when after despair of safety, a Tempest drives them upon the shore.[33]

This imagery may have been chosen due to its religious connotations—in the Bible, shipwreck is a symbol of terror, insecurity, and financial disaster; the apostle Paul was a frequent victim.[34] There was also a broader cultural reason at play: mariners' tales were widely disseminated in early modern England, the subjects of innumerable ballads, so it is likely that even those patients with no personal experience of shipwrecks felt some affinity with the plight of sailors.[35] Indeed, accounts of these seafaring calamities bear striking similarity to those of survival

---

[28] Rogers, *Practical discourses*, 44–5.

[29] See the Introduction, note 93, on the meaning of 'friend'.

[30] See Hannah Newton, ' "Rapt up in Joy": The Dying Child in Early Modern England', in Kimberley Reynolds, Katie Barclay, and Ciara Rawnsley (eds.), *Death, Emotion and Childhood in Premodern Europe* (Basingstoke, 2017), 87–107, at 93–4.

[31] Baxter, *A treatise of death*, 11. He was speaking about the reunion of the body and soul in Heaven, but the statement is equally applicable to the interaction that occurred when death had been escaped.

[32] Edward Lawrence, *Christ's power over bodily diseases* (1672, first publ. 1662), 268.

[33] Jean-François Senault, *The use of passions*, trans. Henry Earl of Monmouth (1671, first publ. 1649), 469.

[34] For instance, see Psalm 48:7; 1 Kings 22:48; 2 Chronicles 9:21; Ezekiel 27:1–9; 2 Corinthians 11:25. See *DBI*, 785–6.

[35] My thanks to Dr Richard Blakemore for this information. A search on the UCSB English Broadside Ballad Archive for 'seaman' produces 220 results. A typical example is *The mariners delight, or the seaman's seaven wives* (1662–92): <https://ebba.english.ucsb.edu/> (accessed 13/6/17).

from illness. When Daniel Defoe's protagonist, Robinson Crusoe, was delivered safely on shore, he mused:

> I believe it is impossible to express... what the extasies... of the soul are, when it is so sav'd,... out of the very grave... I walk'd about on the shore, lifting up my hands,... wrapt up in the contemplation of my deliverance.[36]

The physiological understandings of the passions mentioned earlier explain why Crusoe lifted his arms up: joy and praise drove the spirits, the instruments of animation, in a centrifugal motion, towards the hands and feet.[37]

As well as the natural reason for patients' relief to escape death, there was a pressing soteriological factor: survival provided time to 'work out the Salvation of thy soul', which meant finding proof that one was destined for Heaven.[38] An anonymous female diarist, a relative of Oliver Cromwell, recorded in 1699 that God took away her fever 'to help me... [in] getting my Evedences clearer for Heaven, that when Death shall come, I may be in a Readiness'.[39] This woman was referring to the doctrine of election, which held that Christians were able to discern signs of salvation in their daily lives; she hoped to find more of such proofs before she died.[40] For those individuals who had become convinced that they would go to Hell, the escape from death was even more welcome: it spared them from eternal damnation, at least in the short-term, and offered 'soul-saving opportunities' for altering this judgement.[41] The ejected Presbyterian minister from Shropshire, Edward Lawrence (d. 1695), warned sinners, 'if thou hadst dyed in thy last sickness, thou wast in great danger to be damned; and now thou hast time to labour to be saved'.[42] One patient who would have agreed was the Cambridge student Isaac Archer (1641–1700), who went on to become a minister: sick of smallpox in 1657, he believed, 'verily I should have dyed, and gone to hell'. He rejoiced at his escape, addressing God, 'let mee praise thee... with joyfull lipps in the land of the living, Oh God my God!'[43] Women too might undergo these experiences. In the late 1670s, the Hertfordshire Quaker Alice Hayes (1657–1720) was 'brought... near to Death' by a great 'fit of sickness'. To her '*Horrour and Amazement*' she realized she was about '*to step out... into... the Lake that burns with Fire and Brimstone for evermore*'. When God raised her 'from the Brink of the Grave', she cried with relief, '*Oh! the boundless Mercies of God; how shall they be sufficiently set forth by me.*'[44]

---

[36] Daniel Defoe, *Robinson Crusoe* (2012, first publ. 1719), 43–4. For a real shipwreck example, see Ralph Thoresby, *The Diary of Ralph Thoresby*, ed. Joseph Hunter, 2 vols. (1830), vol. 1, 25–6.
[37] See B.A., *The sick-mans rare jewell* (1674), 30.   [38] Lawrence, *Christ's power*, 263.
[39] BL, Additional MS 5858, fol. 219v (Religious diary of a female cousin of Oliver Cromwell, 1687/90–1702). See also Oliver Heywood, *The Rev. Oliver Heywood, B.A: His Autobiography, Diaries, Anecdote and Event Books*, ed. Horsfall Turner, 4 vols. (1883), vol. 3, 254–7.
[40] Ryrie, *Being Protestant*, 39–41; Leif Dixon, *Practical Predestinarians in England, c.1590–1640* (Abingdon, 2014), ch. 7.
[41] Rogers, *Practical discourses*, 63–4.   [42] Lawrence, *Christ's power*, 264.
[43] Isaac Archer, 'The Diary of Isaac Archer 1641–1700', in Matthew Storey (ed.), *Two East Anglian Diaries 1641–1729*, Suffolk Record Society, vol. 36 (Woodbridge, 1994), 41–200, at 54–5.
[44] Alice Hayes, *A legacy, or, widow's mite, left by Alice Hayes* (1723), 24–6. See also Anne Halkett, *The Autobiography of Anne Lady Halkett*, ed. John Gough Nichols, Camden Society New Series, vol. 13 (1875–6), 32–3.

Such experiences were not confined to divinity students and zealous minorities—
even those with a reputation for their more 'scientific' attitudes thanked God for
sending sickness to save them from 'the Flames and Shriecks of Hell'.[45] It is more
difficult to discern whether the poorer sectors of society shared these reactions, but
some evidence is provided in the Proceedings of the Old Bailey, wherein defendants described how they felt about the prospect of a reprieve from the death sen-
tence. Although these individuals were not sick, and their responses were mediated
by scribes, such accounts provide the closest insights available. Seventeen-year-old
John Culverwell, accused of stealing a horse in 1686, told the Ordinary that 'if he
might escape Death at this time he hoped that he should Reform his Life, and not
Commit any Crime', thus implying that he wished to improve his spiritual state
and future.[46] Relief to escape damnation continued to shape experiences of survival in the early eighteenth century, contrary to the views of those who have
argued that belief in Hell was declining at this time.[47]

One only has to cast a glance at contemporary accounts of damnation to understand why patients were relieved to avoid this destiny. The theologian Henry
Greenwood (b. 1544/5), described Hell as a 'wofull place of torment, where there
shall be scretching and screaming, weeping, [and] wayling...for eternity...easelesse,
endlesse, remedylesse'.[48] Religious authors emphasized the comparative mildness
of the pains experienced during illness compared to the sufferings of the reprobate.
In his treatise *Hells terror* (1653), the London minister Christopher Love (1618–51)
told his readers:

> Upon earth, you have diseases haply;...though some parts are afflicted, other parts are
> free...though ill in your head, yet vitals free; though in your vitals, yet arms and legs
> free; there is no disease that puts the whole body in pain at once: but in hell...all the
> parts of your bodies, and powers of your souls[,] shall be tormented.[49]

In their restless slumbers, the sick were haunted by visions of this place, a tendency
aggravated by high fevers and hallucinations.[50] In his late teens, the fishmonger
apprentice Richard Norwood (1590–1675) from Hertfordshire complained that
he 'had horrible dreams and visions...[and] verily thought that I descended into
Hell, and there felt the pains of the damned'. He was relieved when he woke up,
and realized it was only a dream; he had time to change his fate.[51]

By expressing relief to have escaped Hell, the above patients implied that it was
possible to influence their eternal destiny. While such thinking was unproblematic

---

[45] Robert Boyle, *Occasional reflections upon several subjects* (1665), 213.

[46] POB, ref: OA16861217 (accessed 19/12/16).

[47] See note 3 in this chapter on this historiography. An eighteenth-century example is provided in
the memoirs of John Cannon, an officer of the excise from West Lydford, Somerset: SHC, DD/SAS
C/1193/4, p. 102.

[48] Henry Greenwood, *Tormenting tophet; or a terrible description of hell* (1650, first publ. 1615),
239–41.

[49] Christopher Love, *Hells terror: or, a treatise of the torments of the damned* (1653), 42–3.

[50] Hallucination was recognized as a concept—see Thomas Blount, *Glossographia, or, a dictionary*
(1661), image 154.

[51] Richard Norwood, *The Journal of Richard Norwood, Surveyor of Bermuda*, ed. Wesley Frank
Craven and Walter Hayward (New York, 1945), 26, 68–70.

for Arminians, Protestants who emphasized the power of man to resist sin, we might have expected supporters of the Calvinist doctrine of predestination to have been more troubled by such a notion.[52] Predestinarianism taught that God had already decided whether a person would be damned or saved, and there was nothing anyone could do to alter His decree.[53] As the nonconformist minister Eusabius Pagit (1546/7–1617) confirmed, 'God chooseth either to Salvation or refuseth to Damnation: for he doeth predestintate as well the wicked as his children'.[54] In the light of this belief, it is somewhat surprising to find that even puritan patients—the 'hotter sort of Protestants' normally associated with this doctrine—were amongst those who seem to have thought that they could improve their soteriological chances. Perhaps these individuals reconciled the contradiction by assuming that God had foreseen a near-death spiritual reforma-tion, and built it into His original plan.[55]

The escape from damnation was described using dramatic imagery, an examination of which provides further insights into patients' experiences. Reminiscing about a nearly fatal fall as a youth, the puritan clothier Joseph Lister (1627–1709) con-sidered, 'O how near was I to death at this time! and had I died then, surely I had gone down to the pit.'[56] The word 'pit' was a metonym for Hell: it was conceived as a bottomless black hole, located in the core of the Earth.[57] Patients also referred to 'the Gates' of Hell, sometimes hinting that they had caught a glimpse of what lies behind the imposing doors.[58] In biblical phraseology, gates were places of judi-cial assembly, which made sense given that final Judgement took place at death.[59] The third metaphor used in this context referred to the jaws or mouth of Hell. After an illness in 1699, the Suffolk minister Thomas Steward (1668/9–1753) told his parishioners, 'behold a Man...snatch'd out of the very Jaws of Death; which... even gaped upon me, and stood ready to...devour me as it's lawful Prey'.[60] He imagines death as a terrifying monster, with an enormous mouth. These metaphors would have been familiar to most people in society, down to the very poorest, since they were conveyed through visual and sound media, such as songs and woodcuts, as well as literary texts.[61] For example, the popular ballad *The great assize* (1672–96), is illustrated with a woodcut of the mouth of Hell, into which a queue of sinners

---

[52] On Arminianism, see Nicolas Tyacke, *Anti-Calvinists: The Rise of English Arminianism, c.1590–1640* (Oxford, 1987).

[53] For historiography on this doctrine, see Chapter 4, note 8.

[54] Cited in Dixon, *Practical Predestinarians*, 2.

[55] Alexandra Walsham suggests that 'thorny' doctrinal niceties of this kind could be easily forgotten at moments of crisis: *Providence in Early Modern England* (Oxford, 2003, first publ. 1999), 152–3.

[56] Joseph Lister, *The Autobiography of Joseph Lister of Bradford, 1627–1709*, ed. Thomas Wright (Bradford, 1842), 4.

[57] For example, James Allen (born in Oxford), *Serious advice to delivered ones from sickness* (Boston, 1679), 13.

[58] John Hall, *Select observations on English bodies*, trans. James Cooke (1679, first. publ. 1657), 49.

[59] Job 38: 17; Matthew 16:18.   [60] Steward, *Sacrificium laudis*, 1–2.

[61] On images of Hell in woodcuts, see Tessa Watt, *Cheap Print and Popular Piety 1550–1640* (Cambridge, 1991), 110–12, 171, 283–9.

is entering.[62] Although we do not know how people responded to these images—whether they 'Tremble' or 'cheerfully laugh'—the fact remains that Hell was part of everyone's cultural repertoire in early modern England.[63]

Implicit in the use of the above metaphors, besides the obvious terror of damnation and relief of survival, is the impression that the escape from death was a moment of physical and aural contact with God. The Lord called, stretched out His hand, and plucked the patient from the danger zone. The Cambridgeshire Presbyterian Elizabeth Bury (1644–1720) recorded that 'the Lord was entreated to spare' her, 'and say *Return*'.[64] The Anglican judge Matthew Hale (1609–76) told his newly recovered son that God, 'by his own hand brought you back from the very threshold of the Grave'.[65] Theologians attributed this anthropomorphizing tendency to the Bible itself, which speaks of God 'as if he had eyes, eares, [and] hands', in order to 'have us...fully perswaded, that he hath sight, hearing, knowledge, power, etc'.[66] The sense of intimate contact with God conjured by these sensory metaphors may have been cherished by patients as a way to foster feelings of intimacy and love for the Lord, emotions known as 'holy affections' in this period, and regarded as essential religious responses to divine deliverance.[67]

Having discussed the natural and soteriological factors that lay behind patients' joyful responses to the escape from death, we can turn to the so-called earthly reasons. Rogers declared that death is:

> [A]n End of all the World[:]... When his Eyes are once clos'd by Death, he is no more to behold the Sun, Moon and Stars...nor his Fields and Gardens, his Shops and Houses...He quits for ever all those Earthly things on which he...set his Heart;...he will not awake to pursue...Business...He must no more frequent his *Exchange*, nor read Books, nor discourse with his Relations and Friends...All the Affairs of... Trade,...all his projects...all these things are at an end with him for[-]ever.[68]

Thus, all earthly delights, activities, and interactions cease with death, a prospect that filled many patients with fear during illness, and jubilation upon survival. Here, the most regularly cited of these factors will be discussed: relief not to be separated from loved ones.[69] In his 1618 treatise on death, the Anglican clergyman Nicolas Byfield (1578/9–1622) mused, 'I cannot willingly goe from my kindred[:] ... life is sweet in respect of their presence, and love, and society... this is the greatest contentment of life'.[70] Over a century later, the theatre director Aaron Hill

---

[62] Minister Stevens, *The great assize; or, Christ's certain and sudden appearance to judgment* (1672–96). The metaphors of pit, mouth, and jaws all feature in this ballad.

[63] Walsham, *Providence*, 39.

[64] Elizabeth Bury, *An account of the life and death of Elizabeth Bury* (Bristol, 1720), 122.

[65] Matthew Hale, *A letter from Sr Matthew Hale...to one of his sons, after his recovery from the smallpox* (1684), 18.

[66] Richard Kilby, *Halleluiah: praise yee the Lord, for the unburthening of a loaded conscience* (Cambridge, 1635), 3.

[67] See Chapter 4, pp. 146–55, on the holy affections.

[68] Rogers, *Practical discourses*, 48–9; see also Hardy, *Two mites*, 26–7.

[69] Attitudes to work, wealth, and the outdoors are discussed in Chapter 6.

[70] Nicolas Byfield, *The cure of the feare of death* (1618), 153–4.

(1685–1750) echoed, 'the one Thing, which makes Death terrible, and triumphs' over all other causes,

> [Is] that we are torn from our Friends' Society.—That we are divided...from what Love has made dearer to us than our Life is! It is this Blending...of Two Hearts...which is the Spirit of all human Blessings![71]

As this author hints, the fear of parting was due to love. Coeffeteau explained that this passion has a 'uniting vertue', which causes 'him that loveth to aspire to unite himselfe to the thing beloved'. Hence, 'the presence of the party beloved is so deare and pretious unto us..., that we feele our selves filled with content...whereas his absence and separation gives us a thousand torments'.[72] Since death 'is as it were a perpetuall absence', it inevitably evoked fear in the sick, and joy at its escape. In fact, when the patient 'sees himself imbraced and entertained by the party beloved' upon his survival, 'hee recovers his life doubly', since being loved is a source of further joy.[73]

Patients' memoirs show that these ideas about love and separation were not confined to published philosophical works, but were borne out in daily experience. When Lady Judith Isham (1590–1625) from Northamptonshire fell gravely ill at the age of 34, she cried out, 'death is terrible to mee', and pleaded to God, 'O let me live with my husband and my Children'.[74] Husbands reciprocated these feelings. Robert Viscount Yarmouth told his wife Rebecca in 1677, 'My dearest deare[,]... you are the subject for which I desire to live, [it is] the hopes you give mee that things may mend'.[75] Children were particularly anxious about the prospect of parting from parents, and relieved when relationships continued, a finding that would come as no surprise to modern child psychologists.[76] Of course, it is worth remembering that not everyone married or bore children in this period: historical demographers have estimated that around 20 per cent of the population remained single, and about a fifth of married couples were childless.[77] These individuals did not live 'empty lives', devoid of love, however: as Amy Froide has shown, unmarried people usually enjoyed particularly strong ties with friends, siblings, and cousins.[78] It is therefore likely that single or unmarried people who escaped death would have experienced similarly intense emotions.

An analysis of patients' words when they realized they would not be compelled to 'bid adieu to Wife, Children, Friends', reveals that their experiences were gendered.

---

[71] Aaron Hill, *The plain dealer: being select essays on several curious subjects* (1724), 184–5.
[72] Coeffeteau, *A table*, 161–2.   [73] Ibid., 167–8.
[74] Elizabeth Isham, *Diary and Confessions: Constructing Elizabeth Isham, 1609–1654*, Warwick University Online Editions, ed. Elizabeth Clarke, Nigel Smith, Jill Millman, and Alice Eardley: <http://web.warwick.ac.uk/english/perdita/Isham/index_bor.htm> (accessed 14/01/17), fol. 19 r–v. Isham died in this illness. See also BL, Additional MS 36452, fol. 37r (Private letters of the Aston family, 1613–1703).
[75] Robert Paston, *The Whirlpool of Misadventures: Letters of Robert Paston, First Earl of Yarmouth 1663–1679*, ed. Jean Agnew, Norfolk Record Society, vol. 76 (2012), 287.
[76] Newton, '"Rapt up in Joy"', 94. For a child psychologist's viewpoint, see Grace Hyslop Christ, *Healing Children's Grief* (Oxford, 2000).
[77] See the Introduction, note 94.
[78] Amy Froide, *Never Married: Singlewomen in Early Modern England* (Oxford, 2005), 44–86.

In 1625, the royalist gentlewoman Lady Margaret Harrison (d. 1640) nearly died from fever; at this time, her daughter, Ann, was only three months old. Margaret recalled that 'the sence of leaving my girl...remained a trouble upon my spirits', and begged of God, 'O let me have the same grant given to Hezekiah', the biblical king of Judah, 'that I may live fifteen years [more], to see my daughter a woman'. To her extreme joy, she was granted these extra years.[79] Margaret's response was typical of mothers' reactions to surviving disease—they expressed joy to see their children grow up, and were relieved that they would not have to leave young infants without maternal care. While men were also glad not to be parted from their families, their precise preoccupations differed. After a fifteen-day illness in 1620, Richard Carpenter, a clergyman from Cornwall, told his father-in-law, 'in regard of the needful dependency of my loving wife and poore chyldren on my temporary life, I must confesse that I have mainly strivyen...against many violent pangs...opposing death'.[80] He was worried about the financial position of his dependants. Such anxieties were expressed more than a hundred years later by Aaron Hill, as he imagined the thoughts of a gravely sick husband:

> Can a Husband sit Easie...when he is straining his dying Eyes, for the last, afflicting Sight of a Wife, who deserv'd his Tenderness, and was intitled to his Protection; but [she is] whom he is, that Moment, compell'd to leave, to struggle with the Bitterness of Want...[C]an there be a Strength...to sustain a dying Father, whose Heart is tourt'd with the burning Uncertainty, of what shall become of his helpless Orphans... without Guide, Support, or Prospect?[81]

Hill's empathetic reading, perhaps inspired by thinking of his own wife Mary and their nine children, reveals that a man's inability to fulfil his divinely ordained role as provider and protector could be a cause for great anxiety. Such a finding supports Alexandra Shepard's reminder that the doctrine of patriarchy, traditionally regarded as the source of unmixed satisfaction to men, had a flipside.[82] These responses also show that the 'obligation' and 'affect' functions of marriage—seen by the likes of Lawrence Stone as mutually exclusive—were in fact inseparable, since a husband might wish to fulfil his duties out of love for his wife.[83] Nevertheless, there may also have been a more selfish reason behind men's anxieties: some husbands seem to have been more preoccupied with their own reputations than their wives' well-being. The Lancashire Presbyterian minister Henry Newcome (c.1627–95), sick of ague in 1660, admitted that his 'constant fear' was that he would 'die and...leave nothing for my wife and children'; he worried that 'men will say, ["]This was his strictness, and this is Puritanism! see what it gets them! what it leaves to wife and

---

[79] Ann Fanshawe, *Memoirs of Lady Fanshawe*, ed. Richard Fanshawe (1829), 27–8. Hezekiah's recovery is narrated in 2 Kings 18–20; Isaiah 36–9; 2 Chronicles 29–32.

[80] SHC, DD\WO/55/7/47-1 (Trevelyan Papers).   [81] Hill, *The plain dealer*, 185.

[82] Alexandra Shepard, *Meanings of Manhood in Early Modern England* (Oxford, 2003), 5. See also Mark Brietenberg, *Anxious Masculinity in Early Modern England* (Oxford, 1996).

[83] The 'problematic dichotomy' between interest and emotion is discussed by Tadmor, 'Early Modern English Kinship', 26–7.

children!["]'[84] Keith Thomas has suggested that the growing concern about 'post-humous remembrance' may be indicative of 'a weakening confidence in the Christian promise of life after death'—reputation on earth was 'an alternative to heaven as a way of overcoming mortality'.[85] This could not have been so for Newcome, since he professed strong faith in the existence of an afterlife. In any case, there is no reason why the two preoccupations—reputation on earth and one's own life after death—could not coexist comfortably.

It is more difficult to discern the reactions of poorer patients to the prospect of separation from loved ones, owing to a lack of direct written evidence. But if popular ballads are anything to go by—texts that were supposed to resonate with the values of people throughout society—we can infer that their feelings were no different. *The lamented lovers* (1675–96?), tells of a love-struck gallant who falls into a mortal fever; expecting death, he cries to his sweetheart, 'I now shall never see thee more, Whom I so dearly did adore', and with these words 'his heart did break'.[86] Further glimpses are provided in legal documents, in which defendants were faced with possible execution. The Old Bailey Proceedings report that a man known as R.O., accused of murdering a sea-surgeon in 1675, told the court that he did not want to die because of 'his wife and Children', and desired his friends 'to take care' of them after his decease.[87] Although these documents convey 'the words of scribes, not the voices of the past', to doubt the veracity of this statement would be to suggest that poorer families did not enjoy loving relationships, a view which has been thoroughly repudiated by Patricia Crawford.[88]

The discussions so far have concentrated on happy responses to the escape from death. Not everyone feared dying, however—some patients had positively looked forward to it during sickness. For these individuals, survival could be cause for disappointment rather than joy! When the minister Robert Blair (b. 1593), 'apprehended death to approach' during a burning fever in the 1610s, he was 'not at all dismayed but on the contrary...began to rejoice greatly upon the consideration that shortly I might...enjoy God eternally'. After several hours of happy contemplation, however, his fever lessened, 'and the vehemence of my rejoicing also abated'.[89] Similar experiences were reported at the end of the century. The non-conformist Halifax minister Oliver Heywood (*c*.1630–1702) admitted that during his illness in 1691, 'I was not afraid of death, nay I longed for it, and when many judged me a gone man, I was afraid it was too good to be true, and was loath to be sent back'.[90] It was not just godly ministers who responded in this way. In 1665,

[84] Henry Newcome, *The Autobiography of Henry Newcome*, ed. Richard Parkinson (Manchester, 1852), vol. 1, 135–6.
[85] Thomas, *The Ends of Life*, 234–5.
[86] *The lamented lovers: or the young men and maiden's grief* (1675–96?).
[87] POB, Ref: t16751013-3 (accessed 16/12/16).
[88] Patricia Crawford, *Parents of Poor Children in England 1580–1800* (Oxford, 2010), 27.
[89] Robert Blair, *The Life of Mr Robert Blair, Minister of St Andrews (1593–1636)*, ed. Robert McCrie, Wodrow Society (Edinburgh, 1848), 17–18. See also Bury, *An account*, 122; Bulstrode Whitelocke, *The Diary of Bulstrode Whitelocke, 1605–1675*, ed. Ruth Spalding (Oxford, 1990), 764.
[90] Heywood, *The Rev. Oliver Heywood*, vol. 3, 245; see also John Shower (ed.), *Some account of the holy life and death of Mr Henry Gearing* (1699), 113–14.

twelve-year-old Alice Thornton told her mother that during her illness she had been 'overjoyed...with the glorious sights she then saw, as if heaven opened to receave her, and she was angry to be disturbed from that happinesse' upon her revival.[91] Children seem to have had especially vivid imaginations of what Heaven would be like, which perhaps explains their distress when they escaped death.[92]

The above responses may seem scarcely credible. It is possible that patients may have exaggerated their disappointment in their survival as a way to elicit praise and esteem from their families and friends, since such a response was evidence of a person's election to Heaven. The art of death, the dominant model of deathbed carriage in early modern England, taught that willingness to die was essential for salvation; patients may therefore have feared that to express too much joy upon survival would expose their previous statements of resignation as false.[93] Emotions scholars would interpret these expressions as careful performances, designed to tread a fine balance between longing for death and gratitude for life.[94] Nonetheless, patients' disappointment begins to seem more plausible once we examine contemporary comparisons of earthly and heavenly existence. From their infancy, English churchgoers were taught about the 'vanity of life' compared to the 'infinite joys' of Heaven, a message espoused in sermons, ballads, and imaginative literature. 'As our life is very short so is it very miserable, and therefore it is well it is short', summed up Jeremy Taylor in one of the most popular devotional guides of the seventeenth century.[95] He elaborated:

> Our dayes are full of sorrow and anguish, dishonoured...with many sins,...insnared with passions, amazed with fears, full of cares...warne away with labours, loaden with diseases, daily vexed with dangers..., and in love with misery.

He continued, even 'Mens joyes are troublesome', since 'the fear of losing them takes away the present pleasure', while 'his very fulnesse' from sensual delights, 'swells him and makes him breath[e] short upon his bed'.[96] By contrast, Paradise was 'all joy and no sorrow'.[97] Patients often agreed with these comparisons. After reading a treatise on death, the Manchester wigmaker Edmund Harrold (b. 1678) wrote, 'I[']le reflect thus, that...we al[l] have our exercise in this world, one by sickness, another by death of chil[dr]en...So that we are always troubling our selves about one object or other'.[98] The poetry and prose of Alathea Bethell (1655–1708)

---

[91] Alice Thornton, *The Autobiography of Mrs Alice Thornton*, ed. Charles Jackson, Surtees Society, vol. 62 (1875), 151.

[92] See Newton, '"Rapt up in Joy"', 99.

[93] Richard Wunderli and Gerald Broce, 'The Final Moment before Death in Early Modern England', *Sixteenth Century Journal*, 20 (1989), 259–75. See Chapter 3, note 7 on the art of death.

[94] The idea that emotions are performed was developed by Fay Bound Alberti, in her thesis, 'Emotion in Early Modern England: Performativity and Practice at the Church Courts of York, c. 1660–1760' (D.Phil., University of York, 2000).

[95] Jeremy Taylor, *The rule and exercises of holy dying* (1651), 36, 44; this text went through nineteen editions.

[96] On the imperfections of earthly pleasures, see Senault, *The use of passions*, 308–9, 475.

[97] Henry Gearing, *A prospect of heaven* (1673), 246–7.

[98] Edmund Harrold, *The Diary of Edmund Harrold, Wigmaker of Manchester 1712–15*, ed. Craig Horner (Aldershot, 2009), 30.

from Basingstoke is full of sayings about how 'no Earthly Happyness was Ever trusted to without a disapoyntment', and 'this world nothing in it is of any Reall worth'.[99]

Lived experience as well as reading and reflection lay behind patients' disappointment not to die. Assailed by financial troubles and a loveless marriage, the London gentlewoman Elizabeth Freke (1642–1714) bewailed, 'God spared my life to know [suffer] more misery'.[100] One can only imagine how terrible patients in real poverty would have felt.[101] Another woman whose love-life precipitated these thoughts was the ailing Londoner Anne Halkett (1623–99), when she discovered that her fiancé was already married: she welcomed death, saying, 'I expected now an end to all my misfortunes...butt itt seemes the Lord...thought fit...to spare mee'.[102] These examples testify to the extreme impact romantic relationships exerted on women's attitudes to life and death, an influence from which men were not immune.[103]

Other powerful circumstances that left some patients disgruntled not to die were old age and bereavement. In her mid-sixties, the Hertfordshire gentlewoman Sarah Cowper (1644–1720) considered that while 'life in its self [is] a Blessing,... He that lives Long do's many times outlive his Happiness', due to the 'Decays that Age make on him'.[104] Although speaking in the third person, these sentiments seem to have reflected Cowper's own feelings about life and death. For the bereaved, survival meant the postponement of a joyful reunion in Heaven. Six months after the loss of his wife, the lawyer and politician Bulstrode Whitelocke (1605–75) fell sick of a fever, during which illness he was 'full of...desire of death, & to goe to his deare wife'.[105] When he recovered, he was not altogether happy. Amongst the poorer groups in society, these responses were also reported, though the evidence is indirect and possibly fictional. A ballad from 1675–96, describes how a young man from Wolverhampton longs for death following the decease of his sweetheart:

> [M]y very Soul's opprest:
> I'd fain surrender up my Breath, to give me ease...
> For Life is worse to me than Death.[106]

Further evidence of patients' distress at survival is the fact that whole books were dedicated to this predicament. William Hooke (1600/1–78), a minister in Bishopsgate, published a treatise about the unique 'opportunities thou hast... on this side of Heaven, beyond what are to be enjoyed there'. His aim was to convince people they 'should not so passionately desire death...but prize life'.

[99] Lambeth Palace Library, London, MS240, fols. 33v, 28r; see also fols. 3r–4r, 39r, 45r–45v, 51v (Prose and verse meditations of Alathea Bethell). Other examples from poetry are Brotherton Library, Leeds, MS Lt 36, fol. 12v (Edmund Waller's poetry); Bod, Ashmole MS 718, fol. 137 (Edward Lapworth, 'Verses Written by Dctr Latworth in an Extreamity of Sicknes wch he Suffered').

[100] Elizabeth Freke, *The Remembrances of Elizabeth Freke*, ed. Raymond Anselment, Camden Fifth Series, vol. 18 (Cambridge, 2001), 61.

[101] Poignant accounts of the financial straits of poor families are provided in Crawford, *Parents of Poor Children*.

[102] Halkett, *The Autobiography*, 35–6, 65.

[103] Dudley Ryder, *The Diary of Dudley Ryder*, ed. William Matthews (1939), 294–5; see also 343.

[104] Cowper, *Diary*, vol. 5, 43–4.   [105] Whitelocke, *The Diary*, 248.

[106] *An answer to the maiden's tragedy* (1675–96?); see also *The lamented lovers*.

These opportunities included 'reproving Sin, confuting Errors, instructing the Ignorant,... feed[ing] the hungry...cloth[ing] the naked, visit[ing] the sick', none of which could be performed in Heaven because 'there is no Sin, no Error, no Ignorance..., none Afflicted'.[107] A patient who failed to cherish his survival was like 'a lazy servant', who 'will be often listening to the Clock,... and longing for the Evening, not minding so much his Work as his Wages'.[108] There was clearly an appetite for this advice, as can be discerned from the fact that some patients requested prayers on their behalf to make them 'content to live'.[109] In sum, while the escape from death was usually a cause for celebration, there were also occasions when patients felt a degree of disappointment: it depended on one's soteriological confidence and life circumstances.

FAMILY AND FRIENDS

The second half of this chapter examines the reactions of families and friends to the patient's survival. This investigation yields insights into the strength of affection between these parties, as well as the relationship between different passions. Our story begins with loved ones' feelings while the patient was still in danger of death, a time during which their minds oscillated between the dichotomous passions of hope and fear. The clergyman Philip Henry (1631–96) was 'full of cares & fears', and 'betw[een] hope & fear' for his 'dear Child' Matthew in 1673.[110] Hope was defined as a motion of the soul which 'with fervency seeks after an absent, difficult, possible good', while fear was the fervent recoiling of the soul from *some approaching Evill, wherewith man is threatned, without any apparence to be able to avoyd it easily*.[111] These two passions were inextricably linked—in the words of Senault, they 'go hand in hand, and seldom apart: they march together as do the prisoners with their Guards'.[112] Both 'hold a man in suspense', but whereas the 'object of hope is good', the object of fear is bad.[113] These polarized 'objects' made the two passions torturous to experience—relatives and friends felt their minds were being stretched 'on the rack'.[114]

The precise balance of hope and fear depended partly on whether or not the individual was physically present during the illness. For those who were present, emotions tended to correspond with the patient's changing condition, directly observable to onlookers. When possible signs of death appeared, fear overcame all hope, and loved ones practically went into mourning. One evening in 1671, the ailing Bulstrode Whitelocke was sitting by the fire with his wife, son, and friend

---

[107] William Hooke, *The priveledge of the saints on earth beyond those in heaven* (1673), 12–13.
[108] Ibid., 108.   [109] Heywood, *The Rev. Oliver Heywood*, vol. 2, 104.
[110] Philip Henry, *The Diaries and Letters of Philip Henry of Broad Oak, Flintshire, A.D. 1631–1696*, ed. M. H. Lee (London, 1882), 256. See also Paston, *The Whirlpool*, 164.
[111] Senault, *The use of passions*, 320; Coeffeteau, *A table*, 430. See also W. Ayloffe, *The government of the passions* (1700), 91.
[112] Senault, *The use of passions*, 314.   [113] Coeffeteau, *A table*, 515.
[114] BL, Additional MS 70115, unfoliated manuscript letter from Lady Abigail Harley to her husband Edward about their infant son Brian, c.1680s (Portland papers, 1688–98).

Mr Pearson; suddenly Bulstrode's 'sight & speech began to fayle him, & stretching down his hands, his eyes sett, his throat ratled, & he fell down out of his chayre'. His son Samuel cried out in panic, 'O mother looke to my father[!]' These extracts indicate that the fear of death was a deeply sensory experience: the sight of the staring or cast up eyes, and the sound of rasping breath—two of the most notorious 'messengers of death'—provoked terror in loved ones.[115] When the patient seemed to revive, however, hopes started to outstrip fears. Alice Thornton noted that God 'did begin to give us better hopes, the smale pox then comeing out and appeare[ing]' on her daughter's skin, signs that the venomous humour was leaving the body.[116] Clearly, laypeople were familiar with the prognostic signs of life and death, perhaps helped by the many vernacular books available on the subject.[117]

The experiences of absent relatives and friends seem to have been less variable—almost always, their fears outweighed their hopes, regardless of any optimistic reports from the patient's household. The politician from Buckinghamshire Ralph Verney (1613–96) wrote to the wife of his old family friend Lord Lee in 1639, saying, 'Sweet Maddame, I heard a rumour of your husband's sicknesse...and though the same letter told me the physitions were confident' about his prognosis, 'yet I shall not be satisfied untill I heare it confirmed by yourself, for when my freinds are ill my feares I confesse overcome my hopes'.[118] It is easy to see why Verney was so suspicious—he knew that it was common for the sick to be falsely reported as better, only to find out later that they had already passed away.[119] These individuals were commonly 'soe terrified and frightned' that they could 'take noe rest' at night, and in the daytime waited, 'tremblingly afraid of some worse news'.[120] Just before dinner, the famous diarist and naval officer Samuel Pepys (1633–1703) heard that a man from Huntingdon had come to speak with him; he recorded, 'how my heart [did] come into my mouth [fearing]...that my father, who had been long sicke, was dead. It put me into a trembling'. Luckily, 'it was no such thing, but a countryman come about ordinary business'.[121] Not being present left loved ones in a state of helpless suspense—they wanted to be able to check with their own senses that the patient was still alive, but instead had to depend on the often unreliable postal system.[122]

Once the patient was out of danger, fears were quenched, and hopes melted into joy. Joy was understood to be the fulfilment of the heart's hopes: it was 'the enjoying

[115] John Macollo, *XCIX canons, or rules learnedly describing an excellent method for practitioners in physic* (1659), 58–9; Nicolas Culpeper *Semeiotica uranica: or, an astrological judgement of diseases* (1651), 151–2.

[116] Thornton, *The Autobiography*, 159. See Chapter 1, pp. 51–2 on this theory.

[117] For example, Culpeper lists numerous signs of life or death in his *Semeiotica uranica*.

[118] Frances Verney (ed.), *The Verney Memoirs, 1600–1659*, vol. 1 (1925, first publ. 1892), 148.

[119] Ibid., 149; Anne Clifford, *The Diaries of Lady Anne Clifford*, ed. D. D. H. Clifford (Stroud, 1990), 35–6.

[120] Freke, *The Remembrances*, 68; Paston, *The Whirlpool*, 164.

[121] Samuel Pepys, *The Diary of Samuel Pepys*, ed. Henry B. Wheatley (1893), Project Gutenberg, managed by Phil Gyford: <http://www.pepysdiary.com/archive/1667/03/01/> (accessed 9/12/16).

[122] On developments in the postal system, see James Daybell, *The Material Letter in Early Modern England: Manuscript Letters and the Culture and Practices of Letter-Writing, 1512–1635* (Basingstoke, 2012), 109–47.

of a pleasing Good, which renders the soul content, and which interdicts... desires...and fear'.[123] These feelings were so intense they were difficult to articulate. The Suffolk politician John Hervey (1665–1751) told his convalescing wife, '[it] gives me joy inexpressible...for thy precious life is of so inestimable value to me'.[124] Shouts, embraces, and tears, rather than words, were the best way to convey these feelings. The survival of eleven-year-old Martha Hatfield from 'Spleen-winde' in 1652 occasioned 'many tears of joy', and her friends and relations' 'hearts were mightily ravished with the appearance of God in this Businesse', wrote her uncle James Fisher.[125] In Galenic medical theory, crying was regarded as a therapeutic measure through which the body's internal healing agent, 'Nature', expelled the superfluous humours generated in extreme passions like joy, thereby preventing disease, or even death. The Sheffield physician Timothy Bright (c.1551–1615) explained that happy tears 'most commonly falleth out, when he whom we love hath escaped daunger', by reason of the 'fulnesse of the spirits, & heat', and the 'enlargement of the heart', which 'for[c]eth out...the moysture...of the eyes & distilleth into drops'.[126]

The happy responses of family and friends to survival varied once more according to how they found out about it—whether in the flesh or by letter. Those who were present in the household witnessed with their own senses the extraordinary shift in the patient's appearance, from the 'affrightful Spectacle' of a deathlike state to a more lively condition, a change that occasioned blissful relief.[127] The Essex minister Anthony Walker (c.1622–92) recorded that when he and his wife were both taken ill together:

> I recovered first, and when I first could leave my Bed, and creep into her Chamber, the sight of me was like Life from the Dead. She hath oft[en] told me, she could not express what alteration it made in her[:] the joy so revived her Spirits it helped to cure her.[128]

Elizabeth's joy at seeing her husband's lively looks was so great that it contributed to her recovery: this passion multiplied the body's spirits, the instruments used by Nature to remove disease.[129] Even when temporarily out of the sickroom, the patient's sudden escape from death could be a sensory experience for loved ones, though aural rather than visual. Alice Thornton recalled that at three in the morning, the very hour the doctor expected her husband's death, she was 'wakened...out of sleepe' by the sound of his voice calling for 'toste and butter'. Speaking was proof of life, but what made his words all the more welcome was that an appetite

---

[123] Senault, *The use of passions*, 442–3.

[124] John Hervey, *Letter-Books of John Hervey, First Earl of Bristol, vol. 1, 1651–1715* (Wells, 1894), 300.

[125] James Fisher, *The wise virgin, or, a wonderful narration of the various dispensations towards a childe of eleven years of age* (1653), 149.

[126] Timothy Bright, *A treatise of melancholie* (1586), 150.

[127] *Heraclitus Christianus, or the man of sorrow* (1677), 168.

[128] Elizabeth Walker, *The vertuous wife*, ed. Anthony Walker (1694), 55–6. See also Archer, 'The Diary', 150.

[129] See Chapter 1 on the role of Nature and the spirits in recovery.

for food was a sign of growing health.[130] A common feature of families' experiences was 'how fast' acute illnesses 'gallop out', often occurring overnight.[131] In 1630, the London woodturner Nehemiah Wallington (1598–1658) recorded that his 'sweet Sonne Samuel' suffered 'sore fites of convultion', so that:

> I sayd unto my selfe (over night)...I should not see him alive in the morning: But behold the greate goodnes of my God which of his grate mercy gave him unto mee againe in the morning...Though sorrow may abide in the evening yet joy comes in the morning.[132]

The last line, taken from Psalm 30, was quoted regularly in this context—the verse seemed to capture perfectly the wonderful change in emotions.[133]

Even more dramatic experiences were reported by those relations who had been away during the illness, but made a special journey to see the patient upon recovery. One night in 1730, the minister and medic James Clegg (1679–1755), received a message from his brother 'to call me to my son James, dangerously ill of a Fever', from which he 'feard I should scarce find him alive'. At bedtime, 'sleep departed from me...and my heart was filld with fears and trouble'. When morning came, he 'set out for Manchester in heavy rain and with an heavy heart'. Arriving by noon, 'I...found my son alive, for ever blessed be God'. He declared, 'May I ever retain a thankful sence of the goodness of God in these instances of my heart'.[134] The need to remember divine mercies was one of the spiritual duties of recovered patients and their families, necessary for sustaining holy affections, such as love for the Almighty.[135] These religious feelings were augmented when, after a delayed or hazardous journey, God brought the loved one safely to the patient's bedside. This was the case for Elizabeth Freke in 1705: late at night, she received news that her husband was in 'great Hazard of his Life...which filled my Heart with Sorrow, and banished all Sleep frem my Eyes'. She spent the night 'labouring for a Conveyance to *London*', but only succeeded at two in the morning, thanks to prayers 'cry'd to God'. By ten o'clock, 'I came safe to *London*, to a living Husband!' Her soul 'filled with Praise...after such Experience of his Power'.[136] In both these examples, it was the terrible uncertainty—not knowing if the patient was dead or alive—that enhanced the proceeding joy. As the philosopher Senault confirmed, 'Joy measureth it self so justly by sorrow, that...nothing adds more to Pleasure than the Pain that hath gon before it'. He gave an example of an only son, whose mother was in fear of his death: 'her joy ariseth from her sorrow; and the contentment of enjoying him would not be so great, had she not fear'd to have lost him'.[137]

---

[130] See Chapter 2, pp. 78–9.

[131] Robert Harris, *Hezekiahs recovery. Or, a sermon, shewing what use Hezekiah did, and all should make of their deliverance from sicknesse* (1626), 46.

[132] London Metropolitan Library, MS 204, p. 433 (Nehemiah Wallington, 'A Record of the Mercies of God: or A Thankfull Remembrance').

[133] Psalm 30:5; see also Newcome, *The Autobiography*, 96–7.

[134] James Clegg, *The Diary of James Clegg of Chapel-en-Frith 1708–1755*, vol. 1 (1708–36), ed. Vanessa Doe, Derbyshire Record Society, vol. 5 (Matlock, 1978), 97–9.

[135] See Chapter 4 on these duties.   [136] Bury, *An account*, 153–4.

[137] Senault, *The use of passions*, 469.

Given that 'joy was measured by sorrow', it may come as no surprise that amongst the most ecstatic reactions were from those relatives who had been led to believe that the patient was already dead, and thought they were travelling to see what they assumed would be the corpse. In 1618, the clerk of the chancery, Paul D'Ewes (1567–1631), was dining in Chancery Lane, when several of his junior colleagues expressed their condolence for the 'abortive loss' of his eldest son Simonds, aged 16. Shocked by this news, D'Ewes set out immediately towards Cambridge where his son was studying at the University, stopping overnight in Ware; the next morning, as he entered the outskirts of the city, he met a student, of whom he asked, 'what was the news there'. The young man replied 'None sir,... but that a fellow-commoner of St. John's College, whose name I know not' died 'two days since', a report which 'banished all' lingering hope, and filled [his] heart only with sorrow; so he now thought of nothing else... but that he should come time enough to see [Simonds] interred'. A few miles further on, Paul D'Ewes passed another student, and asked again of his son; he received the following reply: 'I am of that college, and know [your son] very well; and heard but this morning... that he was fully recovered'. This father's hopes were rekindled, and he 'rode on more cheerfully'. Finally, entering his son's chamber, he found him alive and well, to his immense joy; the two expressed their 'mutual congratulations' and took supper together.[138] Simonds had been brought up mainly by his grandparents, so this example reveals that such arrangements did not necessarily inhibit parents' love for their children, as was once assumed.[139] We might think that Paul D'Ewes' happiness was enhanced by Simonds' status as first-born and heir, but the survival of younger children also elicited extreme joy, as will be demonstrated below.[140]

Even when relations knew that they would arrive to find their loved one alive, the joy could be extreme. This was the case for the Leeds wool merchant and former parliamentarian soldier John Thoresby (1626–79). His second-born son, Ralph, aged 20, was sick of ague while sailing back to England from Rotterdam in 1678, and the ship was nearly wrecked during a storm. The young man recorded that his father 'was extremely full of fears, alarms, and disturbances during that storm, [even] though he knew nothing of my being in it'. As soon as he heard of his son's safe arrival, he 'came in person' to meet him at the port in Hull, 'and what a meeting we had[,] which shall never be forgotten by me'. Usually 'full of rhetoric', his father 'could not express his joy otherwise than by tears, (not usual from a soldier) and embraces that would have moved an adamant', that legendary rock of diamond-like hardness.[141] Besides revealing the immense affection between a

---

[138] Simonds D'Ewes, *The Autobiography and Correspondence of Sir Simonds D'Ewes, Bart.*, ed. J. O. Halliwell, 2 vols. (1845) vol. 1, 129–30. Simonds had suffered an injury to his head from an accident involving the chapel bell.

[139] Stone, *The Family, Sex and Marriage*, 84–6. Stone refers to D'Ewes here.

[140] Stone assumed heirs monopolized their parents' affections, ibid., 87. Ralph Houlbrooke has produced a more balanced picture, showing that while 'Primogeniture... reinforce[d] the bond between fathers and... eldest sons,... this did not mean that fathers were indifferent to... younger offspring': *The English Family, 1450–1700* (1984), 179–82, at 180; see also Linda Pollock, 'Younger Sons in Tudor and Stuart England', *History Today*, 39 (1989), 23–9.

[141] Thoresby, *The Diary*, vol. 1, 27–8.

father and his adult son, this example shows that even members of the most masculine of professions shed tears on occasions.[142]

The most varied emotional experiences were those of relatives and friends who learned of the patient's survival not in person, but by letter or messenger. At one end of the spectrum were those individuals who heard this news before they had even realized the patient had been in danger. When suffering from a 'grievous sicknes...which I thought would have put an end to my days', eighteen-year-old Oliver Heywood sent to his 'friends in the country to signify my condition, yet by miscariage of letters they heard not of my sicknes til they heard of my recovery'. He was grateful to God for 'preventing...my indulgent mother[']s sorrow' had she known his true state.[143] Some forty years later, Heywood himself was party to this experience: when his sons Eliezer and John were sick in 1692, he 'never knew one syllable of it' until one of the boys came home, and 'told me of the tragicomedy of both their ilnes and recovery'. This experience bolstered Heywood's trust in his 'prayer-hearing god' by fulfilling the pledge in Isaiah 65, 'before they call I will answer'.[144] Given that joy was enhanced by preceding fear, we might expect these relations—shielded from the terror of death—to have responded with more muted joy when they heard the news. But this seems not to have been so: relatives found that the knowledge God had tenderly protected them from sorrows made the situation doubly joyful, since it encouraged feelings of mutual love between themselves and the Lord, keenly desired holy affections.

Similar experiences were reported by relatives and friends who heard the news of sickness and survival in close succession. In 1688, Dr John Tillotson (1630–94), who soon after became archbishop of Canterbury, 'received...two letters' from his wife, 'who in the first told me she feared my child was dying, which troubled me much; in the other that she was perfectly well, which amazed me more...so soon can God when he pleases turn our mourning into joy'.[145] Fortunately, this father's fears were short-lived, and rapidly gave way to happiness, a transformation once again attributed directly to God. It was not only parents who partook in these experiences. In 1698, the Yorkshire vicar Thomas Brockbank (1671–1732) received a letter from his cousin Rowland Tatham, stating:

> [W]e were all in sore trouble of mind when we heard of your sickness. I was at Your Fathers house the next day after your Tutors Letter got thither so...I was the messenger of that unacceptable newes to your...Grandfather and the rest of your Relations & wellwishers with us...We were all Jealous your good Tutor had not writ of the worst til we had the happiness to see a confirmation of Your own writing, which your good Father took the pains to bring over the next day as soon as he'd received it, knowing it to be satisfaction to us allso.

[142] On attitudes to crying in males, see Chapter 3, note 203.

[143] Heywood, *The Rev. Oliver Heywood*, vol. 1, 162.

[144] Ibid., vol. 3, 348–9. For another example, see Cambridge University Library, Buxton MS 104/35 (Family archive of Buxtons of Channons).

[145] Russell, *Letters*, 249. See also William Lawrence, *The Pyramid and the Urn: Life in Letters of a Restoration Squire: William Lawrence of Shurdington, 1636–1697*, ed. Iona Sinclair (Stroud, 1994), 55.

Tatham added that his own mother—Thomas' aunt—was 'not a little glad to hear the certainty of your good recovery'.[146] This letter reveals the reciprocal love between son and father, as well as grandparents, cousins, and aunts. It also shows that it was not always the 'miscarriage of letters' that lay behind the delayed news of illness: rather, patients or their carers sometimes decided to defer the correspondence until they could give better tidings in order to avoid creating unnecessary anxiety.

Less fortunate were those correspondents who, rather than hearing of the patient's safety before ever learning of the danger, were informed—incorrectly—that their loved one was already dead. Elizabeth Freke received in 1710 'a fattall letter of the death of my deerst sister the Lady Norton from my cosin Mills in London'. She thanked God that 'affter my being allmost a week destracted for her,...I heard shee was recovered'.[147] This woman had been plunged into 'distraction', an early stage of mourning characterized by spells of delirium and weeping, before she eventually experienced blissful relief.[148] These misreported deaths were common.[149] Doctors and philosophers believed that the emotional transformation that took place in this situation was so extreme that it could kill! Coeffeteau explained that,

[I]f...joy proceed from an unexpected thing which concernes us much, it [the heart] may be so mooved and agitated, as death may follow. As it happened to those women of [the ancient city of] *Carthage*, who having newes of their sonnes had beene slaine in battaile, when as they saw them living before their eyes: this joy happening contrary to their [expectations], they dyed suddainely.[150]

This thinking might seem to contradict the earlier statement that sudden joy could cure illness, but in fact, it does not, because the timing and depth of the emotion differed. Sudden, unexpected joy made the heart propel all the spirits to the body's extremities, leaving the heart 'abandon'd and destitute of strength'. By contrast, joy that developed slightly more gradually—the kind that came on as a relative witnessed in person their loved one's revival from a deathlike state—caused a less violent movement of spirits, so that the heart did not lose all its vital juice.[151]

Why did these cases of misreported deaths occur? One explanation relates to the Church's insistence on the need for Christians to resign themselves to the possible decease of their loved ones, a reaction which signified respect for God's providence.[152] Pious individuals may have sought to achieve this necessary acceptance by telling themselves that the person was dying, if not already dead.

---

[146] Thomas Brockbank, *The Diary and Letter Book of the Rev. Thomas Brockbank 1671–1709*, ed. Richard Trappes-Lomax, Chetham Society New Series, vol. 89 (Manchester, 1930), 25–6.

[147] Freke, *The Remembrances*, 154.   [148] Newton, *The Sick Child*, 139–40.

[149] For example, Christopher Hatton, *Correspondence of the Family of Hatton being Chiefly Addressed to Christopher, First Viscount Hatton, 1601–1704*, ed. Edward Maunde Thompson, Camden Society, vol. 22 (1878), 58–9; BL, Additional MS 28050, fol. 62r (Domestic correspondence of the Osborne family, 1637–1761).

[150] Coeffeteau, *A table*, 253. See also James Hart, *Klinike, or the diet of the diseased* (1633), 397, 400.

[151] Timothy Nourse, *A discourse upon the nature and faculties of man* (1686), 141–2.

[152] On resignation, see Newton, *The Sick Child*, 149–51.

A rather more practical explanation is provided in the memoirs of Simonds D'Ewes. Recovering from a violent fever in 1625, Simonds 'slept so long and soundly the next morning' that his nurse decided to keep

> [T]he chamber doors shut, and not suffering anyone to come to enquire how I did, divers began to doubt, not knowing my partial recovery, whether I were alive or dead. Nay, after my father and the rest of the family [had] ascertained my well-doing, yet most of the neighbouring towns who knew of my sickness, hearing the knell-bell to ring the same morning...for a poor workman, then newly dead in my father's house, thought verily I had been departed out of this life...by which means the report of my death was falsely spread...many miles off from the place where I lay sick. So that I may say that I did, after a manner, outlive myself.[153]

A series of coincidences, together with gossip, were the reasons that people started to believe D'Ewes had died. In a society that recognized the danger of words, and took very seriously such things as slander and scolding, gossip was a powerful medium of communication, which could spread news far and wide.[154] A condemnatory view of such rumours was given by Oliver Heywood, who had been 'confidently reported... dead' in 1700 by five or six letters 'writ up to London': he was not amused, writing, 'Alas what a lying world is this! some raise a groundles report, [and] others tell it confidently without examining the grounds therof'.[155] In sum, while loved ones shared in common a transition from fear and hope, to joy, the balance and timing of these emotional changes varied according to how they learned about it.

While emotions cannot be quantified, it is possible to identify several factors which seem to have augmented the depth of loved ones' responses to survival. The first was the age or life-stage of the patient. The survival of children and youths tended to elicit particularly effusive expressions of joy from parents and other relatives, since they wished to see them enjoy a long life and fulfil their potential. When Elizabeth Egerton's (1626–63) little daughter Frances was ill, she asked God to 'raise my deare Babe to long life, that she may enjoy the Honour of Age'.[156] Old age was an 'honourable estate', despite its associated weaknesses.[157] Parents also expressed a desire for their offspring to grow up to be 'a great comfort to my gray haires', referring to both the financial and emotional support provided by children.[158] For young male survivors of middling status, hopes were usually directed at

---

[153] D'Ewes, *The Autobiography*, vol. 1, 260. See also Izaak Walton, *The lives of Dr John Donne, Sir Henry Wotton, Mr Richard Hooker, Mr George Herbert written by Isaak Walton* (1670), 68–70.

[154] Laura Gowing, *Domestic Dangers: Women, Words, and Sex in Early Modern Oxford* (Oxford, 1996); Bernard Capp, *When Gossips Meet: Women, Family and Neighbourhood in Early Modern England* (Oxford, 2004).

[155] Heywood, *The Rev. Oliver Heywood*, vol. 3, 302.

[156] BL, MS Egerton 607, pp. 18–23 ('True coppies of scertaine loose Papers left by the Right honourable Elizabeth Countesse of Bridgewater, Collected and Transcribed together here since her Death Anno Dm 1663'). See also Newcome, *The Autobiography*, vol. 1, 105.

[157] For a defence of old age, see Thomas Sheafe, *Vindiciae senectutis, or, a plea for old-age* (1639), *passim.*

[158] Ralph Josselin, *The Diary of Ralph Josselin 1616–1683*, ed. Alan Macfarlane (Oxford, 1991), 308. See also Robert Woodford, *The Diary of Robert Woodford, 1637–1641*, ed. John Fielding, Camden Society, vol. 42 (2012), 103; Freke, *The Remembrances*, 244.

their budding career potential. In 1680, Isaac Lawrence had just been admitted into the East India Company before falling dangerously ill; his older brother wrote how he longed for him to live, so that he can 'shine' in his new career, 'increase in wealth and title, grow rich abroad and great at home'.[159] The equivalent ambition for young women was to see them on their wedding days, or as new mothers. The Countess of Manchester expressed her relief that her niece, 'for whom I have soe tender an affection', was out of danger in 1681, adding, 'I pray God she may…in His time, bring a son into [the] family'.[160] Not surprisingly, fathers of young children expressed special joy when their wives survived illness, knowing that their offspring were highly dependent on their mothers for care. In turn, wives were relieved when their husbands survived to fulfil their allotted gender roles as breadwinners.[161] 'Make her a joyfull mother', cried the attorney Robert Woodford (1606–54) when his wife Hannah lay very ill in 1637, so that 'she may bring up the poore infant with comfort'.[162] The reproductive roles of men were also celebrated in this context. James Clegg's joy at the preservation of his adult son from fever was enhanced by the consideration that, the day before, his daughter-in-law had been delivered of a baby daughter: he was relieved that the newborn 'should [not] be deprivd…of its Father'.[163] Such reflections could also take place retrospectively. About thirty years after her son's recovery from a nearly fatal accident, Elizabeth Freke thanked God that he went on to become 'the father of two lovely boys'.[164] These examples are useful reminders that parenthood was an important component of masculine, as well as feminine, identity.[165]

The other major factor to influence the intensity of emotional responses to survival was the depth of affection between the two parties. Men and women who were in love—courting or married—were amongst those who professed the greatest joy upon survival. When Ralph Josselin's wife Jane was ill in 1648, he lamented that his house would not be a home without her; on another occasion, when she was well, he was 'sensible of the comfort of my wife, my love', noting that 'every[-]thing [is] more pleasant because I have her'.[166] Wives often felt the same. The Wiltshire gentlewoman Joan Thynne (1558–1612) told her husband John that in his 'well-doing consists my only joy and comfort', and desired him to preserve his health 'for the good of me'.[167] The word 'comfort' is ubiquitous in these accounts—it referred to the enjoyment couples took in each other's company, as well as the practical support they provided.[168] Another familial relationship which gave rise to these intense feelings was the parent–child connection, deemed by some moralists

---

[159] Lawrence, *The Pyramid*, 55.   [160] Hatton, *Correspondence*, vol. 2, 5.

[161] On the financial repercussions of illness, see Chapter 6, pp. 222–4.

[162] Woodford, *The Diary*, 100, 125. See also Archer, 'The Diary', 139.

[163] Clegg, *The Diary*, 97–9 (also 14–15).   [164] Freke, *The Remembrances*, 42.

[165] On men's sadness at not being able to have children, see Helen Berry and Elizabeth Foyster, 'Childless Men in Early Modern England', in their edited volume, *The Family in Early Modern England* (Cambridge, 2007), 158–83.

[166] Josselin, *The Diary*, 433. See also Russell, *Letters*, vol. 2, 90–1.

[167] Alison Wall (ed.), *Two Elizabethan Women: Correspondence of Joan and Maria Thynne 1575–1611*, Wiltshire Record Society, vol. 38 (Devizes, 1983), 30. See also Thornton, *The Autobiography*, 168.

[168] OED, 'comfort' (noun): 'Pleasure, enjoyment, delight, gladness' (accessed 19/10/16).

to be the 'second strictest tie' implanted by God after conjugal love.[169] When fourteen-year-old Mary Glover from London survived diabolical possession in 1602, her father 'tooke her by the hand, as not beinge able to speake a word: and the mother went...with like watery cheekes kissed her'.[170] Since 'mighty Joys' as well as grief were said to 'exceed all our Words', these inarticulate gestural responses convey the extreme happiness of Mary's parents.[171] Offspring seem to have felt the same when their parents escaped death, though in the case of young children, we have to go by indirect evidence owing to a lack of written accounts by this age group.[172] After conjugal and parental love, 'the third...strictest tie' of affection was the love between siblings, a relationship which has only recently begun to attract historical attention.[173] Alice Hatton told her 'deare brother' in 1687 'I cant but dread' his possible death 'which would, I am sure, be the greatest [affliction] that can happen to me in this world'. If he recovered, she said 'what ever ellse God pleases to lay upon me, I will never repine, but thinke myself happie soe long as I have my dearest brother'.[174] Brothers frequently returned these feelings.[175]

Although the Church held that the love God implanted between spouses, parents, and siblings was the most extraordinary, lived experience taught that unrelated individuals also felt intense emotions upon the patient's potential death and eventual survival.[176] When the Norfolk MP Robert Paston survived a violent attack in 1675, his friend John Hildeyard, rector and JP, told him that the news of his survival

> [G]ave me an happy allay to my griefe and now the very remaynes thereof are van-guished and by your prefect recovery wholy swallowed up into joy...all your friends are much joyed at your deliverance.[177]

Language of combat and liquid is used here to describe the way one passion is usurped by another, a fitting choice given that the emotions were imagined as powerful fluids, which competed with each other.[178] Work colleagues purported to share these feelings. Paston's attorney, Thomas Bulwer (*c.*1612–94), told him that his jeopardy did 'cast us upon the brinke of confusion', but that his escape occasioned 'joy & gladnes of harte for soe signall, soe gracious, & soe wonderfull a deliverance'.[179] This somewhat obsequious expression could be dismissed as an

---

[169] *The fathers legacy: or counsels to his children* (1677), 173.

[170] *A true and briefe report, of Mary Glovers vexation* (1603), 51.

[171] Rogers, *Practical discourses*, 156.

[172] Paston, *The Whirlpool*, 164. On difficulties and possible solutions to accessing children's view-points, see Newton, *The Sick Child*, 24–6.

[173] *The fathers legacy*, 173. On siblings, see Naomi Miller and Naomi Yavneh, *Sibling Relations and Gender in the Early Modern World: Sisters, Brothers and Others* (Aldershot, 2006); Patricia Crawford, *Blood, Bodies, and Families in Early Modern England* (Harlow, 2004), ch. 7; Richard Grassby, *Kinship and Capitalism: Marriage, Family, and Business in the English Speaking World, 1580–1740* (Cambridge, 2001), 210–15.

[174] Hatton, *Correspondence*, vol. 2, 65.

[175] For example, see Robert Boyle's letters to his sister Katherine, in his *Occasional reflections*.

[176] *A declaration of the principall pointes of Christian doctrine* (1647), 242–3; Lancelot Andrewes, *The pattern of catechistical doctrine at large* (1650), 31, 339.

[177] Paston, *The Whirlpool*, 167.

[178] See the Introduction, note 92, on the 'hydraulic' model of emotions.

[179] Paston, *The Whirlpool*, 169.

epistolary convention, helpful for lubricating professional relationships, but given that work was an important context in which friendships developed, such affection is plausible.[180] While these examples demonstrate that friends and colleagues as well as relatives could feel hearty joy upon the patient's survival, their reactions may not have been identical to those of families. The very fact that they were able to put their emotions into words would have signalled to contemporaries that their joy was not so extreme as those felt by relatives. As Coeffeteau stated, the afflictions and prosperities of 'those of our blood . . . touch us so neere' that they 'deprive us of our speech . . ., whereas the miseries of our other friends' yield words.[181]

So far the discussions have concentrated on the happy responses of loved ones. We might expect that those individuals who disliked the patient would have reacted with emotions of a different kind, but few admitted to such feelings. Indeed, the reverse seems to have been the case—enemies' vitriol towards the patient was sometimes tempered by a life-threatening condition, a tendency connected to the injunction not to speak ill of the dead. In 1672, the alchemist Thomas Henshaw commented that when his friend Harry Germin recovered from a dangerous state:

> [T]his advantage he hath had by it[:] that pitty hath soften[ed] most men's harts to speake as good words of him as ever I heard of any young gallant which perhaps if his prosperity had continued they would not have afforded him.[182]

Patients themselves were aware of this change of heart. Simonds D'Ewes observed dryly that when he was misreported as dead, 'such as perhaps envied me whilst I lived, were yet heard to lament and condole my immature decease in the very flower of my youth'.[183] The only examples found in this study of overtly negative responses to survival come from those who had stood to gain financially from the patient's death. The London law student Dudley Ryder (1691–1756) recorded that when his elder brother was 'very ill' in 1716, 'I was concerned with myself to find that . . . I found a little kind of pleasure rising in my breast at the thought of my gaining his estate by his death'. He was ashamed of this response, but reassured himself with the thought that 'it is entirely involuntary and I am angry with myself'. When his brother began to get better, Dudley did not voice any gladness.[184] Such a response confirms Joan Thirsk and Patricia Crawford's observation that primogeniture—the inheritance custom whereby the firstborn son was sole heir to the estate—sometimes created resentment in younger brothers.[185] Samuel Pepys expressed similar sentiments, though in relation to his uncle: one morning he awoke to the news that 'uncle Robert is dead'. He confided in his diary that while he was 'sorry in some respect', he was 'glad in my expectations in another respect'. He was 'greedy to see the will, but did not ask to see it till to-morrow', presumably

---

[180] Thomas, *The Ends of Life*, 99.
[181] Coeffeteau, *A table*, 369. See also Ayloffe, *The government*, 119.
[182] Paston, *The Whirlpool*, 141.   [183] D'Ewes, *The Autobiography*, vol. 1, 260.
[184] Ryder, *The Diary*, 341–2.
[185] Joan Thirsk, 'Younger Sons in the 17th Century', *History*, 54 (1969), 358–77; Crawford, *Blood, Bodies, and Families*, 215–16. For a more positive assessment of the effects of primogeniture on fraternal relations, see Grassby, *Kinship and Capitalism*, 210–15. See note 139 in this chapter for further relevant literature.

out of respect for his grieving aunt, whom he noted rather disrespectfully he found 'in bed in a most nasty ugly pickle'.[186] Had his uncle survived, Pepys would probably not have been best pleased. Only the most candid of diarists were prepared to admit to these shameful feelings, but it is likely that such a response was not uncommon—as in any era, some relatives did not get on, and would have preferred financial gain to their relation's continued life.

CONCLUSION

For many patients, recovery was experienced as a narrow escape from death. 'I was snatch'd out of the very Jaws of Death!', exclaimed Thomas Steward in 1699.[187] This close shave usually brought about an emotional transformation from fear to joy, a reaction put down to a combination of natural, soteriological, and earthly factors. These included the instinctive love between the body and soul, a concern about avoiding damnation, and the desire to continue relationships with family and friends in this world. While scholars have examined the fear of Hell, little has been said about these other factors.[188] The personification of the body and soul as 'loving playmates', who were '*loath to depart*', enhances our understanding of how people conceptualized their own beings at this time—they saw themselves as two, intimately connected parts.[189] Patients felt grateful to God for their survival, and saw the 'addition of days' as a gift, or the renewal of '*the lease* of their lives'.[190] However, we have noticed that this joyful response was not universal: for those who were convinced that they were destined for Heaven, or who were undergoing difficult life circumstances, death could seem welcome, and survival, a vexing postponement of eternal happiness. Rather than escaping death, these patients were deprived of 'their escape *by* Death from so manifold hazards and evils of Life'.[191] Ultimately, they felt that all of the joys of survival were inferior versions of what would happen in Heaven—reunion of body and soul, of family and friends, and everlasting life.[192] The great paradox of Christianity is that life is the beginning of death, and death the beginning of life: the biblical phrase, 'I shall not die, but live', thus applies more properly to dying than to surviving.[193] These findings shed fresh light on attitudes to life and death, revealing that these estates were viewed ambivalently. Life was both a gift from God, to be celebrated, and a curse, crossed with sorrows; likewise, death was an affront to nature, the king of terrors, but it was also the pathway to everlasting bliss.

[186] Pepys, *The Diary*, <http://www.pepysdiary.com/archive/1661/07/06/> (accessed 9/12/16).
[187] Steward, *Sacrificium laudis*, 2.
[188] On the fear of Hell, see note 2 in this chapter.
[189] Thomas Fuller, *Life out of death a sermon preached at Chelsey, on the recovery of an honourable person* (1655), 3–4.
[190] Lawrence, *The Pyramid*, 127; Samuel Cradock, *Knowledge and practice: or a plain discourse... [on] salvation* (1673, first publ. 1659), 108.
[191] *A handkercher for parents wet eyes, upon the death of children* (1630), 51.
[192] George Berkeley, *Historical applications and occasional meditations* (1667), 17–18.
[193] Psalm 118:17.

Families and friends usually shared the experience of the patient, undergoing such an extraordinary transformation of emotions that they found it difficult to describe. The most apposite words came from Scripture, especially Psalm 30:5, 'weeping may endure for a night, but joy cometh in the morning', a verse which captured the rapidity at which the patient could revive. Like patients, relatives saw the survival as a divine gift, or the extension of a loan—God has 'given me him againe', wrote Robert Woodford when his son Sam 'suddenly recovered' in 1638.[194] Relatives' reactions varied subtly according to whether or not they were present at the patient's home, and were able to witness with their own senses their loved one's changing condition. For those who *were* present, the sights and sounds of life after witnessing the sinister tokens of death were wonderful, eliciting joyful tears. Family and friends living further away, reliant on second-hand news from letters or messengers, waited 'tremblingly afraid' of false reports, a concern which prompted many to take a journey to visit the patient. Suspense was then followed by wonderful relief when they arrived to find their loved one alive. In an age of instant communication, it is easy to forget what it must have been like for people at this time.

What has emerged most strikingly in this chapter is the warmth and depth of family bonds and friendships in early modern England. Patients' relief not to be parted from their nearest and dearest was matched by the great joy expressed by their loved ones for survival. Such responses were attributed to the passion of love: a sign of true love was its 'uniting vertue', which made loved ones wish to be 'continually together...and...as little absent as may bee'.[195] On the whole, the most acute emotions were professed by husbands and wives, parents and children, and siblings, a finding which fits with the notion that God had created a hierarchy of love. The popular saying, 'blood is thicker than water', suggests that this notion may have resonated with many people.[196] Nonetheless, such a pattern was not hard and fast—those who had been bereaved, estranged, or embittered from their immediate relations were likely to have enjoyed closer relationships with their friends and wider kin. Nor was it necessarily a question of 'either/or'—many patients enjoyed loving relationships with both their closest relatives *and* their friends and wider kin.[197] Finally, the patient's survival did not always elicit joy from families—some 'interested Persons', wrote Robert Boyle sardonically, could be seen during the illness, 'hover[ing] about the...Man's Bed, as Birds of Prey that wait for a Carcass'.[198]

As well as illuminating personal bonds, the chapter has clarified the relationships between different passions in early modern perceptions, an overlooked question that yields insights into how individual feelings were defined. During serious

---

[194] Woodford, 'The Diary', 165.   [195] Coeffeteau, *A table*, 157–8.

[196] Cited by Crawford, *Blood, Bodies, and Families*, 209. Michael MacDonald's study of mental illness also concludes that the 'emotional lives of ordinary men and women were centred primarily within the nuclear family': *Mystical Bedlam: Madness, Anxiety, and Healing in Seventeenth-Century England* (Cambridge, 1981), 105.

[197] Tadmor reminds us that when considering relationships with family and wider kin/friends, we should not 'formulate either/or questions, but rather...investigate how diverse [were] kinship and family patterns': 'Early Modern English Kinship', 25.

[198] Boyle, *Occasional reflections*, 231.

illness, loved ones were racked between hopes and fears, dichotomous passions that held the soul in suspense, only differing in the nature of the anticipated object. If death was suspected to have happened, fear turned to grief, a passion defined as the realization of the soul's fears.[199] However, when the basis behind sadness was proved to be unfounded—the patient was alive—sorrow turned to joy, wherein the soul 'enjoys the happiness it sought for' during its former hopes.[200] These inter-relationships highlight a central feature of the early modern taxonomy of the emotions, which has not been recognized by historians: passions could be classified according to movement or rest: in fear and hope, the soul strove away from, or towards, the object (death or survival), whereas sadness and joy were the 'rest of the soul', since the anticipated event had happened.[201] Nowadays in Western culture, we are more likely to divide emotions into binaries of negative or positive—we would put fear and sorrow in one column, and hope and joy in another, rather than organizing emotions by level of movement. By highlighting these distinctive characteristics of the early modern passions, this chapter has sought to show how emotions are liable to change over time, a key question in the field of emotions history.[202]

Given the entrenched historiographical view that the doctrine of providence was beginning to lose its hold by the close of the seventeenth century, we might expect to find that patients and their relatives were less likely to regard survival as a form of divine rescue by the close of the period.[203] It would also be reasonable to suppose that reactions to escaping death would have become increasingly joyful, as individuals began to see life on earth as the only form of existence.[204] Neither of these trends are visible, however, a finding that adds to revisionist work which questions this particular form of secularization.[205] While this continuity might partly be a consequence of the pious nature of many of the sources used in this study, it may also reflect just how entrenched were Christian ideas about life and death in English culture.

---

[199] Senault, *The use of passions*, 442.
[200] Ibid., 442–3. See also Ayloffe, *The government*, 113.
[201] Senault, *The use of passions*, 440.
[202] For an introduction to this debate, see Peter Stearns, 'Modern Patterns in Emotions History', in Susan Matt and Peter Stearns (eds.), *Doing Emotions History* (Urbana IL, 2014), 17–40.
[203] See Chapter 4 note 16 for historiography on the decline of belief in providence.
[204] See note 3 in this chapter for the apparent decline of belief in the afterlife.
[205] For this literature, see Chapter 4, note 18.

6

'All is Returned':
Resuming Life

In 1709, the Somerset doctor and musician Claver Morris (*c*.1659–1727) tracked his gradual resumption of normal life after 'spotted fever' as follows:

3 August	So sick of a Fever…that I could not get out of bed.
10	All doubted my recovery…
17	I left off Watchers [nurses].
18	I began to eat Flesh.
20	I writ a Letter to my Daughter Bettey the first I was able to write.
23	I went to Church, & first abroad after my Sickness.
6 September	At the Music-Meeting…
9	I din'd & my Daughter at Mr Brockwell's.
17	I visited Mrs Goold, who was Ill of a Tertian Ague.[1]

These entries reveal that Morris returned to three overlapping spheres of life after his illness: spatial life—his physical location; social life—interactions with family and friends; and working life, as a physician and musician. Organized around these several areas, this chapter asks what it was like to resume everyday life after serious illness: it traces the patient's journey from the sickbed to the wider world of society and work. The overarching argument is that the transition was often found to be physically liberating, socially bonding, and mentally stimulating.[2] Ultimately, patients felt they regained not just their bodily faculties, but all the other aspects of life that they cherished, which sickness had rendered impossible, such as the enjoyment of company, the outdoors, and work. There were, however, downsides: in the early days of recovery, residual weakness rendered daily tasks difficult for some patients, certain actions were thought to precipitate relapse, and for those who disliked their work, or did not get on well with their relations, returning to former interactions and employments could be troublesome. By following the patient out of the sickchamber, this chapter attempts to contribute to historiographical territories normally debarred to medical historians, such as house layout, hospitality, and work.

---

[1] Claver Morris, *The Diary of a West Country Physician, 1648–1726*, ed. Edmund Hobhouse (1935), 55–6.

[2] On the connection between work and socializing, see Bernard Capp, *When Gossips Meet: Women, Family and Neighbourhood in Early Modern England* (Oxford, 2004), 321, 330; Keith Thomas, *The Ends of Life: Roads to Fulfilment in Early Modern England* (Oxford, 2009), 99–101, 108.

The ensuing discussions contribute to debates about whether or not patients took up 'the sick role' in early modern England. This term was coined by the American sociologist Talcott Parsons in the 1950s to denote the special exemptions from routines commonly afforded to patients in mid-twentieth-century Western societies, such as sick-leave and bed-rest.[3] Using the Josselin family as a case study, Lucinda Beier implied that 'tak[ing] up a sick role' was often avoided in the early modern period, on the grounds that it 'would have been financially and professionally disastrous'.[4] More recently, in a ground-breaking study of healthcare in early modern Wales, Alun Withey has argued that while 'withdrawal to the sick-bed' was '*the* defining element of full-blown sickness', in practice many individuals were unable or unwilling to adopt such behaviour, due to a combination of economic, religious, and social pressures.[5] While not denying the reality of these pressures, the present study suggests that we have perhaps underestimated the frequency with which patients *did* adopt the sick role. This is evident in the plentiful accounts of recovery by patients like Claver Morris, which are structured around the gradual resumption of daily activities and employments—such descriptions indicate that illness necessarily did involve withdrawal from daily life.

A recurring theme in the chapter is gender: we will see that although the basic trajectory of recovery was the same for men and women, there were some subtle differences, both in terms of the particular occupations to which they returned, and in the ways in which they experienced these changes. The other major variable—even more important than gender—is socio-economic status. Since the lives of people at different ends of the social spectrum were very different, their experiences of returning to their situations must have diverged considerably.[6] Poorer people, living in multi-occupied dwellings of few rooms could not have made the same spatial and social transitions as wealthier individuals, nor would they have been able to afford to be away from paid employment for long.[7] Owing to a lack of detailed, qualitative evidence of the personal lives of the illiterate majority, the story told in this chapter is skewed towards the experiences of the middling and

[3] Talcott Parsons, *The Social System* (1951), ch. 5. In recent years, this concept has come under much criticism, and is no longer seen as applicable to twenty-first century patients' experiences—see John Burnham, 'The Death of the Sick Role', *SHM*, 25 (2012), 761–76.

[4] Lucinda Beier, *Sufferers and Healers: The Experience of Illness in Seventeenth-Century England* (1987), 193, 205. Although Beier acknowledges that there were occasions when patients retired to bed, the emphasis is on their resistance to the sick role. Writing around the same time, Roy and Dorothy Porter draw attention to the advantages of the sick role—it brought attention, and provided opportunities to shirk duties—see *In Sickness and in Health: The British Experience 1650–1850* (1988), chs. 11, 12.

[5] Alun Withey, *Physick and the Family: Health, Medicine and Care in Wales, 1600–1750* (Manchester, 2011), 124–8. Others who have shown that withdrawal to bed did happen on occasions include Philip Wilson, *Surgery, Skin and Syphilis: Daniel Turner's London (1667–1741)* (Amsterdam, 1999), 49; Ann Stobart, *Household Medicine in Seventeenth-Century England* (2016), 22–3.

[6] Poignant insights into the lives of impoverished families are provided in Patricia Crawford, *Parents of Poor Children in England 1580–1800* (Oxford, 2010), especially ch. 4.

[7] On the houses of the poor, see Antony Buxton, *Domestic Culture in Early Modern England* (Woodbridge, 2015), 217–19, 221, 247–50; Vanessa Harding, 'Families and Housing in Seventeenth-Century London', *Parergon*, 24 (2007), 115–38; Crawford, *Parents of Poor Children*, 124–6.

upper echelons, though I have attempted where possible to bring in examples from people lower down the social spectrum.

PRISON TO LIBERTY: SPATIAL LIFE

Recovery was experienced as a process of increasing movement in space. During severe illness, the sick were usually confined to bed, unable to stir; but as health returned, they gradually expanded their spatial horizons, until eventually they could go outdoors.[8] The ensuing paragraphs explore what it was like to make this transition, arguing that it was immensely liberating. The underlying supposition to these discussions, derived from the now well-established interdisciplinary field of spatial studies, is that physical locations are not 'unhistorical... static structure[s]': rather, social actors 'attribute different meanings to space at different times', which leads to 'differential and temporal experience'.[9]

Since the patient's feelings of liberty were contingent on the preceding confinement, it is necessary to start by examining what it was like to be sick in bed. In Galenic medical theory, the act of taking to bed was often interpreted as the beginning of illness; so important was it as a marker of sickness, it had its own special name, 'decumbiture'.[10] Doctors saw decumbiture as a natural inclination, instigated by the body's internal healing agent, Nature, to aid recovery: by prostrating the patient, Nature and her spirits—the vehicles through which this agent operated—could devote all their energies to the task of healing, rather than to keeping the body upright.[11] From the patient's perspective, it was usually sheer exhaustion and weakness that drove them to their beds. Roger North (1653–1734), a lawyer and politician from Suffolk, recorded in his diary that he had initially tried to carry on as normal during his fever, but eventually, 'I was then not able to conceal my illness longer, but was so bad, that... [I felt] dejected and ready to dy[e]...I came home, and satt downe...and had a mind to goe to bed'.[12] This example demonstrates that bed-rest was inevitable in serious illness, even amongst those patients who did not wish to 'own themselves sick'.[13]

Despite the physical necessity of bed-rest, patients seem to have found this aspect of sickness unpleasant, especially if it continued for longer than a few days. The terms that abound in contemporary accounts are 'tedious' and 'troublesome'. In 1711, a North Yorkshire coal trader, Henry Liddell (c.1673–1717), complained, 'Methinks the time of my confinem[ent] very tedious...which is now near 5 weeks

---

[8] David Turner has shown that disabled people, as well the sick, complained about spatial confinement, in *Disability in Eighteenth-Century England* (Abingdon, 2012), 109–10.

[9] Amanda Flather, *Gender and Space in Early Modern England* (Woodbridge, 2006), 2–3. Flather provides a useful introduction to this field on 2–9.

[10] See Chapter 2, note 184, on decumbiture.

[11] See Chapter 1, p. 45 on the importance of peaceful rest during illness.

[12] Roger North, *Notes of Me: the Autobiography of Roger North*, ed. P. Millard (Toronto, 2000), 202.

[13] North confessed that he was 'disposed to endure any thing rather then submit, and owen my self sick': ibid., 205.

and may be as much longer'.[14] It was the lack of mental stimulation, together with the monotony of sights, that made bed so boring—enclosed in a curtained bed-stead, there was little to see beyond the surrounding drapes.[15] Jeremy Taylor (*c*.1613–67), an Anglican bishop from Cambridge, described the scene as 'dressed with darknesse and sorrow', the patient's eyes, 'dim as a sullied mirror' for want of light.[16] Particularly unpleasant, was the feeling of limited bodily movement, a con-sequence of the loss of strength. Peg Verney, aged seven, was 'soe weake that she cannot turne herselfe in her Bed', lamented her father in 1647.[17] To describe this experience, the Oxfordshire minister Robert Harris (*c*.1581–1658) used the meta-phor of a lame horse, an analogy that would have made sense in an era reliant on horse-transport: 'The bodie is deprived of activitie...the soule disappointed, like the Traveller that rides a tyred horse...Its even stifled within it selfe for want of motion'.[18] Metaphors of imprisonment were also used: the sick felt trapped in their own bodies, and longed for the moment when 'those fetters...which...bound our souls in prison' were 'knocked off', either by death or recovery.[19]

As well as being kept in bed, those suffering serious illness were often confined to a room. Such an arrangement obviously depended on the size of the house and number of occupants, but where possible, the sick were assigned an upstairs bedchamber.[20] While there were good reasons for confining the patient in this way—it helped stop the spread of the disease, and shielded the sick from 'noisome noise'—life in the sickchamber was often described unfavourably, and likened once more to imprisonment. 'I have bin confined now a prisoner neer eighteen monthes with a rhumatisme', complained the Norfolk gentlewoman Elizabeth Freke (1642–1714).[21] Addressing the sick in 1683, Everard Maynwaringe (b. 1627/8), a physician from Kent, echoed, 'The want of *health* converts your House into a *Prison*; and *confines* you to the narrow compass of a *Chamber*'.[22] Like prisoners, the

---

[14] Henry Liddell, *The Letters of Henry Liddell to William Cotesworth*, ed. J. M. Ellis, Surtees Society, vol. 197 (Durham, 1987), 48. See also Bulstrode Whitelocke, *The Diary of Bulstrode Whitelocke, 1605–1675*, ed. Ruth Spalding (Oxford, 1990), 766–7.

[15] Sasha Handley has shown that some bed hangings were decorated, which may have lessened the monotony of sights: *Sleep in Early Modern England* (2016), 44, 104–5, 133–4. The tedium may also have been mitigated by reading to the sick: Andrew Cambers, *Godly Reading: Print, Manuscript and Puritanism in England, 1580–1720* (Cambridge, 2011), 62–4. Patients who mention the closed curtains include John Cannon, in SHC, DD/SAS C/1193/4, p. 101; Robert Boyle, *Occasional reflections upon several subjects* (1665), 218–19.

[16] Jeremy Taylor, *The rule and exercises of holy dying* (1651), 72.

[17] BL, M.636/8, unpaginated manuscript; letter from Ralph Verney to Dr Denton, 13 October 1647 (correspondence of Ralph Verney on microfiche). Other aspects of being in bed, such as sleeplessness and the sensation of the mattress, are discussed in Chapter 3, pp. 103–5.

[18] Robert Harris, *Hezekiahs recovery. Or, a sermon, shewing what use Hezekiah did, and all should make of their deliverance from sicknesse* (1626), 29–30. On the importance of horse-travel, see Peter Edwards, *Horse and Man in Early Modern England* (2007), *passim*.

[19] Taylor, *The rule*, 36. This positive conception of death was used by Taylor to comfort patients from the fear of the separation of their bodies and souls; see Chapter 5 for a discussion of this fear.

[20] On the rise of bedchambers, see Handley, *Sleep*, ch. 4; Mark Overton, Jane Whittle, Darron Dean, and Andrew Hann, *Production and Consumption in English Households, 1600–1750* (2004), 133.

[21] Elizabeth Freke, *The Remembrances of Elizabeth Freke*, ed. Raymond Anselment, Camden Fifth Series, vol. 18 (Cambridge, 2001), 157.

[22] Everard Maynwaringe, *The method and means of enjoying health* (1683), 29.

seriously ill could be prevented from leaving the room by 'keepers', the term used for both nurses and jail-wardens.[23]

One explanation for the use of the prison metaphor is that incarceration was a common experience in this period: the early 1600s saw a rise in imprisonment for debt, and during the Civil Wars many religious and political dissidents found themselves in prison.[24] A significant number of the individuals in this study had first-hand experience of imprisonment, or at least knew others who had.[25] However, this explanation becomes less convincing when we consider the actual conditions of prison life in early modern England. Molly Murray has shown that incarceration at this time 'did not inevitably imply strict physical confinement': prison buildings were often 'permeable to the world outside' owing to poor upkeep, and the practice of day-leave.[26] The reason for these lax arrangements was that English prisons in this era did not usually fulfil a punitive function; instead they were primarily holding places for those awaiting trial.[27] If patients' choice of metaphor was not inspired by real prison environments, it must have sprung from the imagined conditions, which in turn were probably derived from two of the most widely diffused texts of the period, the Bible and the popular martyrology *Acts and Monuments*, by the sixteenth-century Protestant theologian John Foxe. Together, these texts make over six hundred references to imprisonment, many of which suggest constraint and gloom.[28] Psalm 107, for instance, describes the prisoner as sitting 'in darkness... being bound in affliction and iron', his heart 'bowed down', while Foxe writes of one man 'cast in prison', where he became 'weake and feable'.[29] Undoubtedly, the connection between incarceration and sickness was galvanized by the Crown's policy of 'locking up' plague sufferers in their homes, an intervention designed to halt the spread of the disease.[30] Ballads lamented the misery induced by this practice in ways resembling ordinary patients' accounts of confinement to the sickroom. *The shutting up of infected houses* (1665) bewails the 'sad and dismal restraint' of being 'shut up from all our comfort[,] ... from free and wholsome air'.[31]

---

[23] Margaret Pelling, *The Common Lot: Sickness, Medical Occupations and the Urban Poor in Early Modern England* (1998), 186.

[24] Amanda Bailey, *Of Bondage: Debt, Property, and Personhood in Early Modern England* (Philadelphia PA, 2013), 118.

[25] For example, Richard Allestree, John Bunyan, Jeremy Taylor, Thomas Tuke, Adam Martindale, Joan Barrington, and William Waller were all imprisoned at some point. Those whose relatives were imprisoned include Ann Fanshawe, Anne Halkett, and Mary Penington.

[26] Molly Murray, 'Measured Sentences: Forming Literature in the Early Modern Prison', *Huntingdon Library Quarterly*, 72 (2009), 147–67, at 152–3; see also Bailey, *Of Bondage*, 119–20; Jerome De Groot, 'Prison Writing during the 1640s and 1650s', *Huntingdon Library Quarterly*, 72 (2009), 193–215, at 200. On the gap between the imagined and real conditions, see Cambers, *Godly Reading*, 215–16.

[27] Ruth Ahnert shows that conditions varied considerably; some prisons *were* punitive: *The Rise of Prison Literature in the Sixteenth Century* (Cambridge, 2013), 11, 17–18.

[28] *DBI*, 112, 657–9; John Foxe, *The Unabridged Acts and Monuments Online* or *TAMO* (1583 edition), HRI Online Publications, Sheffield, 2011, <http//www.johnfoxe.org> (accessed 14/09/16).

[29] Psalm 107:10, 12; Foxe, *Acts and Monuments*, 836.

[30] Paul Slack, 'The Response to Plague in Early Modern England: Public Policies and their Consequences', in John Waller and Roger Schofield (eds.), *Famine, Disease, and the Social Order in Early Modern Society* (Cambridge, 1991, first publ. 1989), at 169–71, 183.

[31] *The shutting up infected houses as it is practised in England* (1665), 8–9.

Experiences of confinement were influenced by gender. This is illustrated through a comparison of the illness narratives of a married couple, the Quaker from Kent, Mary Penington (*c.*1623–82), and her first husband, William Springett (1621/2–44). Sick of fever in 1682, Mary wrote, 'the Lord hath graciously stopped my desires after every pleasant thing, that I have not been at all uneasy at my long confinement, for the most part to my bed, and to this present day to my chamber'.[32] Women like Mary were familiar with bed-rest, due to frequent childbearing: it was customary for new mothers of middling or elite status to be confined to a bedchamber for up to a month after childbirth, a period of rest known as 'her confinement' or 'lying-in'.[33] Owing to these regular experiences, some women felt they had become experts at turning spatial restraint to their spiritual advantage, which in turn helped them to cultivate both their Christian and feminine identities.[34] Mary's experience contrasts strikingly with that of her husband, the young parliamentary colonel William Springett, whom she reported 'knew not how to yield to confinement'.[35] During an acute fever in 1644, he was so unwilling to be kept to his chamber that his fellow officers 'were obliged to sit round his bed to keep him in it'.[36] She attributed his reluctance to stay in bed to the fact he was 'so young and strong, and his blood so hot', a reference to the Galenic medical notion that young men abound in hot and dry humours, which makes them active, strong, and restless, qualities not conducive to lying down for long periods.[37] There was also a powerful cultural reason for William's aversion to confinement: the indoors was regarded as a feminine sphere, despite the fact that in practice women routinely left the house.[38] Conduct book writers insisted that, 'The dutie of the husband, is to dispatch all things without dore: and of the wife, to ... give order for all things within the house'.[39] Popular proverbs concurred: for example, 'A House and a Woman suit excellently'.[40] As such, confinement to the sickchamber was potentially emasculating for males.[41] This might explain why William eventually forced his way to the window, from where he shot 'birds ... with his cross-bow', an attempt, perhaps, to rescue his masculine identity by performing an archetypally manly act.[42]

Having explored experiences of confinement, we can now investigate what it was like to extend one's spatial horizons, a process that apparently began with sitting up. The cover illustration depicts a woman about to make this move—she is propping herself up, and looking out through the bed-curtains, her face full of hope and

---

[32] Mary Penington, *Experiences in the Life of Mary Penington Written by Herself*, ed. Norman Penney (1992, first publ. 1911), 69.

[33] On lying-in, see the Introduction, p. 9.

[34] For example, see Brilliana Harley, *Letters of The Lady Brilliana Harley*, ed. Thomas Taylor Lewis (1853), 52.

[35] Penington, *Experiences*, 90.

[36] Another example of a young man held down during illness is John Cannon, in SHC, DD/SAS C/1193/4, p. 100.

[37] Penington, *Experiences*, 90–1.   [38] Flather, *Gender and Space, passim*.

[39] John Dod and Robert Cleaver, *A godlie forme of household government* (1621, first publ. 1598), 167–8.

[40] N.R., *Proverbs English, French, Dutch, Italian, and Spanish* (1659), 3.

[41] Turner agrees that confinement 'posed a threat' to manhood, but in relation to those who were disabled: *Disability*, 110–11.

[42] Penington, *Experiences*, 190.

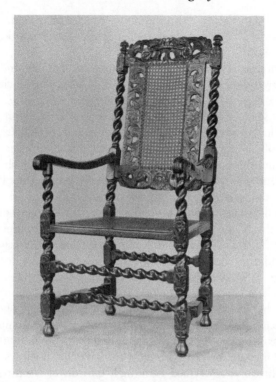

Figure 8. Armchair with floral scrollwork, *c.*1685; © Victoria and Albert Museum, London; W.17-1911. Armchairs rose in popularity in the 1600s; the use of cane for the back and seat is an innovation from Asia. With a high back, and long arms, this chair would have provided good support for the sitter's shoulders and back, an essential requirement for the weak convalescent. A cushion would have been placed on the seat for comfort.

expectation.[43] Such minor movements might not seem noteworthy, but to early modern patients they were highly significant, providing evidence that the disease was gone, and strength was beginning to return. Accordingly, patients expressed relief when they were able to sit up, and monitored the length of time they could do so. The Buckinghamshire gentlewoman Brilliana Harley (*c.*1598–1643) told her son Edward in 1639, 'I thanke God I am now abell to site up a littell. This day I sate up...allmost an ower'.[44] This milestone was recognized throughout the period, but there was a change in its material culture: new types of armchairs were becoming available during the seventeenth century, some of which may have been designed with convalescents in mind (Figure 8).[45] These seats were usually positioned

[43] 'A Woman in Bed', by Rembrandt Harmensz van Rijn, *c.*1647; National Galleries of Scotland; accession number: NG 827. Little is known about the subject of this painting, or even if she was supposed to be recovering, but her expression of hope, and the paleness of her face, match patients' accounts of the beginnings of recovery nicely.

[44] Harley, *Letters*, 80.

[45] Buxton, *Domestic Culture*, 139–46; Sandra Cavallo and Tessa Storey, *Healthy Living in Late Renaissance Italy* (Oxford, 2013), 122–3. On the rise of chairs see Overton et al., *Production and Consumption*, 93–4, 126.

between the bed and fireplace to protect the patient from cold, with the sitter assisted into position.[46] For those who could not afford such luxuries, the bed itself functioned as a seat.

The next movements performed by patients were standing and walking. The biography of eleven-year-old Martha Hatfield (b. 1640), by her uncle, James Fisher, a Sheffield vicar, provides a detailed account of these movements. In 1652, after nine months of sickness, Martha told her father 'she felt strength come into her legs[,] ... trickl[ing] down, ... into her thighs, knees, and ancles, like warm water'.[47] After a quarter of an hour, Martha's older sister, Hannah, 'took her up, and set her upon her feet, and she stood by her self without holding, which she had not done for three quarters of a year'.[48] Her relatives were 'afraid to trust her strength, it being so long a time since she had any use of her Legs', but to their amazement, 'she went up and down the room beyond all expectation'. Her mother asked her, 'Childe, is not thy minde full of apprehensions of the Lords wonderfull dealings with thee?' Martha replied, 'Yes ... but I cannot expresse it so largely as I desire'. [49] This example indicates that rising and walking generated excitement and spiritual wonder, the like of which was difficult to verbalize. In Martha's case, her family played a vital role in her spiritual and spatial rehabilitation, helping her stand up, and reminding her to acknowledge God's role. Alec Ryrie has shown that early modern Protestants engaged in 'extemporal meditations', spiritual musings triggered by daily actions: rising and walking, for instance, brought to mind the resurrection of Christ, and his command to 'Arise and walk' when healing the sick and lame.[50] Given that meditation was deemed 'dauntingly difficult' at this time, especially for children, patients like Martha may have cherished these physical actions as useful spurs to this vital exercise.[51] It is more difficult to uncover how poorer patients felt as they took their first steps after illness, but miracle accounts provide some, albeit indirect and stereotyped, insights. In 1666, Joseph Warden, a 'stout Seaman belonging to the *Royal Charles*', was healed by the famous 'Irish stroker' Valentine Greatrakes.[52] Previously lame due to 'grievous [pains] in his hip, thigh, ham and ankle', he was now able to walk 'lustily to and fro in the Garden', tossing his crutches 'triumphantly upon his shoulders'.[53] Clearly, this man was delighted with his achievement. The speed at which strength returned was one of the principal

---

[46] For example, BL, Additional MS 36452, fol. 128r (Private letters of the Aston family, 1613–1703).

[47] This simile may have been derived from the Galenic notion that movement and sensation was driven by the flow of warm vapours called 'animal spirits', through the muscles: Levinus Lemnius, *The touchstone of complexions*, trans. Thomas Newton (1576), 82, 738–9.

[48] James Fisher, *The wise virgin, or, a wonderful narration of the various dispensations towards a childe of eleven years of age* (1653), 158–9.

[49] Ibid., 160–1.

[50] Alec Ryrie, *Being Protestant in Reformation Britain* (Oxford, 2013), 112. 'Arise and walk' features in Matthew 9:5–6; Mark 2:9–11; Mark 5:41–2; Mark 9:27; Luke 5:22–5; Luke 8:54–5; Luke 17:19; John 5:8–12; Acts 9:34.

[51] Ryrie, *Being Protestant*, 117. Examples of adult patients who used these spurs for meditation include Timothy Rogers, *Practical discourses on sickness & recovery* (1691), 268; John Donne, *Devotions upon emergent occasions and severall steps in my sicknes* (1624), 560.

[52] For historiography on Greatrakes, see the Introduction, note 152.

[53] Valentine Greatrakes, *A brief account of Mr. Valentine Greatraks* (1666), 70.

ways in which supernatural recoveries were distinguished from natural ones, hence this sailor's sudden capacity to walk 'lustily'.[54]

Once patients were up, they could get dressed. During illness, it was customary to wear nightclothes or underwear—long linen shirts called 'shifts', together with caps to keep the head from cold.[55] Patients expressed great satisfaction when they could finally change into their day-clothes. During his recovery from fever in 1720, Claver Morris recorded:

> I got up, and after my Breeches only were slipped on...I put on everything [else] excepting my shoose, & completely dress'd my self in 2 Minutes, by my Wife'[s] Watch which I desired her to observe.[56]

Besides revealing something about female clock ownership, this extract suggests that male patients sometimes approached getting dressed as a race, hoping perhaps to inject a degree of manly competitiveness into what could be construed as a rather mundane happening. Morris' use of the passive voice to describe the putting on of his breeches implies that someone assisted him with this action; this choice of grammar is significant because it suggests he did not want to draw attention to the fact that he was being helped—such assistance carried connotations of child-like dependence, which were at odds with his masculine identity. No comparable evidence of women's dressing has been found, which may be due to contemporary concerns about modesty and decency.[57]

After dressing, patients could leave the room and go downstairs. Historians have shown that over the course of the early modern period, beds migrated from ground-floor multipurpose 'halls', to first-floor chambers, devoted to the function of sleep.[58] The majority of the homes featured in this study contained upstairs bedchambers, as attested by the fact that patients almost always went downstairs during recovery. A typical entry, provided by the royalist MP Christopher Hatton (*c.*1632–1706), reads: 'I have kept my chamber since Tuesday, falling very ill...of a feavor...but I thanke God am now got down staires againe'.[59] Hatton was evidently relieved to go downstairs: it symbolized re-entrance into the realm of normal life, and proved that the body had regained considerable strength.[60]

Once downstairs, the patients normally mention entering the hall or parlour. The former space was transformed over our period from a multi-functional area for sitting, eating, and sleeping, to an entrance lobby, out of which the staircase

---

[54] See Chapter 2, p. 71.

[55] Handley, *Sleep*, 52–7; Susan North, 'Dress and Hygiene in Early Modern England: A Study of Advice and Practice' (unpublished PhD thesis, Queen Mary, University of London, 2012), 30–3. A number of smocks have survived—for example, item T.243–1959 at the Victoria and Albert Museum: <http://collections.vam.ac.uk/item/O137793/smock-unknown/> (accessed 30/06/16); my thanks to Alice Dolan, Sasha Handley, and Kevin Siena for assistance on this subject.

[56] Morris, *The Diary*, 78.

[57] On the taboo of nakedness/dressing in women, see Sarah Toulalan, *Imagining Sex: Pornography and Bodies in Seventeenth-Century England* (Oxford, 2007), 233, 263–5; Patricia Crawford, *Blood, Bodies and Families in Early Modern England* (Harlow, 2004), 34.

[58] Handley, *Sleep*, 110–17; Overton et al., *Production and Consumption*, 133.

[59] Hatton, *Correspondence*, vol. 1, 51.   [60] Stobart, *Household Medicine*, 22.

arose.[61] This development was linked to the rising popularity of the parlour, a room designed specifically for dining and socializing.[62] Generally, entrance into these two areas elicited gladness and divine praise in patients and their relatives. When his family was recovering from bad colds in 1648, the Essex clergyman Ralph Josselin (1617–83) wrote in his diary, 'This morning was comfortable and cheerly to us all, the lords name bee praised for it; wee removed...downe into the hall'.[63] On another occasion, when Josselin's wife Jane was convalescing from a disease resembling smallpox, he wrote, 'my wife came down into the parlour, very well'.[64] This man implies that the joy of these spatial movements sprung partly from the social interaction that occurred in these rooms after a period of isolation; these aspects of resuming life will be explored later in the chapter.[65] In middling and upper-class homes, parlours and halls were usually well-appointed rooms, with colourful furnishings, upholstered chairs, and paintings.[66] These new sights, after the monotony of the sickchamber, were a source of delight to patients. The parliamentary army officer William Waller (c.1598–1668) described the paintings in his home as '*artificial miracles*', since, 'without taking the pains to go abroad [i.e. outdoors] I can go abroad within doores, and in a small [frame] see, a whole Contry, diversified with Hills, and Dales...Rivers, Sea's'.[67] Such paintings transported convalescents imaginatively to the outdoors, where they could enjoy a variety of sensory stimuli from which they had been deprived during sickness.

Intriguingly, patients rarely mentioned what historians have labelled the 'female rooms'—the kitchen, buttery, and washroom—places for domestic chores. This was probably because it was not deemed safe for women to undertake physical tasks too soon: such actions could cause relapse.[68] In the case of wealthy women, domestic work may have been delegated to servants.[69] More so than gender, it seems to have been patients' socio-economic status and residential arrangements that made a difference to room-to-room movements. Amanda Flather has shown that servants and apprentices enjoyed less spatial freedom within their masters' homes than family members, from which we can infer that they may not have made the same transitions.[70] Instead of entering the parlour, they would probably have returned to the kitchen or other work-rooms. For poorer individuals, living in single-storey dwellings of only one or two rooms, the spatial transitions were obviously much more limited. These variations are depicted in Figure 9.

[61] T. J. Cliffe, *The World of the Country House in Seventeenth-Century England* (1999), 24; Overton et al., *Production and Consumption*, 129–30.

[62] Overton et al., *Production and Consumption*, 130–2.

[63] Ralph Josselin, *The Diary of Ralph Josselin 1616–1683*, ed. Alan Macfarlane (Oxford, 1991), 118.

[64] Ibid., 617. For other examples, see Robert Paston, *The Whirlpool of Misadventures: Letters of Robert Paston, First Earl of Yarmouth 1663–1679*, ed. Jean Agnew, Norfolk Record Society, vol. 76 (Norwich, 2012), 229; Arthur Searle (ed.), *The Barrington Family Letters, 1628–1632* (1983), 242; Anton Bantock (ed.), *The Earlier Smyths of Ashton Court From their Letters, 1545–1741*, ed. Anton Bantock (Bristol, 1982), 116.

[65] On halls and parlours as sociable places, see Cambers, *Godly Reading*, 87–110.

[66] Buxton, *Domestic Culture*, 219–28.

[67] William Waller, *Divine meditations upon several occasions* (1680), 95–6.

[68] On the danger of exertion, see Chapter 2, pp. 87–9.   [69] Flather, *Gender and Space*, 79.

[70] Ibid., 48–9.

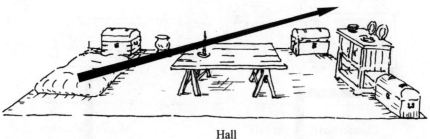

Hall

Dwelling and furnishings of Thomas Franklin, labourer, 1611

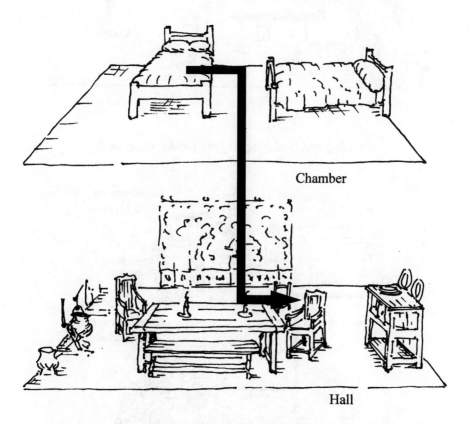

Chamber

Hall

Dwelling and furnishings of John Simons, husbandman, 1605.

Figure 9. House layouts, with patients' spatial movements during recovery; kindly supplied by Anthony Buxton, *Domestic Culture in Early Modern England* (Woodbridge: Boydell and Brewer, 2015). The floorplans are based on the probate documents of four individuals from Thame, Oxfordshire. The arrows show the typical movements made by patients during recovery, from which it is evident there would have been considerable variation between people of different socio-economic levels and occupations.

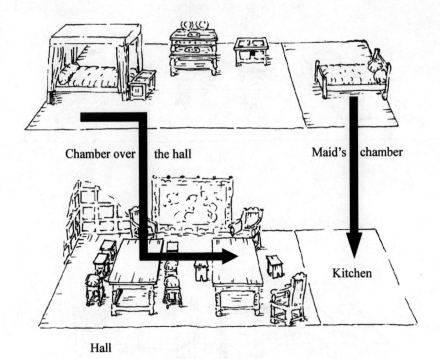

Chamber over the hall

Maid's chamber

Kitchen

Hall

Dwelling and furnishings of John Trinder, vicar, 1629

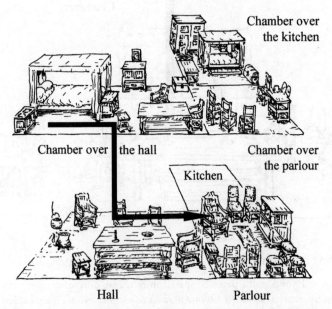

Chamber over the kitchen

Chamber over the hall

Chamber over the parlour

Kitchen

Hall   Parlour

Dwelling and furnishings of Richard Somers, gentleman, 1665

The final spatial transition was 'going abroad', which meant leaving the house. Patients usually found this movement wonderfully liberating, as indicated by their use of imagery of release from prison. Ralph Josselin recorded in 1648, 'This weeke after a long restraint…god was pleased to sett mee at liberty againe[;] I went abroad'.[71] So familiar was this language that it appears in all sorts of texts, including advertisements for medicines. William Atkins' 'gout-balsam', for example, describes how one Mr Clifton of Old-Fishstreet, London, 'had been confined by the Gout for the whole Winter…but was set at liberty about *Christmass*'.[72] The most striking parallel between leaving the house and prison was the sensory transformation that took place: individuals emerged from the dark and musty confines of the indoors, to the bright, fresh, and fragrant outdoors.[73] The Gloucestershire preacher and agricultural expert Timothy Nourse (1636–99) provides a vivid picture of these sensory delights. He reflected, when a man finds himself suddenly 'surrounded with all the pleasant Scenes and Beauties':

> [W]ith what Gust does he tast the…Delights of Nature? How Acute are his Senses[?]…At once he sees all the Varities of shady Woods, of lofty Trees,…of flowry Meadows… How…every flower [is]…admirable in its Contexture[,]…Colour…[and] Smell? How refreshing is it to him to…hear the…Melody of Birds, together with the Murmuring of Chrystal Waters.[74]

The outdoors thus filled all five senses with delight. Particular emphasis was placed on the contrast between the 'thick darkness' of the indoors, and the 'sweet light' of outside, together with the relief to breathe in 'sweet air' after being cooped up.[75] Henry Liddell informed a friend in 1726, 'Yesterday was the first day I gott into the Fields for a mouthful off fresh air' since his 'stout feavor' had begun.[76] He felt nourished by the intake of breath, an idea that would have made sense to contemporaries, since the air was thought to contain nutritious particles—in the form of scents—which could be digested in the blood.[77] Carole Rawcliffe has shown that the combination of 'Delectable Sightes and Fragrant Smelles' was thought to 'delight [and] invigorate' the patient's spirits, thereby triggering happy emotions, and strengthening the body.[78] Of course, not every patient would have been greeted with sensory delights when leaving the house: those living in crowded cities

---

[71] Josselin, *The Diary*, 119.

[72] William Atkins, *A discourse shewing the nature of the gout* (1694), 79.

[73] Having said this, doctors did recommend that bedchambers were well-ventilated: see Handley, *Sleep*, ch. 2.

[74] Timothy Nourse, *A discourse upon the nature and faculties of man* (1686), 324–6.

[75] Waller, *Divine meditations*, 1–2, 5. On the darkness of interiors, see Mary Thomas Crane, 'Illicit Privacy and Outdoor Spaces in Early Modern England', *Journal for Early Modern Cultural Studies*, 9 (2009), 4–22, at 6, 10.

[76] Liddell, *The Letters*, 235. See also Paston, *The Whirlpool*, 231.

[77] Evelyn Welch, 'Scented Buttons and Perfumed Gloves: Smelling Things in Renaissance Italy', in Bella Mirabella (ed.), *Ornamentalism: The Art of Accessories* (Ann Arbor MI, 2011), 13–39, at 19–20.

[78] Carole Rawcliffe, '"Delectable Sightes and Fragrant Smelles": Gardens and Health in Late Medieval and Early Modern England', *Garden History*, 36 (2008), 3–21, at 9, 11. See also Leah Knight, *Reading Green in Early Modern England* (2014).

were more likely to notice the smells of sewage than the scent of flowers![79] Nonetheless, this was the era of the 'garden city': urban areas contained plenty of green spaces, so we can assume that most people would have had access to an urban garden, or the semi-open country.

For pious patients, the joy of going outdoors sprang partly from its spiritual connotations. One of the 'evils of sickness' was the patient's deprivation from the sights of God's beautiful creation: entering the outdoors thus inspired praises to God for His wonderful works. 'A man is... constrained to commend, to praise and magnify the Lord', wrote John Mirfield, a late medieval theologian, when he is 'gazing far and near, and upon the sky, the sea and the green landscape'.[80] Although the Lord was supposed to be omnipresent, preachers implied that his actual location was the heavens, for which reason the outdoors was the best place for prayer and praises—Christians could send forth their words directly to God above, unconstrained by ceilings.[81] Alexandra Walsham has pointed out that the outdoors also 'provided manifest evidence' of God's existence.[82] Given the intense religiosity of many of the individuals in this study, we might suppose that they would not have needed any such confirmation, but even the pious were vulnerable to doubts on occasions.[83]

Going abroad was enjoyed by patients of both sex, but it carried additional premium for men, owing to prevailing cultural connections between masculinity and the outdoors.[84] Popular ballads ridiculed males who spent too much time inside. *Advice to batchelors* (1685) scorns those 'weaker sort' of men, who let their wives 'wear the Breeches', forcing them to stay inside, washing 'Pots and dishes' and 'childrens clouts'.[85] Bombarded with such messages, some male patients may have suffered the loss of part of their masculine identity during prolonged stints indoors, and relished the first opportunity to leave the house. This is implied by the common tendency for men to make this spatial transition prematurely, ignoring their relatives' kindly cautions. Anne Clavering from Durham reported in 1708 that she 'scolded' a male neighbour of hers 'for going [out] of the house... so soon after his illness'. She added, 'If he plays the fool with his health 'tis not the fault of his friends for... he often has a lecture'.[86]

Having presented a largely positive picture of the spatial transition from the sickbed to the outdoors, it must be noted that there were some downsides. Namely,

[79] On the sensory environment of cities, see Emily Cockayne, *Hubbub: Filth, Noise and Stench in England 1600–1770* (2007).

[80] Cited by Rawcliffe, '"Delectable Sightes"', 13.

[81] Ryrie, *Being Protestant*, 162–4. On outdoor religious contemplation/reading, see Cambers, *Godly Reading*, 111–16.

[82] Alexandra Walsham, *The Reformation of the Landscape: Religion, Identity, and Memory in Early Modern Britain and Ireland* (Oxford, 2011), 331.

[83] See the Introduction, note 166, on atheism.   [84] Flather, *Gender and Space*, ch. 1.

[85] *Advice to batchelors, or the married mans lamentation* (1685). See also *The woman to the plow and the man to the hen-roost* (1675).

[86] James Clavering, *The Correspondence of Sir James Clavering*, ed. Harry Thomas Dickinson, Surtees Society, vol. 178 (Gateshead, 1967), 22.

the joy of increasing temporal movement was often countered by exhaustion and weakness, together with fears that such actions might cause relapse. 'One warm day' in 1657, during his convalescence from ague, the Yorkshire shopkeeper Joseph Lister (1627–1709)

> [D]esired to be helped down the stairs; and being down, I longed to go into the garden... and did so for a few minutes, but soon repented my folly, for next morning I was confined to my bed, and much worse than before.[87]

This extract reminds us that the resumption of normal spatial life did not always follow a linear motion—patients might return to bed after leaving the house too soon, or in the words of Alun Withey, they 'crossed and re-crossed the... boundary of sickness'.[88] There was also a pressing spiritual concern: the 'gorgeous dresse' of the outdoors, with its delightful 'colour, shape, and scent' might tempt the Christian to fall in love with the world again, so that when death eventually occurred, it would be resisted.[89] Preachers sought to prevent this from happening by reminding their flocks of the transience of everything 'under the sun': flowers, for example, 'Now... flatter, and seem beautfiull to the eye, and suddenly they wither [and] vanish'.[90]

ISOLATION TO INTEGRATION: SOCIAL LIFE

The next section explores the social dimensions of recovery, proposing that the return to health was experienced as a transformation from isolation to integration. This interpretation complicates the common view that before the rise of the isolated hospital ward in the nineteenth century, sickness was a highly sociable affair—patients were cared for at home, surrounded by family and friends.[91] While it was common for the sick to receive visitors, we will see that such interactions did not always counter their loneliness. After identifying the ways in which illness could be isolating, the discussions turn to the incremental stages of reintegration that took place during recovery.

'As Sicknesse is the greatest misery, so the greatest misery of sickness is *solitude*... it is an *Outlawry*, an *Excommunication* upon the *patient*', declared the poet and Dean of St Paul's Cathedral, John Donne (1572–1631), during his convalescence

---

[87] Joseph Lister, *The Autobiography of Joseph Lister of Bradford, 1627–1709*, ed. Thomas Wright (Bradford, 1842), 43–4.

[88] On the reason going outdoors led to relapse, see Chapter 2, pp. 87–8.

[89] Edward Bury, *The husbandmans companion containing one hundred occasional meditations* (1677), 61–2.

[90] Ibid., 61–5.

[91] For example, Porter and Porter, *In Sickness*, 195; Hannah Newton, *The Sick Child in Early Modern England* (Oxford, 2012), 100–1, 166–70; Michael Stolberg, *Experiencing Illness and the Sick Body in Early Modern Europe* (Basingstoke, 2011, first publ. in German in 2003), 53–5; Withey, *Physick and the Family*, 172–6.

from spotted fever.[92] The most obvious form of isolation was spatial segregation, discussed earlier: the sick were usually separated physically from the rest of the household in a designated bedchamber. Even in small, one-storey houses, some degree of segregation could be achieved through partitioning off part of a room with a panel screen.[93] Sickness also disabled patients from 'travelling abroad' to visit loved ones, and for those who fell ill while away from home, it prevented them from returning. Speaking of his recent illness in 1618, the courtier and poet Robert Sidney (1563–1626) told his wife '[what] rankles me worst is that it hath taken from me the means to see you'.[94] 'Your absence... causes a sofring... beyond sickness', echoed Katherine Aston (b. 1620s) to her husband Henry.[95] Such sentiments were also voiced by parents, children, and close friends.[96] Aristotelian philosophers attributed these reactions to the 'uniting vertue' of the passion of love, which makes 'the presence of the party beloved... deare and pretious unto us', and 'his absence' the cause of 'a thousand sorrowes'.[97]

The usual solution to the patient's inability to visit loved ones was for loved ones to visit the patient.[98] This did not always lessen their feelings of loneliness, however, because patients often felt they could not appreciate their visitors' company. The Presbyterian minister from Durham, Timothy Rogers (1658–1728), dedicated a sermon to the gentleman who had visited him during his sickness. It opens with an apology:

> I thank you for Visiting me in my low Estate, tho[ugh] the greatness of my Pain, and the anguish of my Thoughts allowed me not to take such notice of so great an Honour as otherwise I should have done.[99]

He reflected, 'Sickness... deprive[s] us of all our... Friendships [and] Conversations,... it... will not allow us to take any Delight in... the Society of our Friends'.[100] Part of the difficulty was communication, a consequence of the temporary loss of rational powers or speech. This was the case for the nonconformist Lancaster minister Adam Martindale (1623–86), who grew light-headed during a fever in 1650. He was 'tormented with thoughts' that he had squandered his estate, but his friends refused to discuss the matter with him, knowing it was a delusion springing from 'the weaknesse of body and braine'.[101] It is possible that men like Martindale

---

[92] Donne, *Devotions*, 92–3.   [93] Overton et al., *Production and Consumption*, 122.

[94] Robert Sidney, *Domestic Politics and Family Absence: The Correspondence (1588–1621) of Robert Sidney, First Earl of Leicester, and Barbara Gamage Sidney*, ed. Margaret Hannay, Noel Kinnamon, and Michael Brennan (Aldershot, 2005), 219.

[95] BL, Additional MS 36452, fol. 37r.

[96] For parents and children, see Newton, *The Sick Child*, 170–1; for friends/work colleagues, see Liddell, *The Letters*, 118.

[97] Nicholas Coeffeteau, *A table of humane passions*, trans. Edward Grimeston (1621), 157.

[98] On sick-visiting, see Olivia Weisser, *Ill Composed: Sickness, Gender, and Belief in Early Modern England* (2015), ch. 4; Withey, *Physick and the Family*, 174–6, Beier, *Sufferers and Healers*, 245–9.

[99] Rogers, *Practical discourses*, iv.   [100] Ibid., 121.

[101] Adam Martindale, *The Life of Adam Martindale*, ed. Richard Parkinson, Chetham Society, vol. 4 (Manchester, 1845), 100.

found the loss of rationality, and the 'conduit of reason', speech, particularly troubling, as these powers were prized in males.[102]

For many sick people, company was not simply unappreciated: it was the source of sensory discomfort. The royalist clergyman John Kettlewell (1653–95) warned, 'Sometimes sick persons can ill bear noise…[,] or would be troubled, not relieved, by the presence of others'.[103] One patient who would have agreed was twelve-year-old Caleb Vernon, sick of consumption in 1665; he complained to the maid that the 'noise being made among the little ones', his younger sisters, '*hurt[s] me*'.[104] Contributing to patients' distress was their concern that they themselves were not good company to their visitors.[105] Henry Liddell wrote self-deprecatingly:

> [M]y distemper so load[s] my head that I am unfitt for any conversation, and a garrett…
> would be the properest place for me, by which means I should be only burthensome
> to my selfe while my friends happily escape.[106]

He believed a quantity of dense humours had accumulated in his head, which made speaking difficult. Patients were also aware that their irritable moods might prove annoying to their guests. The London law student Dudley Ryder (1691–1756) admitted that when his brother came to see him during his illness, he was 'in a very peevish, angry humour'. He reflected on the irony that when his relations had been absent, he had 'wish[ed] for company', but when he 'had it[, he] wanted to be alone'.[107] This vignette brings to mind the saying that the sick can never be pleased: their friends' 'absence offends him, and so doth their presence'.[108]

Not all patients had the chance to find out if they enjoyed the company of visitors: those suffering from acutely infectious diseases might be avoided on the grounds of potential contagion. Donne stated, 'when the infectiousness of the disease deters them who should assist from coming', the patient is separated 'from all offices not onely of *Civilite, but of…Charitie*'.[109] The archetypal infectious disease was plague—royal proclamations issued throughout the period forbade anyone from visiting infected homes, except doctors.[110] One anonymous critic to this policy pleaded, 'add not sorrow to affliction…O let us not withal be forsaken by men!…[it is] dreadful…to be shut up from all…society'.[111] So unwelcome was the isolation occasioned by infectious diseases that some patients 'deny…their disease, and thrust themselves into all meetings, and drinkings, and feasts, and

---

[102] Alexandra Shepard, *Meanings of Manhood in Early Modern England* (Oxford, 2003), 76; see also 29–30, 56, 67–8.
[103] John Kettlewell, *Death made comfortable* (1695), 56–7.
[104] John Vernon, *The compleat scholler; or, A relation of the life…of Caleb Vernon* (1666), 58–9.
[105] Turner makes this point too, though in relation to disability: *Disability*, 110–12.
[106] Liddell, *The Letters*, 8.
[107] Dudley Ryder, *The Diary of Dudley Ryder*, ed. William Matthews (1939), 45, 134.
[108] Harris, *Hezekiahs recovery*, 29–30.   [109] Donne, *Devotions*, 94–5.
[110] Beier, *Sufferers and Healers*, 252–4.
[111] *The shutting up*, 3, 5. See also J.V., *Golgotha; or, a looking glass for London…With an humble witness against the cruel…shutting-up* (1665), 10.

drink boldly with their pocky lips in the Cups [of] others', bewailed the sixteenth-century Dutch physician Levinus Lemnius.[112]

Over the course of recovery, however, the patient gradually re-entered family and community life, a transition often found to be deeply bonding and mutually joyful. In cases of nearly fatal illness, the first stage of integration took place when the patient's rational powers had been restored, and the danger of death was considered to be over; it involved embraces with relatives, and expressions of love and happiness. A poignant example is provided in James Fisher's biography of his young niece, Martha Hatfield. Fisher recorded that soon Martha 'knew [recognized] her Mother, and rejoyced to see her with laughing and stroaking of her face'. When her father came, and asked her 'if she knew him', she 'did the like to him'. That evening, she recognized 'her sister *Hannah*, and her Grand-Mother', and to each she 'did express [herself] by laughing and stroaking their faces'. Taking her grandmother's and mother's hands in hers, Martha declared, 'Me is pretty well, I praise my God'.[113] Steeped in emotion, these tactile interactions reveal the great intimacy between a variety of family members; the urge to make physical contact was attributed to the aforementioned 'uniting virtue' of love.[114] Relatives and friends also expressed a heightened appreciation for their loved one's life and company, an effect of the recent contemplation of death. Samuel Pepys recorded in 1663 that his 'great terror' that his wife Elizabeth might die proved 'a great tryall of my true love and passion for her'.[115] Strained relationships might be improved in this context. In 1702, the Hertfordshire gentlewoman Sarah Cowper (1644–1720), whose relationship with her husband William had long been unhappy, remarked wryly that during her amendment from a dangerous chest infection, he 'shows some regard...enough to show he cannot hate me'.[116] As with the spatial milestones analysed earlier, godly patients used these moments of social reintegration to spark extemporal spiritual meditation. Preaching in 1672, the Presbyterian Shropshire minister Edward Lawrence (d. 1695), stated:

> Thou art restored to...thy dear bosom-friends...therefore...See the gracious face and presence of God shining upon thee in the face of all thy friends;...look on thy parents, and look upon God; look on thy children, &c. and look upon God.[117]

Lawrence hoped that through seeing their relations' beaming faces, patients would catch a glimpse of the loving countenance of God. Since loving the Lord is the most important commandment in the Bible, recovery was cherished by some patients as an ideal opportunity for fostering this holy affection.[118]

Amongst the literate, the next stage of social reintegration cited by patients was writing a letter, a form of communication that enabled the patient to resume

---

[112] Levinus Lemnius, *The secret miracles of nature* (1658, first publ. 1559), 245.

[113] Fisher, *The wise virgin*,145–6, 152.   [114] See Chapter 5, pp. 173–4.

[115] Samuel Pepys, *The Diary of Samuel Pepys*, ed. Henry B. Wheatley (1893), Project Gutenberg, managed by Phil Gyford: <http://www.pepysdiary.com/diary/1663/09/14/> (accessed 17/08/16).

[116] Cowper, *Diary*, vol. 1, p. 197.

[117] Edward Lawrence, *Christ's power over bodily diseases* (1672, first publ. 1662), 262–3.

[118] On the holy affections, see Chapter 4, pp. 146–55.

relationships with family and friends outside the home.[119] Historians have explored the use of letters in medical consultation, but the role of this medium in the resumption of life after illness has rarely been acknowledged.[120] The clergyman from Westminster Philip Henry (1631–96) wrote to a friend in 1688, 'two or three dayes [I have been] a Prisoner to my Bed under Distempers, & this is the First-fruit of my Recovery, the first time I sett Pen to Paper to write a letter' (see Figure 2, in the Introduction).[121] The length of letters ranges from a few 'scribled lines' to several pages, but they exhibit certain common features: patients usually apologize for the delay in correspondence, reassure their recipient they are now 'out of danger', and give thanks for concern shown during the sickness.[122] 'I cannot but prise that care you have exprest to me, and your ernest desires for my health', wrote Brilliana Harley to her son Edward during her convalescence in 1639.[123]

These letters enabled patients not just to resume their relationships, but to consolidate them, an impression borne out by their affectionate, even obsequious tone. This is illustrated in the correspondence of Thomas Wentworth (1593–1641), lord lieutenant of Ireland. In 1624, he informed his friend, Sir Arthur Ingram, a London merchant:

> I conceaved it would not bee altogether displeasinge unto yow to see my owne hand testimony for the daunger (I praise God) is now escaped; soe as I maie now with this good blessing hope yet to live to give yow demonstracon of that truth and friendship, which I have professed.

Wentworth suggests that a major benefit of his survival is the opportunity it will bring for him to prove his friendship, and goes on to imply that Ingram is honoured to be the recipient of, 'This...the first letter I writte since I was ill'.[124] The same day Wentworth penned two other letters, to Christopher Wandesford and George Calvert, both close friends; he informed Wandesford that his illness had made him realize that the 'greatest comfort' in life is 'from our friends and [the] mutuall and true love wee shold beare one to another, in which number I esteem your selfe a principal one'.[125] He told Calvert that 'writing to soe noble and soe deare a freind' cheers up his 'languishinge spiritts'.[126] These effusive expressions

[119] On the 'epistolary sick role', see Withey, *Physick and the Family*, 133. James Daybell confirms that letter-writing was disrupted by sickness: *Women Letter-Writers in Tudor England* (Oxford, 2006), 68, 112, 136, 149. David Thorley comments that in some cases, letter-writing might continue amongst one's nearest and dearest, but correspondence with wider social relations ceased: *Writing Illness and Identity in Seventeenth-Century Britain* (Basingstoke, 2016), 122.
[120] On letter-writing in medical consultation, see Wendy Churchill, 'Gendered Medical Advice within Anglo-Irish Correspondence: A Case Study of the Cary–Jurin Letters', in Fiona Clark and James Kelly (eds.), *Ireland and Medicine in the Seventeenth and Eighteenth Centuries* (Farnham, 2010), 163–82; Wayne Wild, *Medicine-by-Post: The Changing Voice of Illness in Eighteenth-Century British Consultation Letters and Literature*, Clio Medica, vol. 79 (New York, 2006). On the use of letters for shedding light on illness experiences, see Thorley, *Writing Illness*, ch. 4.
[121] BL, Additional MS 42,849, fol. 6r (Letters of the Henry family).
[122] The scribed lines were by Joan St John in 1631: Searle (ed.), *Barrington Family Letters*, 200.
[123] Harley, *The Letters*, 83–4.
[124] William Wentworth, *Wentworth Papers 1597–1628*, ed. J. P. Cooper, Camden Society, vol. 12 (1973), 204.
[125] Ibid., 204–5.   [126] Ibid., 204.

would come as no surprise to Keith Thomas, who has shown that in this period the 'language of friendship could be extravagant', almost romantic in tone.[127] The preservation and advancement of a person's socio-economic standing depended on the successful cultivation of friendships; letter-writing was a vital mode through which these bonds were fostered.[128] Since the above three recipients were Wentworth's chief contacts at court, he had particular reason to ingratiate himself to them. Nonetheless, we should not doubt his sincerity: after all, work was one of the main forums in which friendships developed.[129] Of course, letter-writing was not a universal rite of passage for patients—those who lacked writing skills may have instead sent news of their recoveries via a messenger. This was the case for Mary Maillard, a thirteen-year-old French interpreter, who was believed to be cured miraculously in 1693. She called out to the maid, Bridget, who 'ran down and told it to the House, and it was noised about the Neighbourhood that Evening'.[130] To reach relatives living further away, these patients may have asked a literate neighbour to write a letter on their behalf.[131]

Once patients were strong enough to go downstairs, they could rejoin the rest of the household in the main living quarters, a transition termed 'being up and down amongst the family'. Reunited in space after a period of separation, patients and their relations often relished one another's company, describing their interactions in happy terms, as 'comfortable' and 'delightful'. Ralph Josselin recorded in 1664, 'my heart rejoyceth' to be with 'my deare wife'.[132] It was partly the abatement of physical suffering that enabled patients to once more appreciate their relations' company. Harris observed that whereas the sick find the conversations of their friends wearying, in recovery 'he sees a wife to be a wife, children to be children, friends to be friends'. No longer in a 'bitter or sowre' mood, the recovered patient 'findes contentment in all'.[133] Another factor that fed into patients' positive experiences was the recent memory of relatives' tender care during illness. The newly married Yorkshire gentlewoman Alice Thornton (1626–1707) recorded in her autobiography that, 'My deare husband, with my mother, was exceeding tender over me, which was a great comfort to my spiritts' during her dangerous illness in 1651.[134] Husbands expressed similar sentiments about their wives' attentions. The lawyer and politician Bulstrode Whitelock (1605–75) wrote appreciatively that during an episode of 'bloody flux' in 1670, his 'wife was very tender & carefull of him . . . his children were affectionate, his wifes maid Betty was very carefull & his other servants ready to doe anything for him'.[135] It was common for patients to single out the attentions of their servants, a tendency which supports Bernard

---

[127] Thomas, *The Ends of Life*, 204.   [128] Ibid., 191–2.   [129] See note 2 in this chapter.
[130] *An exact relation of the wonderful cure of Mary Maillard* (1730, first publ. 1694), 7.
[131] Adam Fox, *Oral and Literate Culture in England 1500–1700* (Oxford, 2002), 37.
[132] Josselin, *The Diary*, 504.   [133] Harris, *Hezekiahs recovery*, 29–30.
[134] Alice Thornton, *The Autobiography of Mrs Alice Thornton*, ed. Charles Jackson, Surtees Society, vol. 62 (1875), 83. See also Elizabeth Walker, *The vertuous wife*, ed. Anthony Walker (1694), 83, 131–2.
[135] Whitelocke, *The Diary*, 764. See also SHC, DD/WO 55/7/47-1 (letter from Richard Carpenter to his father-in-law, John Trevelyan, 24 March 1619).

Capp's assertion that relations between household staff and their employers could be affectionate, despite potential for exploitation.[136] Nonetheless, the positive picture conveyed here may not represent everyone's experiences, as will be shown at the end of this section.

After rejoining the rest of the household, patients were commonly inundated by visitors. Pepys noted in 1663 that one morning during his recovery from 'itching and pimples', he was 'visited by Mr. Coventry and others, and very glad I am to see that I am so much inquired after[,] and my sickness taken notice of'. The next day, several more visitors appeared, including his uncle, Mr Creed, and Sir J. Minnes, who Pepys added, were 'mighty kind to me and careful of me in my sickness'.[137] Clearly this man felt gratified by the attentions of all his callers. Social visits might seem a somewhat mundane occurrence, but they could exert an enormous impact on the patient's personal life. Two examples can be cited, the first from the memoirs of Mary Boyle (1624–78). Newly recovered from measles in the 1630s, the only person prepared to risk infection was a young man from court, Charles Rich; she recorded that his 'frequent visits to me…to a great degree [did] heighten my passion for him'. Upon his knees, he 'did so handsomely express his passion…for me…[that] I consented to be his wife'. The two were later married, despite the initial objections of Mary's family.[138] The second example is from an account of the miraculous healing of the aforementioned Mary Maillard from lameness. Before her cure, this girl had been bullied by children in her neighbourhood: they used to 'flock about' her, and 'abuse her with rude Language', calling her 'opprobrious Names'. This treatment ended abruptly when the culprits, along with what appears to have been most of the neighbourhood, were brought to visit Mary at news of her recovery. Mary recorded, 'Crouds came so thick to see me…[of] Multitudes of…Ages, and both Sexes…and the House was so crouded, that I had hardly time to eat'.[139] When one of her bullies, 'the butcher's girl', entered the room, Mary called out, 'That's she that derided me a while ago'. Shamed in front of her community, the girl and her collaborators ceased their bullying. This rare insight into playground politics shows that recovery was a context in which the realms of public and private coalesced: visitors were arriving in such numbers that the patient's home became a semi-public arena.[140] While miracles may have drawn the greatest crowds, natural healings could also attract numerous visitors. The nonconformist Halifax minister Oliver Heywood (c.1630–1702) noted proudly that in 1691, 'above 40 of our Christian friends and neighbours' came to his home to attend 'a

---

[136] See for example, Pepys, *The Diary*, <http://www.pepysdiary.com/diary/1663/02/10/> (accessed 19/05/17); Capp, *When Gossips Meet*, ch. 4: see also Meldrum, *Domestic Service*, ch. 4.

[137] Pepys, *The Diary*, <http://www.pepysdiary.com/diary/1663/02/11/> (accessed 19/05/17). See also Fisher, *The wise virgin*, 146; Anne Clifford, *The Diaries of Lady Anne Clifford*, ed. D. D. H. Clifford (Stroud, 1990), 81.

[138] Rich, *Autobiography*, 6–7.   [139] *An exact relation*, 9.

[140] Similar numbers visited those diagnosed with diabolical possession: see Newton, *The Sick Child*, 101, 166–7.

solemn day of thankfulness' for his recovery. He added, 'my heart apt to be lifted up with multitudes and quantitys of visitors, the Esteem... of gods people'.[141]

Once patients were strong enough to leave the house, their next social milestone on the road to normal life was attending a thanksgiving church service. Besides the spiritual purpose of thanksgiving, this special service fulfilled important social functions: patients were welcomed back into the community, and were able to return their thanks to fellow parishioners for prayers and visits.[142] Timothy Rogers led his own thanksgiving service in the 1690s, addressing his congregation:

> I am now come to thank... those of you here... for your kind Affection, and for the Requests which... you presented to the Throne of God in my behalf... There are several Persons here, that wept with me when I wept, and that prayed for me when I was in trouble; to these and others... Come, and let us now rejoyce together.[143]

Since the sharing of emotions was a sign of true love, Rogers was effectively reminding himself and his fellow parishioners of the affection that exists between members of the church.[144] Andrew Cambers has shown that collective religious devotion was at the heart of godly Protestant identity; the thanksgiving service was part of this sociability.[145] While it is unlikely that all patients would have been treated to their own special service, we know that church was an important site of sociability across the classes, regardless of the particular type of service on offer.[146] Perhaps, therefore, it is conceivable that the return to church may have been appreciated even by those patients who were not so interested in religion.[147]

Church was supposed to be the first destination to which patients headed after recovery, but in some cases, it was the pub. The aforementioned Rogers complained, 'Some indeed when they recover... the first Visit they make is to their old *Good-fellows*', the alehouse, where 'they are welcomed into the jolly Company with full Bowls and loud Huzzaes'.[148] Predictably, the pious diarists in this study rarely admitted to partaking in these drunken affairs, but they do occasionally castigate the behaviour of their less godly neighbours for doing so. Oliver Heywood wrote of one Jane Thompson, who, 'being something better' from her illness, 'would goe with her husband to... an alehouse... to... chear up her spirits with ale and company'.[149] While we lack first-hand evidence of the experiences of convalescents like Jane, popular ballads suggest that alehouses were merry places, where people could 'laugh and sing'.[150] A lively description of what patients got up to in these venues is provided in a medical text by Levinus Lemnius: 'when men recover of their disease', he wrote, they are joined by 'many witty merry companions', who 'invite them to rejoyce, and make merry... Hence they eat, and drink healths one

[141] Heywood, *The Rev. Oliver Heywood*, vol. 4, 141, vol. 3, 258.
[142] On these spiritual functions, see Chapter 4, pp. 155–7.
[143] Rogers, *Practical discourses*, 2, 268.   [144] See Chapter 3, pp. 113–14.
[145] Cambers, *Godly Reading, passim*.   [146] Thomas, *The Ends of Life*, 220.
[147] On those uninterested in religion, see Capp, *When Gossips Meet*, 360. On the incentives for church attendance amongst the less religious, see Hunt, *The Art of Hearing: English Preachers and their Audiences, 1590–1640* (Cambridge, 2010), 205–6.
[148] Rogers, *Practical discourses*, 210.   [149] Heywood, *The Rev. Oliver Heywood*, vol. 3, 85.
[150] Cited by Mark Hailwood, *Alehouses and Good Fellowship in Early Modern England* (2014), 147.

another round about...and commonly they sing bawdy songs'.[151] He is describing here what was known as 'health drinking', a ritual that has rarely been explored in the context of recovery: friends raised their glasses, offering their congratulations, and expressing their wishes for the patient's continued health; each drinker pledged in turn, draining their glasses in unison, or passing round a 'healthing bowl' from which everyone would take a gulp.[152] Mark Hailwood believes that drinking healths was 'a meaningful social ritual', which served both as 'an expression and reinforcement of...lasting bonds' between friends, particularly for young men.[153] This demographic may therefore have been especially keen to partake in such rituals upon recovery, though as we saw from the example of Jane Thompson above, women were not excluded from this form of sociability.[154] As the period progressed, new venues for recreation emerged, including coffee-houses, theatres, and pleasure gardens.[155] These places do not, however, feature very frequently in accounts of recovery. This does not mean that patients were not resorting to such locations, but rather that they had yet to attain the status of a recognized milestone on the road to health.

The penultimate step to social reintegration involved visiting friends in their homes, a setting which Sasha Handley believes 'allowed for deeper bonds of friendship to be forged' than in public houses.[156] In this period, reciprocity was central to all relationships, human and divine; it was thus vital to repay one's relations and friends for their visits and prayers.[157] Economic and political fortunes depended on informal support in this era, so it is not surprising that the reciprocation of favours was important in many areas of life, including illness and recovery.[158] This is demonstrated in the memoirs of Yorkshire curate Thomas Brockbank (1671–1732): he was supported financially by one Mrs Preston of Holkner, whose patronage propelled him to the position of vicar. During Mrs Preston's illness in 1708, he visited her 'almost every day', and led prayers in church; when this lady eventually recovered, she sent Brockbank a guinea as 'a small acknowledgement of your kindness'.[159] These back-and-forth favours, which helped sustain relationships between patron and client, are reminiscent of

[151] Lemnius, *The secret miracles*, 135.

[152] Rebecca Lemon, 'Compulsory Conviviality in Early Modern England', *English Literary Renaissance*, 43 (2013), 381–414, at 381. On health-drinking in general, see Hailwood, *Alehouses*, 101–2; Lemon, 'Compulsory Conviviality'; Peter Clark, 'The Alehouse and the Alternative Society', in Donald Pennington and Keith Thomas (eds.), *Puritans and Revolutionaries: Essays in Seventeenth-Century History Presented to Christopher Hill* (Oxford, 1978), 47–72, at 64; Shepard, *Meanings of Manhood*, 101.

[153] Hailwood, *Alehouses*, 218; Shepard, *Meanings of Manhood*, 101.

[154] A nuanced discussion of women's presence in alehouses is provided in Flather, *Gender and Space*, 112–21; she shows that women *were* present, but men 'lingered far longer, more freely, and frequently'.

[155] For an introduction to these developments, and their historiographies, see Sasha Handley, 'Sociable Sleeping in Early Modern England, 1660–1760', *History*, 98 (2013), 79–104.

[156] Handley, *Sleep*, 163.

[157] See Chapter 4, p. 148, on the reciprocation of divine attentions.

[158] See note 160 in this chapter.

[159] Thomas Brockbank, *The Diary and Letter Book of the Rev. Thomas Brockbank 1671–1709*, ed. Richard Trappes-Lomax, Chetham Society New Series, vol. 89 (Manchester, 1930), 313, 329, 333, 341, 353. See also Benjamin Rogers, *The Diary of Benjamin Rogers Rector of Carlton, 1720–71*, ed. C. D. Linnell Symcotts, Bedfordshire Historical Record Society, vol. 31 (Streatley, 1951), 25.

the 'three-fold obligation' theory of gifts developed by the anthropologist Marcel Mauss: to give, receive, and repay.[160] The fact that many of the above examples of visits were made by males challenges the common view that neighbourly calls were typically female forms of sociability.[161] Nor were social visits necessarily confined to the wealthy: even those living in subordinate positions, such as servants and apprentices, may have been permitted the freedom to visit their friends on occasions.[162]

After returning friends' visits, the final step of social reintegration occurred: celebratory dinners. In the historiography of hospitality, some work has been undertaken on the feasting that accompanied the rites of passages of birth, marriage, and death, but the festivities that occurred after recovery from illness have not been explored.[163] Meals varied in size and sophistication, from carefully planned, sumptuous feasts to impromptu suppers. Upon recovering from a life-threatening illness in 1691, Oliver Heywood recorded that his many 'Christian friends and neighbours' were 'feasted... nobly' by his wife.[164] Given that hospitality was an important part of a wife's role, it is likely that Mrs Heywood's identity and reputation would have been enhanced by this dinner.[165] A rather more simple supper was described in the autobiography of the Cambridge student Simonds D'Ewes (1602–50): during his convalescence from a head injury in 1618, his university tutor invited D'Ewes, together with his father and friends, 'to sup with him' one evening, to their 'great comfort, and our mutual congratulations'.[166] The meal was hastily arranged when D'Ewes' tutor saw that his father, who had endured a long journey on horseback, was tired and hungry.

Thus far we have seen that recovery was socially bonding, serving to enhance relationships between kin, friends, and neighbours. While this was the case for the majority of the individuals in this study, there do exist some less positive reports. In 1700, Elizabeth Freke travelled 'above two hundred miles in fowre days' to her husband who was 'like to dye'; she recorded in her diary that she found him 'well enough to chid[e] mee', and added with wistful resignation, 'tho itt was nott kind, I expected itt'.[167] The marriage had been unhappy for many years, with the two living apart; she may have hoped that the nearly fatal illness would have renewed

---

[160] Marcel Mauss, *The Gift: Forms and Functions of Exchange in Archaic Societies*, trans. Ian Cunnison (New York, 1967), 7. On gift-giving, see Ilana Krausman Ben-Amos, *The Culture of Giving: Informal Support and Gift-Exchange in Early Modern England* (Cambridge, 2008); Felicity Heal, *The Power of Gifts: Gift-Exchange in Early Modern England* (Oxford, 2014).

[161] Capp, *When Gossips Meet*, 321.

[162] Handley, *Sleep*, 163; Capp, *When Gossips Meet*, 335–7; for example, see Roger Lowe, *The Diary of Roger Lowe of Ashton-in-Makerfield, Lancashire, 1663–1674*, ed. William Sachse (1938), 23, 26, 44.

[163] For example, David Cressy, *Birth, Marriage, and Death: Ritual, Religion and the Life Cycle in Tudor and Stuart England* (Oxford, 1997); Felicity Heal, *Hospitality in Early Modern England* (Oxford, 1990), ch. 9.

[164] Oliver Heywood, *The Rev. Oliver Heywood, B.A: His Autobiography, Diaries, Anecdote and Event Books*, ed. Horsfall Turner, 4 vols. (1883); vol. 4, 141.

[165] Capp, *When Gossips Meet*, 322.

[166] Simonds D'Ewes, *The Autobiography and Correspondence of Sir Simonds D'Ewes, Bart.*, ed. J. O. Halliwell, 2 vols. (1845), vol. 1, 129–30.

[167] Freke, *The Remembrances*, 73–4.

their love, but instead, she was left feeling unappreciated. Freke expressed similar resentment towards one of her servants, Mary Chapman, for failing to show gratitude for her care of this maid during smallpox.[168] Ultimately, whether patients and their relations enjoyed resuming social relationships depended on whether they got on, as well as how attentive and appreciative they had been to each other during the illness.[169]

For individuals who 'love[d] quiett & solitude', and disliked 'the Clatter of Tongues', the social rituals of recovery could be experienced as duties rather than pleasures.[170] This was the case for Robert Paston, a Norfolk MP: when convalescing from gout in 1676, he told his wife, 'I goe now abroad...butt I have a great deale of company dayly heere, and Sir John Hobart, though I have nott...had time to returne his first visitt has made me a second and a long one'. By using the word 'but', Paston hints that the company is undesirable; he also suggests that his visitor has infringed social etiquette by calling twice without an intervening visit. Two days later, Paston told his wife he was about to 'returne one of those too visitts' from Sir John, noting that, 'after halfe an howres dissimulation on both sides I will come home'.[171] Clearly, this man saw visiting as a performance, devoid of real feeling. Such experiences support Felicity Heal's observation that the obligatory nature of sociability could make it 'burdensome to the spirit'.[172]

Convalescents found social activities exhausting on occasions. The Manchester medical practitioner and preacher James Clegg (1679–1755) noted in his diary that 'Mr Kesal, Mrs Creswell and Mrs Waterhouse came to see me. I was glad of their company but talkt too much with them...and found myself weary'.[173] More serious than tiredness, however, was the potential for socializing to precipitate relapse. Alice Thornton recalled that her father, recuperating from fever in 1640, was attended by various 'persons of quality'; but when he entered the dining room, he 'cra[v]ed leave the company to rest himself a little in his bedchamber...but still he grew worse, and...found himself...ill'.[174] Even the more sedate activity of letter-writing could have this effect.[175] When the social rituals of recovery went wrong, the results could be dangerous, as is attested in legal records and popular literature.[176] The Proceedings of the Old Bailey show that in 1683 a quarrel broke out when one Mr Welsh refused to drink the health of his companion, Mr Atkinson; 'Glasses of Wine were thrown...and in the end their [were] Swords drawn, in

---

[168] Ibid., 284–5.
[169] The burden of caring for the sick/disabled could strain relationships, and patients who had felt neglected during their illness also suffered—see Turner, *Disability*, 131–6.
[170] The first quote is from Paston, *The Whirlpool*, 320; the second is from Cowper, *Diary*, vol. 2, 25.
[171] Paston, *The Whirlpool*, 231, 233. [172] Heal, *Hospitality*, 22–3.
[173] James Clegg, *The Diary of James Clegg of Chapel-en-Frith 1708–1755*, vol. 1 (1708–36), ed. Vanessa Doe, Derbyshire Record Society, vol. 5 (Matlock, 1978), 116.
[174] Thornton, *The Autobiography*, 21.
[175] Searle (ed.), *Barrington Family Letters*, 200. See also Christopher Hatton, *Correspondence of the Family of Hatton being Chiefly Addressed to Christopher, First Viscount Hatton, 1601–1704*, ed. Edward Maunde Thompson, Camden Society, vols. 22–3 (1878), vol. 2, 94; BL, Additional MS 28050, fols. 156r–v (Domestic correspondence of the Osborne family, 1637–1761).
[176] Lemon, 'Compulsory Conviviality'.

which Action...Mr Welsh' was killed.[177] Thus, refusal to participate in drinking rituals could have fatal consequences!

For particularly devout individuals, it was the spiritual, rather than the bodily, consequences of socializing that caused most concern. Richard Kilby (d. 1617), a cleric from Kent, admitted that whenever he was in company, he 'fell into a deale of idle unholy communication...merily delight[ing] my selfe with prohane talk'. This sin caused him such anxiety that the mere sound of 'feet coming up the staires' made him 'very fearfull'.[178] Worries of this kind were also expressed when patients found themselves failing to relish their first visit to church after their illness. The usually devout London woodturner Nehemiah Wallington (1598–1658) confessed that after an acute sickness in 1652, 'I take notis[e] of my own base filthy heart in that I could be content to have bin longer sicke that it might have exsempted me from the house of God'. On another occasion, he confessed that the prospect of religious devotion 'is as bitter as gall', and that he would rather 'be sicke in my bed as to goe unto it'.[179] For this patient, sickness was a rare opportunity to miss church. Judging by church court records, Wallington was not alone: in the parish of St Botolph's, one man 'fayn[ed] himselfe sick' in 1598 so that he could avoid the catechism.[180] In sum, while the resumption of social life was in most cases a happy affair, serving to renew and reinforce bonds between patients and their family and friends, it could be the source of emotional, bodily, and spiritual discomfort.

IDLENESS TO OFFICE: WORKING LIFE

Having explored patients' experiences of returning to their normal spatial and social lives, this third and final section investigates how they felt about going back to work after illness. Besides challenging the notion that the sick seldom ceased working in the early modern period, the ensuing discussions contribute to the historiography of attitudes to employment.[181] Scholars have often viewed early modern work in negative terms: amongst the elites, schoolboys were forced into careers based on their parents' preferences rather than their own inclinations.[182] For the lower orders, work is said to have been 'monotonous, dirty and cold', with women's labour singled out for its low status and pay.[183] While not denying that work could

---

[177] POB, Ref: t16831010a-16. See also the case of Phillip Wallis: t16841210-41 (both accessed 19/08/16).
[178] Richard Kilby, *Halleluiah: praise yee the Lord, for the unburthening of a loaded conscience* (Cambridge, 1635), 88–9, 95, 239.
[179] Nehemiah Wallington, *The Notebooks of Nehemiah Wallington, 1618–1654: A Selection*, ed. David Booy (Aldershot, 2007), 163, 321–2.
[180] St Olave Jewry vestry minute-book held at the Guildhall Library, London, MS 4415/1, cited by Hunt, *The Art of Hearing*, 238.
[181] See notes 4–5 in this chapter.
[182] Ralph Houlbrooke, *The English Family, 1450–1700* (1984), 170–1. Houlbrooke believes as time progressed, young men were granted more freedom over their career choice.
[183] Anthony Fletcher, *Gender, Sex, and Subordination in England, 1500–1800* (1995), 223; see also, J. A. Sharpe, *Early Modern England: A Social History* (1997, first publ. 1987), 213. On women's work, see Judith Bennett, '"History that Stands Still": Women's Work in the European Past', *Feminist*

be arduous or demeaning, my study adds to the revisionist scholarship which highlights the more positive attitudes that were also in circulation.[184]

It is first necessary to establish that the seriously ill did in fact stop their usual work. Although it is not possible to provide examples from every sort of employment, a fairly wide selection of callings can be cited. At the upper end of the hierarchy were the landed classes, who spent their time running their estates, and occupying public offices. The politician Sir Horatio Townshend (1630–87) was 'much tak[en]...off his busines' due to a 'dangerous fitt', reported one of his kinsmen in 1665.[185] In the same decade, Bulstrode Whitelocke, keeper of the Great Seal, recorded that he 'durst not attend the busines of the Seale being very weake with his sicknes', ague.[186] It was also usual for members of the middling sectors to abstain from work during severe illness, including clergymen,[187] teachers, traders, and merchants,[188] and those pursuing artistic careers, such as poets,[189] musicians,[190] and architects.[191] The minister Ralph Josselin wrote that he 'preacht twice...after six weeks absence' from the pulpit due to scurvy, while another minister, Richard Baxter, agreed to step in as teacher when the 'old School-master, Mr. *John Owen*, was sick of a Consumption'.[192] Amongst the lower classes—the majority of the population—a range of occupational groups were unable to work during serious disease, including servants,[193] agricultural labourers,[194] seamen and soldiers,[195] shop and alehouse workers,[196] craftsmen and builders,[197] and textile and shoe-makers.[198] In the 1660s, one Thomas Burt, a Buckinghamshire agricultural labourer, fell so ill of fever 'that he was forced to leave his work' until he was miraculously healed.[199]

Studies, 14 (1988), 269–83; Sara Mendelson and Patricia Crawford, *Women in Early Modern England* (Oxford, 2003, first publ. 1998), 260–1, 264.

[184] For example, Thomas, *The Ends of Life*, ch. 3, Alexandra Shepard, *Accounting for Oneself: Worth, Status, and the Social Order in Early Modern England* (Oxford, 2015), and Mark Hailwood, 'Broadside Ballads and Occupational Identity in Early Modern England', *Huntington Library Quarterly*, 79 (2016), 187–200, have shown that work could be a source of self-worth, identity, and pride.

[185] Paston, *The Whirlpool*, 62.   [186] Whitelocke, *The Diary*, 253

[187] Josselin, *The Diary*, 390; John Hall, *Select observations on English bodies*, trans. James Cooke (1679, first. publ. 1657), 275–6.

[188] Liddell, *The Letters*, 1

[189] John Dryden, *The Letters of John Dryden*, ed. Charles Ward (Durham NC, 1942), 132.

[190] Ysbrand van Diemerbroeck, *The anatomy of human bodies ... To which is added ... several practical observations*, trans. William Salmon (1694, first publ. in Utrecht in 1664), 110–11.

[191] John Buxton, *John Buxton, Norfolk Gentleman and Architect: Letters to his Son, 1719–1729*, ed. Alan Mackley, Norfolk Record Society, vol. 69 (Norwich, 2005), 143.

[192] Josselin, *The Diary*, 567; Richard Baxter, *Reliquiae Baxterianae, or, Mr. Richard Baxters narrative* (1696), 5.

[193] Citations in Capp, *When Gossips Meet*, 142.

[194] *A true copy of a letter of the miraculous cure of David Wright, a sheppard* (1694), 1–2.

[195] Greatrakes, *A brief account*, 51; Van Diemerbroeck, *The anatomy*, 85–6. See also Cheryl Fury, 'Health and Health Care at Sea', in Cheryl Fury (ed.), *The Social History of English Seamen, 1485–1649* (Woodbridge, 2012), 193–227, at 211–12, 215, 219, 224.

[196] William Stout, *The Autobiography of William Stout of Lancaster, 1665–1752*, ed. J. D. Marshall (Manchester, 1976), 90–1.

[197] Greatrakes, *A brief account*, 27.

[198] John Harris, *The divine physician, prescribing rules for the prevention, and cure of most diseases* (1676), 143.

[199] Greatrakes, *A brief account*, 50.

An advertisement for a special ointment from 1694 claims that upon taking this medicine, a tapster from a Holborn alehouse, who had been sick of palsy, was able once more to 'draw Drink'.[200] Olivia Weisser's analysis of pauper petitions for monetary relief reveals that illness was a common cause of financial hardship, from which we can infer that poor patients were often unable to pursue their normal work when seriously ill.[201] I should note here that many people in this period undertook multiple employments: there was an 'economy of makeshifts', so the occupational terms mentioned above are imperfect labels.[202]

Besides these socially differentiated groups of workers, were housewives of every social level, who performed or supervised innumerable domestic tasks without remuneration, in addition to any waged work.[203] Historians have tended to assume that domestic duties were even less likely to have been impeded by illness than the sort of formal, paid employments carried out by people of both sex outside the home.[204] Given that 'going abroad' was a major milestone of recovery, and a good proportion—though by no means all—of women's domestic work took place inside, this assumption is understandable.[205] However, I have found that during serious illness, even indoor work was interrupted. This is nicely illustrated in the diary of the ejected minister Henry Newcome (*c.*1627–95): he mentions that he rose at seven in the morning to get the children out of bed, 'my wife beinge ill'.[206] Higher up the social scale, the puritan heiress Margaret Hoby (1571–1633) was at last able to 'talk with some of the sarvants of houshould mattres' following a bout of toothache in 1599; on another occasion, when she was 'somthinge better' from colic, she 'gott dinner for the house'.[207] There seems to have been a concept of being 'abroad in the house', an apparently contradictory phrase which accommodated indoor work within the schema of recovery.[208] Other groups of unpaid workers who ceased their labours when very ill were the young: schoolchildren, apprentices, and students.[209]

---

[200] Atkins, *A discourse*, 101.

[201] Weisser, *Ill Composed*, ch. 6; see also Pelling, *The Common Lot*, chs. 3, 4.

[202] The term 'economy of makeshifts' was coined by Olwen Hufton in 1974; for a more recent discussion of this concept, see Alannah Tomkins and Steve King (eds.), *The Poor in England 1700–1850: An Economy of Makeshifts* (Manchester, 2005).

[203] Alexandra Shepard has shown that in addition to unpaid domestic work, most married women of lower status undertook paid employment, contrary to common assumptions: *Accounting for Oneself, passim.*

[204] Lucinda Beier, 'In Sickness and in Health: A Seventeenth Century Family's Experience', in Roy Porter (ed.), *Patients and Practitioners: Lay Perceptions of Medicine in Pre-Industrial Society* (Cambridge: 2002, first publ. 1985), 101–28, at 123–4.

[205] My thanks to Charmian Mansell and the 'Women's Work in Rural England, 1500–1700' team at the University of Exeter for highlighting the multiple locations of women's domestic work, which included outside spaces. Mark Hailwood has written on this at: <https://earlymodernwomenswork. wordpress.com/2016/06/09/how-domestic-was-womens-work/> (accessed 11/10/17).

[206] Henry Newcome, *The Diary of Rev. Henry Newcome*, ed. Thomas Heywood, Chetham Society, vol. 18 (1849), 173.

[207] Margaret Hoby, *Diary of Lady Margaret Hoby 1599–1605*, ed. Dorothy Meads (1930), 67, 180.

[208] Thornton, *The Autobiography*, 157. Going 'abroad' could be applied to movement from the sickchamber into another room—see Clifford, *The Diaries*, 49.

[209] Newton, *The Sick Child*, 173–5.

Various reasons lay behind patients' inability to work during serious illness. Individuals engaged in manual labour were too weak to perform strenuous tasks, while those pursuing more intellectual pursuits found that disease impaired their mental capacities.[210] These effects were attributed to the reduction in volume of a person's spirits, the special vapours responsible for performing all physical and mental functions.[211] Henry Liddell, a coal trader, told his colleague in 1716, 'my spirits flagg to that degree that I am render'd... utterly incapable off business off any sort...I can't think of business, much less transact any'.[212] Other reasons for stopping work included the irresistible desire to lie down, and the practical need to be close to chamber-pots and other receptacles used for the disposal of the bodily fluids evacuated during illness.[213] For patients whose work involved travel, the inability 'to endure the motion of a coach' was a further impediment to work. The Bishop of Norwich obtained a certificate in 1679 to 'humblie certifie' that he was 'afflicted with the stone', which meant any journey might 'hazard his life'.[214] Likewise, work was hindered by the malfunctioning of the part of the body critical to the person's occupation. John Hugo, a trumpeter, 'could hardly draw his Breath' during his chest condition; he could not speak, let alone 'sound his Trumpet'.[215] Finally, some patients did not offer any explanation for their inability to work, perhaps assuming it was self-evident. The Manchester wigmaker Edmund Harrold wrote laconically, 'Very ill, lay long. Could not work'.[216]

Of course, there were exceptions: some diseases were less debilitating than others, and even severe illnesses did not always stop a determined patient from continuing with work. For clergymen in particular, persevering with preaching could be a way to demonstrate their extraordinary commitment to God. John Donne's biographer described how this man, during 'purple fever', was advised not to preach by his friends, and yet 'passionately denied their requests', and professed '*an holy ambition to perform that sacred work*'.[217] Other workers justified their continued employment on the grounds that they were indispensable. The Stratford physician John Hall (1575–1635) wrote that although he was 'much debilitated' with haemorrhoids, 'yet daily I [was] constrained to go to several places to Patients', due to lack of cover.[218] Nor was it necessarily always a case of either working or not working— some individuals might manage to carry out certain tasks, while omitting the more strenuous, outdoor work. Francis Guybon, a steward, was advised by his master to 'Set somebody [else] to look after your [haymakers] in Meadow Close', but that

---

[210] On physical labour, see Weisser, *Ill Composed*, 173. For an example of intellectual work, see Ralph Thoresby, *Letters Addressed to Ralph Thoresby, FRS*, ed. W. T. Lancaster (1912), 105, 140.

[211] See Chapter 2, pp. 68–71 for an explanation of how disease affected the spirits.

[212] Liddell, *The Letters*, 158, 233.

[213] On the need to lie down in bed, see p. 195 in this chapter; on evacuation, see Chapter 1, pp. 48–56.

[214] Thomas Browne, *The Letters of Sir Thomas Browne*, ed. Geoffrey Keynes (Cambridge, 1946), 423.

[215] Van Diemerbroeck, *The anatomy*, 110–11.

[216] Edmund Harrold, *The Diary of Edmund Harrold, Wigmaker of Manchester 1712–15*, ed. Craig Horner (Aldershot, 2009), 91.

[217] Donne, *Devotions*, 71–2.

[218] Hall, *Select observations*, 149–50. See also Kilby, *Halleluiah*, 106–7.

'While y[o]u are forced to stay indoors[,] write out your accounts for last year'.[219]
Work could thus be adapted to the capacities of the patient. At the bottom of the
social scale, David Turner has shown that in the eighteenth century, chronically ill
or disabled paupers were often required to change, rather than stop, their employment, finding a less physically arduous job.[220] For those in subordinate positions,
there was sometimes no choice but to continue working: cruel masters might force
their servants and apprentices to persist with their tasks, even though such treatment evoked criticism. Equally unlucky were workers who were sacked as soon as
they sickened in order to prevent the spread of infection and escape the costs of
medical care.[221] Nonetheless, the very fact these examples elicited attention indicates
that continuing with work in this context was not normal.

What was it like to resume work after a period of inactivity? A number of common
themes emerge, despite great variations in types of employment. For all but the
wealthiest, the most urgent implications of work, and its resumption, were financial.
Olivia Weisser has shown that the loss of earnings during sickness, coupled with
the expenses accrued from medicines, pushed many families into poverty.[222] This
is evident from the numerous applications for relief received by local parishes, in
which paupers and their relatives emphasized the material toll of illness. William
Smart from Somerset described himself as 'ever laborious and industrious in his
calling', but lately grown 'disabled for labour' by age and disease.[223] Such documents were written by scribes rather than by paupers themselves, but there is no
reason to doubt the level of hardship conveyed.[224] We might assume that the costs
of illness would not have mattered to those higher up the social scale, but this was
not the case. Margaret Pelling has noted that the records of craft companies reveal
'substantial numbers of ex-masters and others of previously important estate sunk
into permanent decay' by sickness.[225] This assertion is corroborated by letters from
individuals of middling status written in pursuit of financial aid. The poet John
Dryden (1631–1700) pleaded for extra cash from his patron in the 1680s due to
his 'extreame wants…& my ill health', an intermitting fever.[226] Even the titled
classes could be affected in this way, as captain John Barrington found in 1629: he
was 'forced by reason of [his] longe sicknes' to ask his mother for 'the releafe of my
greate necessities'.[227] For those to whom money was no object, illness still had
financial repercussions: the saying, 'restore me to health, then talke to me of wealth',

---

[219] William Fitzwilliam, *The Correspondence of Lord Fitzwilliam of Milton and Francis Guybon, His
Steward 1697–1709*, ed. D. R. Hainsworth and Cherry Walker, Northampton Record Society, vol. 36
(1990), 156.
[220] Turner, *Disability*, 128–30. The same has been said about elderly people; rather than retiring
completely from work, they often adapted their work—see Shepard, *Meanings of Manhood*, 236–9.
[221] Capp, *When Gossips Meet*, 148–9.   [222] Weisser, *Ill Composed*, ch. 6.
[223] Ibid., 166–7.
[224] On the level of severity of poverty faced by families, see Crawford, *Parents of Poor Children*, ch. 4.
[225] Ibid., 64.   [226] Dryden, *The Letters*, 20–1. See also SHC, DD/SAS C/1193/4, p. 192.
[227] Searle (ed.), *Barrington Family Letters*, 76. Alexandra Shepard's examination of witnesses'
responses to questions about maintenance reveals that it was not uncommon for members of the
upper echelons to rely financially on their parents in this way: *Accounting for Oneself*, 206–8.

suggests that however rich the patient, disease took away the enjoyment of 'wealth, house, land'.[228] The rhyme of 'health' and 'wealth' is often played on in early modern proverbs.[229]

The return to work was thus a relief to those concerned about their finances. Upon recovering from ague in the mid-sixteenth century, the Somerset composer Thomas Whythorne (1528–96) took on extra work as a servant: he commented, 'I waz behind hand of my welth az [well] of my helth, hoping that in this I shuld rekover them both to their former estate agayn'.[230] Self-employed individuals, such as shopkeepers, were also particularly glad to return to their premises, since their businesses depended wholly on their own efforts. William Stout (1665–1752), a Lancashire grocer, was frustrated when his violent cough halted his plans to renovate his shop; fortunately, within a month he was 'recovred to my former activety', and able to 'help forward my undertakeing', to his immense satisfaction.[231] Even the landed classes were relieved to get better for this reason. The landlord William Fitzwilliam (1643–1719) told his steward in 1707, 'Thank God I am much better' from the stone; his priority was to recoup some of the expenses incurred during his sickness by raising the rents on his land. He instructed his steward, 'Be not too forward in letting the meadow under the usual prices. I want money so much ... [for] my illness has been chargeable'.[232]

The financial aspects of resuming work relate to the second theme to be discussed: gender. For married men, the monetary repercussions of sickness were inextricably tied to anxieties about failure to fulfil their allotted roles as breadwinners.[233] Such was the case for the Somerset schoolteacher John Cannon (1684–1743): during his ague in the 1720s, his wife Susanna gave him 'bad provoking words', and 'mumbled because I could do nothing[,] which fretted me much', telling him that 'she ... must spin ... to support such a lazy indolent fellow as I was'.[234] Spinning was the archetypal occupation of unmarried women ('spinsters'), so Susanna was effectively saying that she might as well be single. Lower down the social scale, inactivity could also be emasculating for men, as Olivia Weisser and David Turner have demonstrated in their analyses of paupers' requests for relief: men sought to counter the stigma attached to economic dependence by emphasizing their 'former ability to sustain themselves without burdening the parish'.[235] There may have been a gender element to women's experiences too: domestic work, including caring for husbands and children, was essential to feminine identity, so anything that hampered these tasks could be distressing. This is exemplified in a poem

---

[228] Thomas Adams, *A commentary ... upon the divine second epistle generall, written by the blessed apostle St. Peter* (1633), 34. For a variation on this saying, see Lemnius, *The secret miracles*, 344; Harris, *Hezekiahs recovery*, 37.

[229] For instance, N.R., *Proverbs*, 49, 61.

[230] Thomas Whythorne, *The Autobiography of Thomas Whythorne*, ed. James M. Osborn (Oxford, 1961), 37.

[231] Stout, *The Autobiography*, 221. [232] Fitzwilliam, *The Correspondence*, 234.

[233] Thomas, *The Ends of Life*, 102, 106. [234] SHC, DD/SAS C/1193/4, p. 182.

[235] Weisser, *Ill Composed*, 166; Turner, *Disability*, 128–34, 139–40.

by the eighteenth-century gentlewoman Jane Winscom, 'The Head-Ache, Or an Ode to Health':

> My children want a mother's care,
> A husband too, should due assistance share.
> Myself for action form'd would fain thro' life
> Be found th' assiduous—valuable wife.
> But now, behold, I live unfit for [n]aught.[236]

This woman professes unhappiness not to be able to fulfil her maternal and wifely roles. The same can be said of poorer women: just as pauper males sought to defend their reputations by highlighting their previous tendency to work hard, female petitioners stressed that prior to their illness they had 'bred up many children'.[237]

Given that the inability to work could undermine one's gender identity, it follows that the resumption of employment was cherished as an opportunity to restore this vital reputation. For men, it was not just the monetary income that was appreciated: work provided the opportunity to exercise a whole array of masculine qualities. Labourers, for instance, could show their physical strength, while those in more managerial positions could demonstrate their capacity to lead and control their subordinates.[238] When John Buxton returned to his work as an architect in the late 1720s, he told his son Robert:

> The building goes forward very well, & I thank God I've yet strength enough to be with the workmen six or seaven hours in the day, & find much occation to be there, not knowing how to depend upon the surveyor, who is often absent & as often ... liable to blunder. I can be on horseback six or seaven [hours], moving from one workman to another, and I find myself very necessary among them all.[239]

Buxton enjoyed the feeling of self-importance and authority that came with managing others; his repetition of the length of time he rode his horse indicates his satisfaction at this achievement. Of course, these masculine benefits might not have been applicable to all jobs—employment that involved subservience to others could harm, rather than enhance, a man's sense of independence.[240] Women as well as men sought to bolster their gender reputations by resuming their allotted roles. Alice Thornton's recovery from pregnancy-related illness in 1666 made her reflect on her purpose in life: she wrote that 'as a Christian wife and mother, [there] was ... a duty incompant upon me to discharge with faithfulnesse and godlinesse towards my deare husband and children ... while I was continued in this world'.[241] Wage-earning women may also have gained some respect for their return to work: in legal records, female deponents asserted proudly that they 'lived honestly by their labour', implying that it was an important component of their identity.[242]

---

[236] Cited by Joanna Bourke, *The Story of Pain: From Prayer to Painkillers* (Oxford, 2014), 33.
[237] Weisser, *Ill Composed*, 167.   [238] Thomas, *The Ends of Life*, 101–2.
[239] Buxton, *John Buxton*, 103.
[240] For example, see Whythorne, *The Autobiography*, 37. He was employed as a serving-man to 'A gentilwoman', and complained it is 'so lyke the lyfe of A waterspannell that must be at commaundement to fetch ... that I cowld not lyke that lyfe'. See Katharine Hodgkin, 'Thomas Whythorne and the Problem of Mastery', *History Workshop Journal*, 29 (1990), 20–41; Shepard, *Meanings of Manhood*, 174, 180.
[241] Thornton, *The Autobiography*, 158.   [242] Thomas, *The Ends of Life*, 105.

Another theme of experience to address is mental stimulation. The lack of work left some patients feeling bored, and its resumption was valued as a welcome 'diversion'. Dudley Ryder, training for the legal profession, complained that he was 'in a restless posture' during his illness in 1715, 'not knowing what to do to keep myself in employment'. On another occasion, he confessed that he 'dread[s] illness upon no other account more than its being likely to bring along with it a turbulency and perplexity of thought and want of fixedness of mind'.[243] Philosophers explained this tendency through metaphors of nutrition: when our thoughts have 'nothing Solid to feed upon', wrote Timothy Nourse, they 'feed upon themselves, or rather than starve, they fasten upon some unsuitable Nutriment, which ripens into Vice'. Far from being relaxing, he believed the lack of work caused weariness: 'One who has neither Books nor a Calling, to employ himself upon, is infinitely more tir'd, than he who groans under all the Fatigues of [working] life'.[244] It was not just those engaged in intellectual pursuits who suffered these effects. A poem by Thomas Gills (d. 1716), a poor disabled labourer from Suffolk, includes the lines,

> Alike uncapable of Work and Play,
> In tiresom idleness he spends the Day.[245]

Ultimately, patients' experiences depended on their habits and inclinations: the expert on melancholy, Robert Burton (1577–1640), mused that when people who are accustomed to activity are 'upon a suddaine come to lead a sedentary life[,] ... it crucifies their soules'.[246] The return to work after a period of boredom could thus be a source of welcome stimulation, as the lawyer Roger North found: he reflected, 'labour... takes off the tedium of life'.[247]

Work could be more than mere diversion, however: for those individuals who were 'in a profession that is agreeable to their genius and inclination', employment was a positive delight.[248] When Ralph Thoresby resumed his work as an antiquary in 1698, he received a letter from a friend, stating, 'you are again reestablish't ... [your] former perfect health, and thereby enabled to pursue your belov'd studies of antiquities'. This correspondent was right: Thoresby wrote in his diary, 'I was able to prosecute my study a little, *Laus Deo*', and 'divert myself a little... amongst my books and coins'.[249] Employment that involved an element of creativity was especially enjoyed. John Buxton, an architect, noted after his illness, 'I am every day more pleased with my [building] schemes at Shadwell', and commented on the 'amusement' it brought.[250] Clergymen were also particularly effusive about their callings. After his fever in 1665, Ralph Josselin recorded, 'its my great joy' to 'have a heart and liberty to preach'.[251] He implies that his eagerness to preach was a source of further joy, an idea which may stem from the Calvinist belief that contentment

---

[243] Ryder, *The Diary*, 44–5.   [244] Nourse, *A discourse*, 330–1.
[245] Thomas Gills, *Thomas Gills of St. Edmund's Bury in Suffolk, upon the recovery of his sight* (1710), 6.
[246] Cited in Keith Thomas (ed.), *The Oxford Book of Work* (Oxford, 1999), 171.
[247] North, *Notes of Me*, 206.
[248] Quotation from Gilbert Burnet (1643–1715), cited in Thomas (ed.), *Work*, 147–8.
[249] Thoresby, *Letters*, 65.   [250] Buxton, *John Buxton*, 103.
[251] Josselin, *The Diary*, 514.

in one's employment is a sign of likely salvation.[252] Part of the pleasure sprung from being good at one's job: it was well known that 'man hath a singular delight to practize those things wherein he thinks to excel'.[253]

Women workers as well as men reported that they took satisfaction in their callings. Constance Pley, a widow who had taken over her late husband's naval supplies company, wrote in 1666 that business was 'all the delight' she took in life.[254] Even domestic chores—which historians usually depict as miserable drudgery—could be the source of pleasure, as is inadvertently revealed in a letter from Mary Ferrar (1550–1634) to her daughters in 1632. She warned them that to make the tasks of housewifery 'your delights, and to pride yourselves in your care…in them, is a great vanitie'.[255] Children might also claim to enjoy resuming their studies or play-time after illness. When twelve-year-old Betty Clavering was 'much mended' in 1707, her older step-sister reported, she '[is] in love with her French and wishes to be mistress of it'.[256] Similarly, a six-year-old patient of the surgeon Daniel Turner (1667–1741) called 'for his playfellows', and was observed 'playing as cheerfully as ever'.[257] Even if this practitioner was exaggerating the boy's newfound capacities—as a way to prove that his treatment had been successful—the extract still reveals that merry play was regarded as a credible behaviour for children after illness.

Most of the above examples come from the middling and upper echelons of society; we might question whether those lower down the social scale, employed in arduous and often monotonous jobs, could have derived much enjoyment from returning to work. However, Keith Thomas has speculated that in some cases, even the poorest paid work could be satisfying. Speaking of ploughmen, the minister and agriculture writer John Flavell (d. 1691) considered, 'Though the[ir] labours… are very great and toylsom, yet with what cheerfulness do they go through them[!]'.[258] Poems and ballads from the period often convey the appealing side of manual employments. George Wither's 1641 poem for labourers reads, 'labour yields me true content…by…pains true pleasures [I] find, And many comforts gain'.[259] A ballad about 'a happy thresher' describes how this man goes

> To his dayly Labour with joy and content
> So jocund and jolly, both Whistle and Sing,
> As blithe and as brisk as a Bird in the Spring.[260]

The cheerful tunes of workers attracted comment higher up the social scale. Dorothy Osborne (1627–95) told her husband she saw 'a great many young wenches keep Sheep and Cow's…singing of Ballads…they want nothing to make them the happiest People in the world'.[261] Of course, these rosy depictions of labour were not written by the workers themselves, and may have been designed to maintain

[252] See pp. 227–8 in this chapter on spiritual attitudes to work.
[253] Coeffeteau, *A table*, 289.   [254] Cited by Thomas, *The Ends of Life*, 95.
[255] Cited by Thomas (ed.), *Work*, 287.   [256] Clavering, *The Correspondence*, 37.
[257] Daniel Turner, *A remarkable case in surgery* (1709), 26–8.
[258] John Flavel, *Husbandry spiritualized, or the heavenly use of earthly things* (1674), 31.
[259] Cited by Thomas, *The Ends of Life*, 93.
[260] *The nob[l]e[-]mans generous kindness* (1672–96).   [261] Thomas (ed.), *Work*, 315.

the status quo, teaching the poor to accept their allotted roles in life, while alleviating any guilt felt by the wealthy for their easier lives. Even so, Thomas warns 'we should not be too quick to dismiss' this evidence, since 'almost any form of work can be satisfying if it requires absolute concentration'.[262]

Other themes of experience are of a spiritual nature: during illness, pious patients seem to have associated time off work with the dreaded sin of idleness, and were glad to resume their vocation upon recovery to stamp out this vice. Alec Ryrie avers that a 'constant drumbeat' in Protestant sermons from the 1580s onwards was the pressure to use time wisely, and avoid idleness.[263] The bishop of Norwich, Joseph Hall (1574–1656) warned, 'The idel man is the divels cushion, on which hee taketh his...ease: who as hee is uncapable of any good, so he is fitly disposed for all evill motions'.[264] While no theologian would accuse the seriously ill of idleness, the link between 'lying abed' and laziness was so strong that some patients could not help but feel guilt or regret during sickness. Richard Baxter declared, 'For all the Pains that my Infirmities ever brought upon me, were never half so grievous...as the unavoidable loss of my time, which they occasioned'. Upon recovery, he was glad to return to his work, exclaiming, 'blessed be the God of Mercies, that brought me from the Grave, and gave me...such sweet Imployment!'[265] Puritan ministers like Baxter may have been especially likely to articulate such thoughts, but the rest of the church-attending population would also have been familiar with the associations between time-wasting and rest, since it was preached from the pulpit regularly.[266]

In addition to the relief of no longer being idle, there was a more positive religious reason for rejoicing when returning to employment: the desire to once more do God's calling. The famous Calvinist theologian from Warwickshire, William Perkins (1558–1602), explains here the concept of callings:

> [E]veryone, rich or poore, man or woman, is bound to have a personal calling, in which they must perform some duties for the common good...the maine ende of our lives,...is to serve God in serving of men in the works of our callings.[267]

Thus, God calls humans to specific employments, which they should pursue willingly and diligently for the benefit of society. This concept was particularly popular amongst Protestant reformers, as Max Weber famously asserted over a century ago: work was a form of divine devotion.[268] Consequently, the return to employment after illness could be cherished as a way to resume one's service to God and man. When Ralph Josselin was sick of fever in 1644, he prayed to God for his recovery, so that 'I might goe on in my calling'. To his joy, 'the Lord...hath heard my cry [and] answered my request', and he returned to the pulpit. It might be expected that these ideas applied only to the clergy, whose occupation was most explicitly

---

[262] Ibid., xxi; Thomas, *The Ends of Life*, 99, 104.   [263] Ryrie, *Being Protestant*, 441–4.
[264] Joseph Hall, *Meditations and vowes* (1606, first publ. 1605), Book 3, 81.
[265] Baxter, *Reliquiae Baxterianae*, 84.   [266] Ryrie, *Being Protestant*, 445–6.
[267] William Perkins, *A treatise of the vocations, or callings of men* (1603), 28–9.
[268] Max Weber, *The Protestant Ethic and the 'Spirit' of Capitalism*, trans. Peter Baehr and Gordon Wells (2002, first publ. 1930), esp. 28–9, 32, 106–7.

spiritual in nature. This was not the case, however: in Protestant thinking, callings encompassed all types of employment, so long as they benefited others.[269] Perkins explained:

> Now if we compare worke to work, there is difference betwixt washing of dishes and preaching…: but as touching to please God[,] none at all…[A]ll…workes that spring from faith…howsoever grosse they appeare outwardly [are holy].

Perkins thought this notion should bring 'marvellous content' to those 'in any kind of calling, though it be but to sweepe the house, or keep sheepe'.[270] Such ideas were rooted in Scripture, wherein readers encounter a whole range of worthy workers, including shepherds, fishermen, tent-makers, and of course, the carpenter Jesus Christ.[271] It is conceivable that this inclusive attitude to callings, widely diffused in early modern society, lent dignity to the employments of ordinary people, and may have shaped how they felt about returning to their occupations after illness. In the words of the poet George Herbert (1593–1633), 'this clause Makes drudgerie divine'.[272] Such positive views of work have been largely overshadowed in the historiography by the more negative religious formulation of labour as a punishment for the disobedience of Adam and Eve in Eden.

Before concluding, it is important to acknowledge that the return to work was not always enjoyed. The anonymous author of a treatise on the sorrows of life, published in 1677, declared, 'who is he among men, who hath betaken himself to any…way of living, that has not at last complained, and been weary of it?'[273] For those who loathed their labour, sickness might be welcomed as a holiday, and the resumption of work, dreaded. In 1659, eleven-year-old James Yonge was apprenticed to a 'morose, ill-natured' surgeon, who had kept him 'perpetually working'; only when he fell ill of a 'malign fever' was he permitted to rest.[274] Some patients were even suspected of feigning, or inducing, illness in order to 'live at ease'.[275] This was so for twelve-year-old James Fraser in 1651: having been 'grievously awed' at school, and 'ordinarily whipt whether I deserved it or not', he decided to 'procure a Sickness'—by binging on unripe fruits—in order to 'rid' himself of this 'grievous bondage'.[276] Adults may have played similar tricks to escape work, as is implied in the rulebook of a Buckinghamshire workhouse from 1725: it states that 'if any Person will not work, pretending Sickness, which may be discover'd by their Stomachs or otherwise, they shall be severely punish'd'.[277] The fact that friends of the sick sometimes felt a need to verify whether the illness was 'reall, & no pretence' further indicates that this was a well-recognized phenomenon.[278] Some individuals

---

[269] Ibid., 28, 32; Ryrie, *Being Protestant*, 442, 447.
[270] Perkins, *A treatise*, 634–5, 39–40.   [271] *DBI*, 965–7.
[272] George Herbert, *The temple: sacred poems* (1633), 179.
[273] *Heraclitus Christianus, or the man of sorrow* (1677), 65. He describes the miseries of different vocations, 64–96.
[274] Newton, *The Sick Child*, 174.
[275] Donne, *Devotions*, 72. See Porter and Porter, *In Sickness*, 188–91 on the 'sweets of invalidism'.
[276] Newton, *The Sick Child*, 173.   [277] Ibid., 174.
[278] George Davenport, *The Letters of George Davenport 1651–1677*, ed. Brenda M. Pask, Surtees Society, vol. 215 (Woodbridge, 2011), 165.

had more pious motivations behind their enjoyment of 'want of diversions'—the gentlewoman Alathea Bethell (1655–1708) commented that her 'most pleasant Refreshment' during illness was 'my Conversation with my selfe and le[i]sure to think of Heaven'.[279]

Even for those who generally liked their occupations, returning to work had its drawbacks. Some believed that the exertion of labour harmed their health. Recovering from a 'sore feaver' in 1650, Adam Martindale strived 'to preach againe too soone', the result of which was 'a dangerous relapse'.[280] If this was the case for preaching, a relatively sedentary role, we can only imagine how it would have been for those in manual jobs, like agricultural labour. Due to their fragility, convalescents were also vulnerable to exploitation by others. On his travels around Europe as a surveyor, Richard Norwood (1590–1675) found himself 'very feeble' after ague; as he resumed his journey, two Irishmen, 'pretending...kindness', said they 'would help me carry a small fardel [bundle] which I had'; immediately, they ran off with his belongings, knowing that he could not catch them up.[281]

CONCLUSION

An extract from Robert Harris' sermon on recovery encapsulates this chapter's argument. He averred, 'Sicknesse put me out of possession of all, but with health all is come back againe; my...friends, my house, my wealth, all is returned...'.[282] The return of health was thus depicted as a re-possession: the patient was able once more to enjoy all the things about life that had been stripped of pleasure during illness, such as home, companionship, and work. Through these discussions, we have seen that withdrawal from normal life and work to the sickbed was more common than has often been assumed. Indeed, this is indicated by the widespread use of the term 'falling sick' to denote the onset of illness: disease prostrated the sick, so that they might cry out, 'O I sinke, I cannot stand'.[283] This chapter has explored what it was like to return to three main areas of life after illness—spatial, social, and working life. Confinement to bed was likened to imprisonment, and the gradual expansion of one's spatial horizons was found to be physically and sensually liberating. Socially, sickness was often isolating, owing to the separation of the sick from the living space of the home; during recovery, integration occurred through conventional social acts and activities, which helped strengthen the bonds between families and friends. Finally, patients seem to have often cherished the return to work after a period of inactivity not just out of financial necessity, but in genuine enjoyment of the employment, together with a conviction that work was an antidote to the sin of idleness. This spiritual theme

---

[279] Lambeth Palace Library, London, MS 2240, fol. 32v (Prose and verse meditations of Alathea Bethell).

[280] Martindale, *The Life*, 100.

[281] Richard Norwood, *The Journal of Richard Norwood, Surveyor of Bermuda*, ed. Wesley Frank Craven and Walter Hayward (New York, 1945), 18.

[282] Harris, *Hezekiahs recovery*, 36–7.   [283] Ibid., 35.

230 Misery to Mirth

runs through all three areas of life: patients could use the various milestones of recovery as triggers to extemporal religious meditation, such as rising and walking, and beholding the happy faces of their relations.

Nonetheless, there were some drawbacks to resuming life. For those who were of a solitary nature, or disliked their vocation, the silver lining to sickness was exemption from society and work; the return to these aspects of life may thus have been distressing. Even more common was for patients to complain that the exertion that accompanied the return to normal life was exhausting, or could trigger relapse. There were also spiritual concerns: the Shropshire minister Edward Bury (1616–1700) considered that the tendency for illness to 'spoil all earthly delights' was actually an advantage, designed by God to wean him from 'setting my affection upon creature-comforts', and instead, set his heart on Christ.[284] Recovery could undo this good work.

The above experiences seem to have undergone surprisingly little change over time—the same themes were mentioned throughout the period, and so too were the main milestones and markers of the resumption of normal life. This might seem strange given the fact that we know that developments *were* occurring in the realms of sociability and work in this period, for instance, with the emergence of new venues for socializing. I think this static picture is a consequence of the conventional nature of the measures of recovery: places like church and the alehouse, for example, were widely recognized milestones on the road to health, whereas the more novel venues of the coffee-house or pleasure garden had yet to attain this status. Thus, even if patients were also resorting to these other places, they chose to mention the traditional ones, in the knowledge that such venues would have sent cues to their contemporaries of their state of health.

While the basic stages in the return to normal life were the same for men and women, we have seen that there were probably some differences in the precise activities to which the two sexes returned, as well as the way they experienced these transitions. For example, leaving the house and resuming paid work may have been especially appreciated by males as ways to re-establish their masculine identities after a period of what could be construed as emasculating confinement and economic dependence. Similarly, since women's identities were heavily dependent on their unpaid work as mothers and housewives, the return to these duties may have been important for their reputations. Another variable considered in this chapter has been socio-economic status. Although we do not possess detailed or direct accounts of poorer patients' experiences, second-hand evidence shows that they too withdrew from life and work during severe illness. There must, of course, have been significant differences in the spatial movements made by patients of humbler means, as well as the degree of social isolation that could have been created in shared homes. For those with no savings, work was more than a mere diversion: it was paramount to survival. Nonetheless, there may also have been some similarities across the social spectrum, such as the conviction that all types of work were forms of divine devotion, and the enjoyment of social relationships after a period of intolerance to noise and interaction.

[284] Bury, *The husbandmans companion*, 460–1.

Conclusion

Disease was not always for life in early modern England, nor did it necessarily lead to death. This book has sought to recalibrate our assessment of early modern health by showing that recovery did exist conceptually at this time, and that it was a widely reported phenomenon. A passage from a letter by the early eighteenth-century Norfolk architect John Buxton to his son Robert, reveals the ubiquity of recovery in everyday life:

> I heard at Norwich on Saturday of your continuing well. You will be pleased to hear we grow better here; your mother has not had any more returns, & your little sister is finerly recovered again... The servants too who have been very bad with this feaver are also like to do well, & even your grandmother Gooch has been for some days below stairs every day... This is the state of my own family & I have the satisfaction to hope in little time we shall all be perfectly well.[1]

Misery to Mirth has asked what families like the Buxtons, and their doctors, meant when they said they were 'perfectly well'. They did not mean, as has been often implied in the historiography, that their bodily functions had been partially restored, or that their pains had been somewhat assuaged.[2] While the sick were certainly glad to attain even the slightest improvement, this book has proposed that they only considered themselves *fully* recovered when their disease had been completely quashed, and its 'footsteps'—weakness and emaciation—erased. This translated into feeling completely better, and being able to resume normal life, unimpeded by weakness or blemishes. Caryl Joseph (1602–73), a London preacher, confirmed that a 'perfect recovery' is when there is '*no scar, nor print, no dregs, nor appearance of his former disease seene upon him*'.[3] Defined as the transition from disease to health, recovery comprised two main stages: the removal of disease, followed by the restoration of strength (or convalescence). This formulation, implicit in medical and lay sources throughout the period, sheds fresh light on the broader concepts of health and illness in contemporary perceptions: it suggests that health was not merely the absence of disease, but the presence of strength, a construction remarkably similar to the modern definition given by the World

---

[1] John Buxton, *John Buxton, Norfolk Gentleman and Architect: Letters to his Son, 1719–1729*, ed. Alan Mackley, Norfolk Record Society, vol. 69 (Norwich, 2005), 119.

[2] See the Introduction, notes 29–30.

[3] Caryl Joseph, *An exposition ... upon the thirty second, the thirty third, and the thirty fourth chapters of the booke of Job* (1661), 416.

Health Organization.[4] As the Worcestershire minister Thomas Doolittle (c.1632–1707) explained in a sermon inspired by the Great Plague, 'when a man is restored from sickness to health, that which made him sick is not onely removed, but that is introduced which maketh him well'—strength.[5] The idea that illness could be 'removed' supports Michael Stolberg's view that disease was regarded as an entity in the early modern period, contrary to the older notion that illness in this period was conceived of non-ontologically.[6] By revealing that recovery comprised several stages, I hope this book will generate greater interest in the constituent phases of illness itself.

   Doctors and laypeople believed that three hierarchical agents were responsible for recovery: God, Nature, and medical intervention. Largely overlooked in the historiography, Nature was a divinely endowed power in the body that performed various essential tasks, including the restoration of health. Personified as both a hardworking housewife and a warrior queen, Nature removed disease through processes that resembled cooking/cleaning and fighting: the 'concoction' and 'expulsion' or 'retention' of the noxious humours. In this scheme, the body was envisaged as a house or a battlefield, and disease as dirt, raw food, or an enemy. After removing disease, Nature could set about the second stage of recovery, the restoration of strength, which involved the replenishment of the body's 'spirits' and 'radical moisture', the instruments of all bodily and mental functions. She did this by inducing certain 'natural' inclinations in the patient, such as cheerfulness, sound sleep, and 'a greedy Appetite' for nutritious food. By placing Nature, rather than the physician, at the centre of early modern therapeutics, this study has shed fresh light on the rationale behind medical treatment at this time: the 'golden Saying' in early modern medicine was that Nature is the healer of disease, the physician just the servant.[7] Medical intervention was designed to promote what this agent was already attempting. This new understanding will help transform our attitudes to pre-modern medical practices, rendering more explicable those treatments which at first glance seem utterly ludicrous, such as taking blood from a patient who is already suffering a nosebleed. Nature's role is also relevant to gender history, serving to illuminate wider cultural attitudes to womankind: while the male physician was supposed to 'act in subserviency' to female Nature, in practice he often 'forget[s] how much Wisdom [he is] wont to ascribe to *Nature*', and 'so far from taking *Nature* for his Mistress', makes her his subordinate.[8] Such a contradictory power balance attests to the ambivalence with which females were viewed—they were kind and caring, but due to their 'very imbecility', needed to be 'always directed and ordered by

---

   [4] The Constitution of the World Health Organization states that 'Health is a state of complete physical, mental and social well-being and not merely the absence of disease or infirmity': <http://www.who.int/about/mission/en/> (accessed 21/04/17).
   [5] Thomas Doolittle, *Man ashiv le-yahoweh, or, a serious enquiry for a suitable return for continued life* (1666), 151.
   [6] Michael Stolberg also questions the non-ontological concept of disease, in *Experiencing Illness and the Sick Body in Early Modern Europe* (Basingstoke, 2011, first publ. in German in 2003), 24–7.
   [7] Everard Maynwaringe, *The catholic medicine, and soverain healer* (1684), 5.
   [8] Robert Boyle, *A free enquiry into the vulgarly receiv'd notion of nature* (1686), 228, 324–5.

others'.[9] In this study, Helmontian theories of recovery have been compared with those of Galenic doctors, as a way to test the prevalence and persistence of belief in Nature's role. I have argued that despite differing in their ideas about the precise mechanisms of recovery, doctors from this rival ideology agreed over the tripartite healing agents. Additional research on other emerging theories of the body, such as the nervous or mechanical body, would be fruitful.[10] This book has focused mainly on the Nature–physician dyad; it invites further investigations into Nature's relationships with other agents, such as God, surgeons, nurses, and empirics. Questions could also be asked about supernatural cures: for instance, what—if any—physiological processes were thought to be happening inside the body during miraculous or magical healings?[11]

It has become apparent that convalescence was not a Victorian invention, but was recognized as far back as antiquity: it was perceived as the period of strengthening that occurred after illness had gone, by which means the patient's fragile frame regained its former vitality and weight. Convalescents were deemed worthy of their own special branch of medicine, 'analeptics', a little regarded concept in medical history, which aimed at promoting the patient's growing strength and preventing relapse. These goals could be achieved through the careful regulation of the 'six non-naturals' in accordance with Nature's intentions: tasty, nutritious food, pure air, and undisturbed sleep 'comforteth and refresheth the body, . . . causing the spirits to wax lively', thereby fattening and invigorating 'the whole man'.[12] The non-naturals also played a crucial, and rarely recognized, prognostic role: the patient's sleeping patterns, appetite for food, mood and emotions, and capacity for exercise and air exposure, acted as measures of growing health. In 1630, James Harrison, town lecturer and chaplain to the Barrington family, announced that Mr Barrington was 'much better . . . but not yet quite so well as that he dares [to] goe much abroad . . . Yet he feeds and sleeps well blessed be God'.[13] Convalescent care seems to have undergone little change over the course of the early modern period, which might lead us to believe that it was based 'more on common sense intuition than theory'.[14] This was not the case, however: its resilience instead rested on the continued belief in the existence of the 'spirits', the source of physical strength.[15] Doctors placed convalescents in the 'neutral' category of human bodies, alongside other individuals who were deemed 'neither sick nor sound', such as the elderly, newborn babies, and lying-in women. By drawing occasional comparisons between the care provided to these various neutral groups, this study has revealed that early modern medicine identified multiple similarities and differences between human bodies, which went beyond the more familiar variables of humoral constitution

---

[9] Richard Hooker (1554–1600) cited in Anthony Fletcher, *Gender, Sex, and Subordination in England, 1500–1800* (1995), 70.

[10] On the rise of nerve theory in the eighteenth century, see Stolberg, *Experiencing Illness*, 170–90.

[11] David Gentilcore has discussed this issue in relation to Italy, but not much has been said on the English context—*Healers and Healing in Early Modern Italy* (Manchester, 1998).

[12] Thomas Collins, *Choice and rare experiments in physick and chirurgery* (1658), 198.

[13] Arthur Searle (ed.), *Barrington Family Letters, 1628–1632* (1983), 158–9.

[14] For this view, see Chapter 2, note 9.

[15] On the persistence of belief in the spirits, see Chapter 2, note 221.

and sex.[16] The interpretive value of this forgotten category is substantial: it brings us to a better appreciation of how early modern people judged ambiguous states of health. As the sixteenth-century Dutch physician Levinus Lemnius confirmed, most people 'ought not to be placed amongst the sick or sound; but partaking in both...[:] the neutrall condition'.[17] This study has concentrated on the care provided to those patients whose 'footsteps of disease' eventually left them; additional work could be undertaken on the treatment and technologies designed to help with the more permanent legacies of disease, such as scars and lameness.[18]

As well as examining the medical perceptions of recovery and convalescent care, this book has investigated the personal experiences of recovering patients, a hitherto neglected piece in our picture of illness. The central argument is encapsulated in the following extended extracts, taken from Robert Harris' sermon on the healing of Hezekiah; it concerns the extraordinary difference between the states of illness and health.

> [In the sickchamber, thou] shall...find silence, solitarinesse, sadnesse, light shut out, misery shut in..., children weeping, wife sighing; the husband groning, ["]Oh my head, O my backe, O my stomach, sicke, sicke, sick,...I cannot stand, I cannot sit, I cannot lye, I cannot eate, I cannot sleepe, I cannot live, I cannot die, O what shall I doe?["]...Sickness at one blow deprive[s] us of the comfort of our meats, beds, houses, grounds, friends, wife, children, &c. [Indeed] it deprives a man of *himself*[:] hee hath wit, but not use of it;...eares, and heares not;...feet, but walkes not...
>
> Now as sickenesse is a great affliction, so health [is] as great a mercie[:]...the healthfull man may...walke when he will, eate when he will, sleepe when he will, worke, play, fast, feast, ride, runne when hee will...Hee enjoyes himselfe, his wits, senses, limbs...the light is pleasant, the ayre sweete, [and] his meate good...[A]nd therefore this motion from sickenesse to health...from sadnesse to mirth, from paine to ease, from prison to liber[t]ie, from death to life, must needs be a happie motion, worthie [of] thankes [to God].[19]

This colourful passage, which inspired the title of the book, sums up what it was like to get better for many patients. At the heart of recovery was contrast—from suffering to ease, misery to mirth, inactivity to activity, constraint to freedom, loneliness to sociability, guiltiness to innocence, and death to life. Playing on the etymology of the word 'recover', Harris presents the return to health as a process of re-possession: 'Sicknesse put me out of possession of all, but with health all is come back againe.'[20] Illness robbed patients not just of their physical ease and bodily functions, but of all the other aspects of life that were usually a source of satisfaction, such as material wealth and work, enjoyment of one's surroundings, and the pleasure of company.[21] With the restoration of health, all these things were returned.

---

[16] See the Introduction, note 17, for literature on sex as a variable.

[17] Levinus Lemnius, *The secret miracles of nature* (1658, first publ. 1559), 244.

[18] Scholarship which touches on this subject is cited in Chapter 2, note 47.

[19] Robert Harris, *Hezekiahs recovery. Or, a sermon, shevving what use Hezekiah did, and all should make of their deliverance from sicknesse* (1626), 30–6.

[20] Ibid., 37.

[21] This trope was common; for instance, see Edward Bury, *The husbandmans companion containing one hundred occasional meditations* (1677), 461.

Through this argument, the book has contributed to debates on sickness behaviour, showing that it was more common for patients to retire from normal life and work to the sickbed than has often been assumed.[22] Since recovery usually involved the gradual resumption of everyday employments and movements, serious illness must have necessitated the relinquishing of these things. Indeed, this is evident in the language of 'falling sick', and 'rising to health': severe illness prostrated the sick, and recovery involved getting up. The exceptions to this happy story will be discussed below.

A compelling feature of patients' accounts is the way they often describe recovery as a 'double joy' of their bodies and souls. Upon recovery, both halves were healed together, since the disappearance of bodily disease was a sign that God had forgiven spiritual sickness—sin. Personified as 'two great Friends', the body and soul rejoiced in one another's newfound ease and health, and felt relieved they would no longer have to part in death.[23] Such accounts enhance our understanding of how people conceptualized their own beings at this time—they lived through two, mutually loving personas. The belief that ultimately it was the Lord who had ordained recovery inspired the outpouring of delightful spiritual emotions called 'holy affections', cheerful responses to divine deliverance which help to counter the largely gloomy picture that dominates the scholarship on the psychological culture of early modern Protestantism.[24] These expressions were part of the 'art of recovery', a set of religious duties incumbent on recovered patients, akin to 'the art of death' with which historians are familiar; it included resisting sin, praising God, and joining together in collective thanksgiving. This forgotten art was the spiritual equivalent to analeptics, the branch of medicine discussed earlier: it was designed to strengthen the soul against sin, and prevent relapse into spiritual sickness. While historians have acknowledged the widespread use of medical metaphors in early modern religious discourse, here we have seen that such comparisons were literal rather than figurative: the soul really was capable of recovery. It might be expected that by the early eighteenth century, the art of recovery would have begun to fade, due to a decline in the popularity of the doctrine of providence, together with an increasing tendency for philosophers to separate the body and soul.[25] This was not the case, however: patients continued to express relief to be eased in both parts of their beings, and showed familiarity with the essential components of the art of recovery into the 1700s and beyond. Indeed, as late as 1836, preachers were still declaring that bodily illness 'has wonderfully worked for our spiritual amendment', and warning of the 'great and solemn' biblical injunction to 'sin no more, lest a worse thing come unto thee'.[26] While this continuity may be partly a reflection of the religious biases of many of the sources, it could also indicate that when it comes to matters of life and death, and health and illness, it is preferable to see a benevolent deity in charge than to hand such things over to the capricious wheels of fortune.[27]

[22] For more information, see Chapter 6, p. 194.
[23] George Berkeley, *Historical applications and occasional meditations* (1667), 16.
[24] For this historiography, see Chapter 4, notes 11–13.
[25] See Chapter 4, note 16, and the Introduction, note 67, for information on these changes.
[26] Robert Milman, *Convalescence, thoughts for those who are recovering from sickness* (1836), 62.
[27] Alexandra Walsham, *Providence in Early Modern England* (Oxford, 2003, first publ. 1999), 21–2.

One of the advantages of this research has been its potential to illuminate not just the experience of recovery and survival, but to provide insights into what it was like to feel ill and face death. The considerable literature on early modern pain has created the impression that this was all there was to illness; but we have seen here that sickness commonly involved various additional components, such as the 'Loathing of Meat', tedium and isolation, 'sleep...labour'd and disturb'd', and confinement to bed.[28] Many other symptoms could be identified, which I hope future studies will explore. Likewise, in the scholarship on emotional responses to death, so much attention has been paid to the reactions to the prospect of Heaven and Hell that other major concerns have been obscured, such as the anticipation of the separation of body and soul, together with worries about what would become of relations. At a more mundane level, it has been possible to unearth many supplementary details about everyday life, such as the fact that most patients slept in upstairs rooms despite the presence of beds downstairs; neighbourly visiting was not an exclusively female form of sociability; and work was more enjoyable than has often been assumed. Cumulatively, these little nuggets help to enhance our picture of what it was like to be alive in early modern England.

Besides investigating medical perceptions and patients' experiences of recovery, this book has examined the reactions of relations and friends to their loved one's restored life and health. I have argued that these individuals usually shared the experiences of patients, undergoing such an extreme transformation of feelings that it was hard to express. The most apposite words came from Scripture, especially Psalm 30, verse 5: 'weeping may endure for a night, but joy cometh in the morning'. This mirroring of experiences, known as 'fellow-feeling' in early modern England, was attributed to the passion of love, a 'true sign' of which was that 'friends rejoyce & grieve for the same things'.[29] So extraordinary were the effects of this emotion, philosophers drew parallels with the magic associated with what would today be called voodoo dolls: just as it is allegedly possible to 'torment men in their absence' by 'touch[ing] nothing but their Picture', so 'love[,] which is as powerful...doth this Miracle every day; when it joyns two souls together, it finds a way to make their sufferings common'.[30] As is implied in this extract, the most striking feature of fellow-feeling was that it was physical as well as emotional, which meant that during illness, loved ones frequently claimed to *feel* something akin to the patient's bodily sufferings, and upon recovery they too experienced blissful ease. This argument challenges the traditional view, associated with Elaine Scarry, that pain is an 'unsharable experience'.[31] Taking a new, sensory approach, I have shown that the main avenues to fellow-feeling were the ears and eyes: the patient's 'doleful Groans' and 'decaying Looks' were replaced by the joyful sounds

[28] Joseph Browne, *Institutions in physick, collected from the writings of the most eminent physicians* (1714), 263–5.
[29] Nicholas Coeffeteau, *A table of humane passions*, trans. Edward Grimeston (1621), 103–5.
[30] Jean-François Senault, *The use of passions*, trans. Henry Earl of Monmouth (1671, first publ. 1649), 480.
[31] See Chapter 3, note 10, on this view and its critiques.

and sights of laughter and smiles.[32] While the senses also played a role in the patient's experience of recovery, it tended to be taste and touch rather than sight and sound that were singled out most frequently by the sick—the sharpness and bitterness of suffering and sin gave way to 'sweet' and 'soft ease', rest, and forgiveness. Such findings have implications for scholarly debates on the ranking of the five senses in early modern culture, supporting recent work which suggests that multiple and overlapping hierarchies were in operation at this time. This study has only scratched the surface of the sensory experiences of sickness: a further, more substantial project on the sensory environment of the sickchamber, and the effects of serious disease and treatment on the five senses, will be necessary to bring these dimensions of illness to life.[33]

Misery to Mirth has showcased the depth of family bonds and friendships in early modern England, thereby confirming recent findings on social networks that suggest that people at this time enjoyed a multiplicity of relationships, both familial and non-familial.[34] This mutual affection has shone through in every context, from the joy of not having to part in death, to the 'great comfort' of 'being up amongst the family' after a period of spatial segregation. Even those relationships which, during health, had become strained, might be rejuvenated upon recovery. When her 'dear Mother' was 'restor'd' in 1721, Anne Dawson, a nonconformist from Manchester, exclaimed, 'Oh wat a sad family had we been' if she had died, and expressed a determination to 'cary [myself] better...to her' in the future.[35] I have shown that while affection was common in many relationships, the most profuse emotions tended to be professed by spouses and lovers, parents and children, and siblings. This claim is supported by early modern philosophical ideas about the 'hierarchy of fellow-feeling', and its effects on a person's capacity to communicate emotion. It was believed that the greater the affection between the two parties, the bigger the challenge of putting feelings into words. During illness, groans, sighs, and tears best expressed loved ones' feelings, inarticulate gestures that gave way during recovery to jubilant shouts, singing, and laughing. Friends and more distant kin might say their emotions were 'indescribable', but they usually went on to contradict such claims by eloquently expressing their sorrows and eventual joys. Of course, these rules were not hard and fast—some patients enjoyed equally intense relationships with non-related individuals, and the primary sources themselves over-represent the happier sorts of family bonds. Inevitably, those patients who were estranged from their families, or suffered abusive relationships, would not have received letters of congratulations upon their restoration to health.

It is important to ask to what extent the findings presented above can be applied to the whole of society. Undeniably, the religious and social skew of the sources in this study has influenced the picture that has emerged. The majority of the authors were devout Anglican or nonconformist Protestants, who interpreted their recov-

---

[32] Timothy Rogers, *Practical discourses on sickness & recovery* (1691), 99.
[33] This is the subject of my current Wellcome Trust University Award (2016–21), *Sensing Sickness in Early Modern England*; reference: 200326/Z/15/Z.
[34] For this historiography, see the Introduction, pp. 18–19.
[35] BL, Additional MS 71626, fol. 11v (Anne Dawson, Diary, 1721–2).

eries in providential terms. More research is needed to find out to what extent Catholics' experiences in England diverged from this Protestant story. People who were not so interested in religion, or who doubted the reality of providence or Heaven were less likely to dwell on the spiritual implications of recovery and survival than their godly neighbours. Socio-economic background also affected patients' and families' experiences. For those who were poor, living in multi-occupied dwellings, or working as apprentices or servants in other people's homes, the spatial, sensory, social, and economic aspects of recovery must have been different. The 'multiplicity of business' of the agricultural labourer, for instance, was 'full of toyl', comprising 'plowing, sowing, harrowing, weeding,...threshing,...planting, graffing' and many more tasks, all of which were known to be far more physically challenging to the weak convalescent than the intellectual pursuits of many middling and elite occupations.[36] Furthermore, the greater financial pressure faced by the lower socio-economic sectors may have led them to return to their employments sooner than their wealthier counterparts, when their bodies were still very fragile. Nonetheless, there is no reason to believe that some of the other dimensions of recovery were not comparable—for instance, the relief not to be separated from one's family at death, and the enjoyment of social celebrations upon recovery, as well as the ease of abated pain and nausea, may have cut across social divides. Other variables that have been considered are gender and age; we have seen that while many features of the return to health were the same for children and adults, and females and males, there were some important distinctions. For instance, young children returned to their toys or schoolwork rather than paid employment, and, owing to the shorter acquaintance between their bodies and souls, infants did not usually express much relief when these two parts of their beings escaped death—their preoccupations centred more on the prospect of remaining on earth with their parents. For young men, recovery brought additional opportunities as well as dangers: the markers of leaving the house, and returning to paid employment, for instance, enabled males to reaffirm their masculine identities, since economic independence and freedom to 'go abroad' were key components of manliness in this period. On the other hand, the allure of the pub, and the return of sexual appetite, were regarded as especially problematic in this sex—the stereotypical 'bad recoverer' was male.

The interpretive thrust of this book has been positive: recovery has been presented largely as a 'happie motion' from misery to mirth, a perspective which I hope may encourage other scholars to embrace the brighter side of the past too. This cheerful picture is partly a consequence of the spiritual function of many of my sources—pious individuals sought to 'excite themselves' to divine praise by juxtaposing the ease and joy of their newfound health with their recent memory of pain and sorrow. The happy picture can also be ascribed to the types of illnesses privileged in this study—it has been concerned with 'serious' diseases, many of which were acute, ending in either complete recovery or death. Nonetheless, the book has not turned a blind eye to the less rosy side of recovery. We have seen that for some

---

[36] John Flavel, *Husbandry spiritualized, or the heavenly use of earthly things* (1674), 2.

individuals, getting better could take a long time, requiring tremendous patience, and of course, not everyone made a full recovery: it depended partly on the nature of the disease, and the strength and age of the patient. Aged about 70, Elizabeth Freke complained that after severe pleurisy, 'I... have... labored ever since under soe violent a cough and weakness as to be uncapable of any business or comfort'.[37] For those who *did* recover, the return to normal life and functioning was not always welcome. In particular, people who enjoyed solitude, or hated their employment, found sickness to be a welcome break, and the resumption of former interactions and work, a source of distress. Nor did recovery always follow a linear motion: patients and their relations and doctors fretted over the possibility of relapse, worrying that the smallest action—even 'putting on a clean Night-cap'—could rekindle illness.[38] This vulnerability extended to the soul: patients might return to their 'former besetting sins' like 'dogs to vomit', with the double calamity of spiritual *and* bodily relapse.[39] In this context, the tendency discussed earlier for illness to dispossess patients of 'all earthly comforts' could be construed as an advantage, since the 'appetite and lust of the weak and sick, are weak and sick as well as they'.[40] Some of the most explicitly negative reactions to recovery come from those individuals who had, during their illness, longed for Heaven. Oliver Heywood lamented in 1691, 'When many judged me a gone man, I was afraid it was too good to be true, and was loath to be sent back'.[41] Ultimately, pious patients believed that all the joys of recovery were inferior versions of what would happen in Heaven anyway. Robert Horne (1565–1640), an Anglican clergyman, described death in language that bears uncanny resemblance to Harris' account of recovery: the Christian goes from 'feare to security, from... paine to ease... prison to libertie, from mortalitie to immortall[ity], and from death to li[f]e'.[42]

Finally, through exploring the diverse experiences of recovering patients and their families, this book has shed fresh light on how emotions were conceptualized and categorized in early modern England. Today in Western culture, we tend to divide up feelings according to whether they are pleasant or unpleasant to experience, creating a negative–positive binary. However, in the period of this study, several additional taxonomies were at play, which together reveal the variability of emotions over time.[43] One relates to direction and temperature: joy and anger, for instance, emotions which we would rarely put together, were thought in the early modern period to have in common a tendency to heat the heart, and fling the

---

[37] Elizabeth Freke, *The Remembrances of Elizabeth Freke*, ed. Raymond Anselment, Camden Fifth Series, vol. 18 (Cambridge, 2001), 280.

[38] Gideon Harvey, *The conclave of physicians* (1686), 109–10.

[39] See Chapter 4, pp. 140–6.

[40] Bury, *The husbandmans companion*, 459–60; Richard Baxter, *A Christian directory, or, a summ of practical theologie* (1673), 57. On gluttony, see Viktoria von Hoffmann, *From Gluttony to Enlightenment: The World of Taste in Early Modern Europe* (Urbana IL, 2016), ch. 2.

[41] Oliver Heywood, *The Rev. Oliver Heywood, B.A: His Autobiography, Diaries, Anecdote and Event Books*, ed. Horsfall Turner, 4 vols. (1883), vol. 3, 245; see also John Shower, *Some account of the holy life and death of Mr. Henry Gearing* (1699), 113–14.

[42] Robert Horne, *Life and death, foure sermons* (1613), 128–9. Harris' extract is given on p. 234 above.

[43] See Chapter 5, note 202, for an introduction to this debate.

body's spirits and humours in an upwards and outwards direction, making '*the eye... lively and quicke sighted, the cheeks of a... ruddy colour*'.[44] By contrast, sorrow and fear cooled the heart, and caused the spirits and humours to zoom inwards, thereby leaving the outer parts of the body pale and shaky. The second classification relates to movement and rest. Hope and fear, for example, were grouped together, on the grounds that the soul was in a state of continual agitation, striving towards or away from the anticipated event. Conversely, sorrow and joy, emotions that we would see as dichotomous, were put in the same category because the anticipated event had now occurred, which 'stoppeth the violence of our' passions.[45] The third taxonomy divides feelings into 'holy affections' and 'passions', a classification based on the spiritual status of the feelings—the former were emotions of a superior quality, elicited by religious considerations, whereas the latter were feelings evoked by 'worldly' things, like getting better. Crucially, recovery was cherished as an opportunity for patients and their relations to upgrade their earthly joys into spiritual ones, since the knowledge that it was God who had ordained recovery was supposed to inspire praise and thankfulness, exquisite spiritual feelings which signified the individual's election to Heaven. Indeed, these experiences could be so moving that they were found to bring about a permanent alteration in a person's emotional disposition. To return to eleven-year-old Martha Hatfield, whose recovery featured at the start of this book, she had, before her illness, been 'much inclined to sadnesse and fretfulnesse'. From the time of her cure, she 'walks on with much cheerfulness... [and] abundance of peace', wrote her uncle, because she now knows that whatever 'new Stormes and Tempests' await her in life, God will 'come with *healing under his wings*'.[46]

---

[44] James Hart, *Klinike, or the diet of the diseased* (1633), 398.

[45] Senault, *The use of passions*, 441.

[46] James Fisher, *The wise virgin, or, a wonderful narration of the various dispensations towards a childe of eleven years of age* (1653), 163–4, 141. He also attributed her changed character to the fact that some of her melancholy humour had been evacuated through the disease process.

Primary Bibliography

MANUSCRIPT SOURCES

London

British Library

Additional MS 5858 (Religious diary of a female cousin of Oliver Cromwell, 1687/90–1702)

Additional MS 27466 ('Recipe-Book of Mary Doggett', 1682)

Additional MS 28050 (Domestic correspondence of the Osborne family, 1637–1761)

Additional MS 34722 (Lady Anne Loules and others, medical and culinary recipes, 1650)

Additional MS 36452 (Private letters of the Aston family, 1613–1703)

Additional MS 42849 (Letters of the Henry family)

Additional MS 45196 (Brockman Papers, 'Ann Glyd Her Book 1656')

Additional MS 45718 (Commonplace book of Elizabeth Freke, 1684–1714)

Additional MS 56248 (Recipe Book of Lady Mary Dacres, 1666–96)

Additional MS 70115, unfoliated manuscript (Portland papers, 1689–98)

Additional MS 71626 (Anne Dawson, Diary, 1721–2)

Additional MS 72619 ('Book of recipes for the Trumbell's household', late 1600s)

Additional MS 74231 (Henry Wotton, 'A Hymn to My God in a Night of my Late Sickness')

Additional MSS 88897/1–2 (Autobiography of Alice Thornton)

Egerton 607 ('True coppies of scertaine loose Papers left by the Right honourable Elizabeth Countesse of Bridgewater, Collected and Transcribed together here since her Death, 1663')

Egerton MS 2214 (Thomas Davies' medical recipes, 1680)

M.636/8 (correspondence of Ralph Verney on microfiche)

Sloane MS 153 (Casebook of Joseph Binns, 1633–63)

Sloane MS 1367 ('Lady Ranelagh's Medical Receipts')

Stowe 962, fols. 56v–57r (Edward Lapworth, 'Verses Written by Dctr Latworth in an Extreamity of Sicknes wch he Suffered')

Lambeth Palace Library

MS 2240 (Prose and verse meditations of Alathea Bethell 1655–1708)

London Metropolitan Library

MS 204 (Nehemiah Wallington, 'A Record of the Mercies of God: or A Thankfull Remembrance')

Royal College of Physicians Library

ALS/F136 A-I (Letters between Henry Watkins and John Freind about illness of Mr Hill)

G62 (Letter from Francis Glisson to Thomas Saunders, Hertfordshire, 25 November 1671)

Wellcome Library

MS 160 (Anne Brumwich, 'Booke of Receipts or medicines', c.1625–1700)

MS 169 (Elizabeth Bulkeley, 'A boke of hearbes and receipts', 1627)

MS 213 (Mrs Corylon, 'A Booke of divers medecines', 1606)

MS 311 (John and Joan Gibson, 'A booke of medicines', 1632–[1717])

MS 1026 (Lady Ayscough, 'Receits of phisick and chirurgery', 1692)

MS 1320 ('A Book of Physick, made in June 1710')
MS 1321 ('A Book of receipts', c.1675–c.1725)
MS 1340 (Boyle Family, c.1675–c.1710)
MS 1795 (Cookery-Books: seventeenth–eighteenth centuries)
MS 2840 (Mrs Elizabeth Hirst and others, collection of medical receipts, 1684–c.1725)
MS 2990 ('Madam Bridget Hyde her receipt book', 1676–90)
MS 3712 (Elizabeth Okeover and others, c.1675–c.1725)
MS 7113 (Lady Ann Fanshawe, recipe book 1651–78)
MS 7851 (English Recipe Book, late 1600s to early 1800s)
MS 8086 (Receipt book, early 1600s)

Cambridge
Cambridge University Library
Additional MS 6843 (The diary of William Coe, 1693–1729)
Additional MS 8499 (The diary of Isaac Archer, 1641–1700)
Buxton 34/11, 49 101, 103; 59/177, 103/66, 3, 104/1–11, 105/9–25, 70 (Family archive
    of Buxtons of Channons)
MS Dd. 3. 64 (Letters of Matthew Poole)

St John's College Library
Miscellaneous Box 7, FA2 (Letter from Thomas Fairfax to his grandfather, 1st Baron, 24 July
    1637)
Miscellaneous Box 16, SH3 (Letter from Mary, Countess of Shrewsbury, to Sir Thomas
    Fairfax, 15 November 1623)
Miscellaneous CA3/10 ('Letters of Cantrell Family', 1683–1748)
Miscellaneous CL3 (Letters of William Clarke, 1724)
Miscellaneous VI1/3 (letter to 'Sr', probably Richard Hill, 1655–1727, a diplomat and
    public servant, 10 May 1698)

Trinity College Library
Additional MS a 331 (Correspondence between Richard Bentley, 1662–1742, Master of
    Trinity College, and Joanna Bernard, 1700)

Leeds
Brotherton Library
MS Lt q 32 (Hester Pulter's 'Poems Breathed forth By The Nobel Hadassas')
MS Lt 36 (Edmund Waller's poetry)
MS Lt 50 (Collection of English religious poetry, possibly by William Tipping, c.1700)

Oxford
Bodleian Library
English Miscellaneous e. 331, 1714–23 (Diary of Sarah Savage)
Ashmole MS 718, fol. 137 (Edward Lapworth, 'Verses Written by Dctr Latworth in an
    Extreamity of Sicknes wch he Suffered')

Taunton
Somerset Heritage Centre
DD/SAS C/1193/4 (Memoirs of John Cannon, officer of the excise, West Lydford, Somerset)
DD/WO/55/7/47-1 (letter from Richard Carpenter to John Trevelyan, 24 March 1620)

Winchester
Hampshire Record Office
44M69/F5/2/2 (Jervoise letters, 1658)
44M69/F6/1/2 (Jervoise letters, 1683–6)
63M84/347 (Letters of Mary Yonge, 1720–1)

Other
MSS D/EP/F29–35 (Sarah Cowper, 'Daily Diary', 7 volumes, 1700–15), housed in Hertfordshire Archives and Local Studies, Hertford; scanned onto microfilm in Amanda Vickery (ed.), *Women's Languages and Experiences, 1500–1940: Women's Diaries and Related Sources: Part 1, Sources from the Bedfordshire and Hertfordshire Record Office* (Marlborough, 1996), reels 5–7; consulted at Cardiff University Special Collections and Archives

PRINTED SOURCES

The place of publication is London, unless otherwise stated
A brief account of Mr. Valentine Greatraks (1666)
A declaration of the principall pointes of Christian doctrine (1647)
A handkercher for parents wet eyes, upon the death of children (1630)
A narrative of the late extraordinary cure wrought in an instant upon Mrs Elizabeth Savage (1694)
A physical dictionary, or an interpretation of such crabbed words… used in physick (1657)
A relation of the miraculous cure of Mrs Lydia Hills of a lameness (1695)
A true and briefe report, of Mary Glovers vexation (1603)
A true copy of a letter of the miraculous cure of David Wright, a sheppard (1694)
A., B., *The sick-mans rare jewell* (1674)
Abernethy, John, *A Christian and heavenly treatise, containing physicke for the soule* (1630, first publ. 1615)
Advice to batchelors, or, the married mans lamentation (1685)
Allen, James, *Serious advice to delivered ones from sickness* (Boston, 1679)
Allestree, Richard, *The art of patience and balm of Gilead* (1694, first publ. 1684)
Allestree, Richard, *The ladies calling* (1673)
Allestree, Richard, *The practice of Christian graces* (1658)
An account of the causes of some particular rebellious distempers (1670)
An answer to the maiden's tragedy (1675–96?)
An earnest exhortation to a true Minivitish repentance (1642)
An exact relation of the wonderful cure of Mary Maillard (1730, first publ. 1694)
Andrewes, Lancelot, *The pattern of catechistical doctrine at large* (1650)
Andrews, John, *Andrewes repentance, sounding alarm to return from his sins* (1631)
Anthony, Francis, *The apologie, or defence of… a medicine called aurum potabile* (1616)
Archer, Isaac, 'The Diary of Isaac Archer 1641–1700', in Matthew Storey (ed.), *Two East Anglian Diaries 1641–1729*, Suffolk Record Society, vol. 36 (Woodbridge, 1994), 41–200
Archer, John, *Secrets disclosed of consumptions* (1684)
Atherton, Henry, *The Christian physician* (1686)
Atkins, William, *A discourse shewing the nature of the gout* (1694)
Ayloffe, W., *The government of the passions* (1700)
Bacon, Francis, *The historie of life and death* (1638)
Bacon, William, *A key to Helmont* (1682)
Banister, John, *A needefull, new, and necessarie treatise of chyrurgerie* (1575)

Bantock, Anton (ed.), *The Earlier Smyths of Ashton Court From their Letters, 1545–1741* (Bristol, 1982)

Barnard, John, *Theologo-historicus, or, the true life of the most reverend divine, and excellent historian, Peter Heylyn* (1683)

Barrough, Philip, *The methode of phisicke* (1583)

Basse, William, *A helpe to discourse. Or, a miscelany of merriment* (1619)

Bauderon, Brice, *The expert physician: learnedly treating of all agues and feavers* (1657)

Baxter, Richard, *A Christian directory, or, a summ of practical theologie* (1673)

Baxter, Richard, *A treatise of death* (1660)

Baxter, Richard, *A treatise of self-denial* (1675)

Baxter, Richard, *Compassionate counsel to all young-men* (1681)

Baxter, Richard, *Reliquiae Baxterianae, or, Mr. Richard Baxters narrative* (1696)

Bayfield, Robert, *Enchiridion medicum: containing the causes... cures of... diseases* (1655)

Bayfield, Robert, *Tes iatrikes kartos... adorned with above three hundred choice and rare observations* (1663)

Beadle, John, *The journal or diary of a thankful Christian* (1656)

Becon, Thomas, *The Catechism of Thomas Becon*, ed. John Ayre (Cambridge, 1844)

Berkeley, George, *Historical applications and occasional meditations* (1667)

Biggs, Noah, *Mataeotechnia medicinae praxeos, or the vanity of the craft of physick* (1651)

Bilson, Thomas, *The survey of Christs sufferings* (1604)

Blair, Robert, *The Life of Mr Robert Blair, Minister of St Andrews (1593–1636)*, ed. Robert McCrie, Wodrow Society (Edinburgh, 1848, first publ. 1754)

Blankaart, Steven, *A physical dictionary* (1684)

Blount, Thomas, *Glossographia, or, a dictionary* (1661)

Boyle, Robert, *A free enquiry into the vulgarly receiv'd notion of nature* (1686)

Boyle, Robert, *Occasional reflections upon several subjects* (1665)

Bradwell, Stephen, *Physicke for the sicknesse, commonly called the plague* (1636)

Braithwaite, Richard, *Essaies upon the five senses* (1635, first publ. 1620)

Breton, Nicholas, *Wits private wealth stored with choise commodities to content the minde* (1612)

Bright, Timothy, *A treatise of melancholie* (1586)

Brockbank, Thomas, *The Diary and Letter Book of the Rev. Thomas Brockbank 1671–1709*, ed. Richard Trappes-Lomax, Chetham Society New Series, vol. 89 (Manchester, 1930)

Brooke, Humphrey, *Ugieine or A conservatory of health* (1650)

Browne, Joseph, *Institutions in physic, collected from the writings of the most eminent physicians* (1714)

Browne, Thomas, *The Letters of Sir Thomas Browne*, ed. Geoffrey Keynes (Cambridge, 1946)

Browne, Thomas, *The Works of Sir Thomas Browne, vol. 6: Letters*, ed. Geoffrey Keynes (1931)

Bruele, Walter, *Praxis medicinae, or, the physicians practice* (1632)

Bryant, Arthur (ed.), *Postman's Horn: An Anthology of the Letters of Latter Seventeenth Century England* (New York, 1946, first publ. 1936)

Bullein, William, *Bulleins bulwarke of defence against all sicknesse* (1579)

Bullein, William, *The government of health* (1595, first publ. 1558)

Bunyan, John, *The life and death of Mr. Badman* (1680)

Burdwood, James, *Helps for faith and patience in times of affliction* (1693)

Burton, Robert, *The anatomy of melancholy* (1621)

Bury, Edward, *The husbandmans companion containing one hundred occasional meditations* (1677)

Bury, Elizabeth, *An account of the life and death of Elizabeth Bury* (Bristol, 1720)

Buxton, John, *John Buxton, Norfolk Gentleman and Architect: Letters to his Son, 1719–1729*, ed. Alan Mackley, Norfolk Record Society, vol. 69 (Norwich, 2005)

Byfield, Nicholas, *A commentary: or, sermons upon the second chapter of the first epistle of Saint Peter* (1623)

Byfield, Nicholas, *The cure of the feare of death* (1618)

Carey, Mary, *Meditations from the Note Book of Mary Carey, 1649–1657*, ed. Francis Meynell (Westminster, 1918)

Caryl, Joseph, *An exposition... upon the thirty second, the thirty third, and the thirty fourth chapters of the booke of Job* (1661)

Case, Thomas, *Correction instruction, or a treatise of afflictions* (1653, first publ. 1652)

Cawdrey, Robert, *A treasurie or storehouse of similies* (1600)

Charleton, Walter, *Natural history of the passions* (1674)

Chudleigh, Mary, *Poems on several occasions* (1713)

Cicero, Marcus Tullius, *Cicero's laelius a discourse of friendship* (1691)

Clavering, James, *The Correspondence of Sir James Clavering*, ed. Harry Thomas Dickinson, Surtees Society, vol. 178 (Gateshead, 1967)

Clegg, James, *The Diary of James Clegg of Chapel-en-Frith 1708–1755*, vol. 1 (1708–36), ed. Vanessa Doe, Derbyshire Record Society, vol. 5 (Matlock, 1978)

Clifford, Anne, *The Diaries of Lady Anne Clifford*, ed. D. D. H. Clifford (Stroud, 1990)

Clowes, William, *A prooved practice for all young chirurgians* (1588)

Cock, Thomas, *Kitchin-physick: or, advice for the poor* (1676)

Cockburn, William, *An account of... the distempers that are incident to seafaring people* (1697)

Coeffeteau, Nicholas, *A table of humane passions*, trans. Edward Grimeston (1621)

Cogan, Thomas, *The haven of health, made for the comfort of students* (1634, first publ. 1584)

Collinges, John, *Several discourses concerning the actual Providence of God* (1678)

Collins, Thomas, *Choice and rare experiments in physick and chirurgery* (1658)

Cotta, John, *A short discoverie of the unobserved dangers of... practisers of physicke* (1612)

Cotton, Charles, *The confinement a poem* (1679)

Cowper, Mary, *Diary of Mary, Countess Cowper*, ed. John Murray (1864)

Coxe, Thomas, *A discourse wherein the interest of the patient in reference to physick and physicians is soberly debated* (1669)

Cradock, Samuel, *Knowledge and practice: or a plain discourse... [on] salvation* (1673, first publ. 1659)

Crooke, Helkiah, *Mikrokosmographia a description of the body of man* (1615)

Cuffe, Henry, *The differences of the ages of mans life* (1607)

Culpeper, Nicholas, *Semeiotica uranica: or, an astrological judgement of diseases* (1651)

D'Ewes, Simonds, *The Autobiography and Correspondence of Sir Simonds D'Ewes, Bart.*, ed. J. O. Halliwell, 2 vols. (1845)

Davenport, George, *The Letters of George Davenport 1651–1677*, ed. Brenda M. Pask, Surtees Society, vol. 215 (Woodbridge, 2011)

Dawson, Thomas *The second part of the good hus-wives jewell* (1597)

De Laune, Thomas, *Tropologia, or a key to open Scripture metaphors* (1681)

Defoe, Daniel, *Robinson Crusoe* (2012, first publ. 1719)

Delaval, Elizabeth, *The Meditations of Lady Elizabeth Delaval, Written Between 1662 and 1671*, ed. D. G. Greene, Surtees Society, vol. 190 (1978)

Diemerbroeck, Ysbrand van, *The anatomy of human bodies... To which is added... several practical observations*, trans. William Salmon (1694, first publ. in Utrecht in 1664)

Digby, Kenelm, *The closet of the eminently learned Sir Kenelme Digbie* (1669)

Dod, John, and Cleaver, Robert, *A godlie forme of household government* (1621, first publ. 1598)

Donne, John, *Devotions upon emergent occasions and severall steps in my sicknes* (1624)

Doolittle, Thomas, *Man ashiv le-yahoweh, or, a serious enquiry for a suitable return for continued life* (1666)

Dryden, John, *The Letters of John Dryden*, ed. Charles Ward (Durham NC, 1942)

Dyke, Daniel, *Two treatises. The one, of repentance* (1616)

Elyot, Thomas, *The castle of health* (1610, first publ. 1534)

Fanshawe, Ann, *Memoirs of Lady Fanshawe*, ed. Richard Fanshawe (1829)

Fisher, James, *The wise virgin, or, a wonderful narration of the various dispensations towards a childe of eleven years of age* (1653)

Fitzwilliam, William, *The Correspondence of Lord Fitzwilliam of Milton and Francis Guybon, His Steward 1697–1709*, ed. D. R. Hainsworth and Cherry Walker, Northampton Record Society, vol. 36 (1990)

Flamant, M., *The art of preserving and restoring health* (1697)

Flavel, John, *Husbandry spiritualized, or the heavenly use of earthly things* (1674)

Flavel, John, *A token for mourners* (1674)

Folkingham, William, *Panala medica vel sanitatis et longaevitatis alumna catholica* (1628)

Framboisière, Nicholas Abraham de la, *The art of physick made plain & easie*, trans. John Phillips (1684, originally publ. in Latin, 1628)

Freke, Elizabeth, *The Remembrances of Elizabeth Freke*, ed. Raymond Anselment, Camden Fifth Series, vol. 18 (Cambridge, 2001)

Fuller, Thomas, *Life out of death a sermon preached at Chelsey, on the recovery of an honourable person* (1655)

Fulwood, William, *The enimie of idlenesse teaching the maner and stile how to… compose… letters* (1568)

Galen, 'On the Causes of Symptoms I', in Ian Johnston (ed. and trans.), *Galen on Diseases and Symptoms* (Cambridge, 2006), 203–35

Galen, *Certaine works of Galens, called methodus medendi… with an epitome… of natural faculties*, trans. Thomas Gale (1586, first publ. 1566)

Galen, *Galen on the Natural Faculties*, trans. Arthur John Brock (Cambridge, 2006, first publ. 1916)

Galen, *Galen's method of physic*, trans. Peter English (1656)

Galen, *Galens art of physic*, trans. Nicholas Culpeper (1652)

Galen, *The epitomie of the third booke of Galen of the composition of medicines*, trans. G. Baker (1579)

Gammon, John, *Christ a Christian's life… preach'd by the author upon his recovery from a fit of sicknss* (1691)

Gearing, Henry, *A prospect of heaven* (1673)

Gesner, Konrad, *The new jewell of health* (1576)

Gills, Thomas, *Thomas Gills of St. Edmund's Bury in Suffolk, upon the recovery of his sight* (1710)

Glisson, Francis, Bate, George, and Regemorter, Assuerus, *A treatise of the rickets*, trans. Philip Armin (1651)

Gouge, William, *Of domesticall duties* (1622)

Gould, Robert, *A poem most humbly offered to the memory of her late sacred majesty, Queen Mary* (1695)

Grataroli, Guglielmo, *A direction for the health of magistrates and students*, trans. Thomas Newton (1574, first publ. 1555)

Greatrakes, Valentine, *A brief account of Mr. Valentine Greatraks* (1666)

Greenham, Richard, *A most sweete and assured comfort of all those that are afflicted in consiscience* (1595)

Greenwood, Henry, *Tormenting tophet; or a terrible description of hell* (1650, first publ. 1615)

Hale, Matthew, *A letter from Sr Matthew Hale… to one of his sons, after his recovery from the small-pox* (1684)

Halkett, Anne, *The Autobiography of Anne Lady Halkett*, ed. John Gough Nichols, Camden Society New Series, vol. 13 (1875–6)

Hall, John, *Select observations on English bodies*, trans. James Cooke (1679, first. publ. 1657)

Hall, Joseph, *Meditations and vowes* (1606, first publ. 1605)

Hall, Joseph, *The remedy of prophanenesse* (1637)

Harcourt, Anne, *The Harcourt Papers in 14 volumes*, vol. 1, ed. E. W. Harcourt (1880)

Hardy, Nathaniel, *Two mites, or, a gratefull acknowledgement of God's singular goodnesse... occasioned by his late unexpected recovery of a desperate sickness* (1653)

Harley, Brilliana, *Letters of The Lady Brilliana Harley*, ed. Thomas Taylor Lewis (1853)

Harris, John, *The divine physician, prescribing rules for the prevention, and cure of most diseases, as well of the body, as the soul* (1676)

Harris, Robert, *Hezekiahs recovery. Or, a sermon, shewing what use Hezekiah did, and all should make of their deliverance from sicknesse* (1626)

Harris, Walter, *Pharmacologia anti-empirica, or, A rational discourse of remedies both chymical and Galenical* (1683)

Harrold, Edmund, *The Diary of Edmund Harrold, Wigmaker of Manchester 1712–15*, ed. Craig Horner (Aldershot, 2009)

Hart, James, *Klinike, or the diet of the diseased* (1633)

Harvey, Gideon, *The conclave of physicians* (1686)

Hatton, Christopher, *Correspondence of the Family of Hatton being Chiefly Addressed to Christopher, First Viscount Hatton, 1601–1704*, ed. Edward Maunde Thompson, Camden Society, vols. 22–3 (1878)

Hayes, Alice, *A legacy, or, widow's mite, left by Alice Hayes* (1723)

Helmont, Jean Baptiste van, *Van Helmont's works containing his most excellent philosophy, physick, chirurgery, anatomy* (1664)

Henry, Philip, *The Diaries and Letters of Philip Henry of Broad Oak, Flintshire, A.D. 1631–1696*, ed. M. H. Lee (1882)

Heraclitus Christianus, or the man of sorrow (1677)

Herbert, George, *The temple: sacred poems* (1633)

Herbert, George, *The Works of George Herbert*, ed. F. E. Hutchinson (Oxford, 2012, first publ. 1941)

Hervey, John, *The Diary of John Hervey, First Earl of Bristol*, ed. S. H. A. Hervey (Wells, 1894)

Hervey, John, *Letter-Books of John Hervey, First Earl of Bristol, vol.1, 1651–1715* (Wells, 1894)

Heywood, Oliver, *The Rev. Oliver Heywood, B.A: His Autobiography, Diaries, Anecdote and Event Books*, ed. Horsfall Turner, 4 vols. (1883)

Hill, Aaron, *The plain dealer: being select essays on several curious subjects* (1724)

Hoby, Margaret, *Diary of Lady Margaret Hoby 1599–1605*, ed. Dorothy Meads (1930)

Hooke, Robert, *The Diary of Robert Hooke (1672–1680)*, ed. H. W. Robinson and W. Adams (1935)

Hooke, William, *The priviledge of the saints on earth beyond those in heaven* (1673)

Horne, Robert, *Life and death, foure sermons* (1613)

Houghton, William, *Preces & lachrymae: a sermon on Acts* (1650)

Jeake, Samuel, *An Astrological Diary of the Seventeenth Century: Samuel Jeake of Rye*, ed. Michael Hunter (Oxford, 1988)

Joannes, de Mediolano, *Regimen sanitatis Salerni: or, the schoole of Salernes regiment of health*, trans. Thomas Paynell (1650, first publ. in Latin in 1497, first English edn. 1541)

Johnson, Robert, *Praxis medicinae reformata: or, the practice of physick* (1700)

Johnstonus, Johannes, *The idea of practical physick*, trans. Nicholas Culpeper and W.R. (1657)

Josselin, Ralph, *The Diary of Ralph Josselin 1616–1683*, ed. Alan Macfarlane (Oxford, 1991)

Joubert, Laurent *Treatise on Laughter*, ed. and trans. Gregory David de Rocher (Alabama, 1980, first publ. in French, 1579)

Kettlewell, John, *Death made comfortable* (1695)

Kilby, Richard, *Halleluiah: praise yee the Lord, for the unburthening of a loaded conscience* (Cambridge, 1635)

Lawrence, Edward, *Christ's power over bodily diseases* (1672, first publ. 1662)

Lawrence, William, *The Pyramid and the Urn: Life in Letters of a Restoration Squire: William Lawrence of Shurdington, 1636–1697*, ed. Iona Sinclair (Stroud, 1994)

Lemnius, Levinus, *The secret miracles of nature* (1658, first publ. 1559)

Lemnius, Levinus, *The touchstone of complexions*, trans. Thomas Newton (1576)

Liddell, Henry, *The Letters of Henry Liddell to William Cotesworth*, ed. J. M. Ellis, Surtees Society, vol. 197 (Durham, 1987)

Lipsius, Justus, *A discourse of constancy*, trans. Nathaniel Wanley (1670, first publ. in Latin 1584, first English edn. 1574)

Lister, Joseph, *The Autobiography of Joseph Lister of Bradford, 1627–1709*, ed. Thomas Wright (Bradford, 1842)

Littleton, Adam, *Hezekiah's return of praise for his recovery* (1668)

Love, Christopher, *A treatise of effectual calling and election* (1653)

Love, Christopher, *Hells terror: or, a treatise of the torments of the damned* (1653)

Lowe, Roger, *The Diary of Roger Lowe of Ashton-in-Makerfield, Lancashire, 1663–1674*, ed. William Sachse (1938)

M.W., *The queens closet opened incomparable secrets in physick* (1659)

Macollo, John, *XCIX canons, or rules learnedly describing an excellent method for practitioners in physic* (1659)

Magrath, John (ed.), *The Flemings in Oxford*, Oxford Historical Society, vol. 44 (Oxford, 1904)

Martindale, Adam, *The Life of Adam Martindale*, ed. Richard Parkinson, Chetham Society, vol. 4 (Manchester, 1845)

Mather, Cotton, *A perfect recovery. The voice of the glorious God, unto persons, whom his mercy has recovered from sickness* (Boston, 1714)

Mather, Cotton, *Mens sana in corpore sano: a discourse upon recovery from sickness* (Boston, 1698)

Mauriceau, François, *The diseases of women with child*, trans. Hugh Chamberlen (1710, first English edn. 1672)

May, Robert, *The accomplish cook, or the art and mystery of cooking* (1660)

Maynwaringe, Everard, *Pains afflicting humane bodies* (1682)

Maynwaringe, Everard, *The catholic medicine, and soverain healer* (1684)

Maynwaringe, Everard, *The method and means of enjoying health* (1683)

Miege, Guy, *A new dictionary French and English* (1677)

Milman, Robert, *Convalescence, thoughts for those who are recovering from sickness* (1836)

Moffet, Thomas, *Healths improvement: or rules... of preparing all sorts of food* (1655)

Moore, Mary, *Wonderful News from the North. Or, a True Relation of the Sad... Torments... on the... Children of Mr George Muschamp* (1650)

Morel, Pierre, *The expert doctors dispenator*, trans. Nicholas Culpeper (1657)

Morris, Claver, *The Diary of a West Country Physician, 1648–1726*, ed. Edmund Hobhouse (1935)

Newcome, Henry, *The Autobiography of Henry Newcome*, ed. Richard Parkinson, Chetham Society, vol. 26 (Manchester, 1852)

Newcome, Henry, *The Diary of Rev. Henry Newcome*, ed. Thomas Heywood, Chetham Society, vol. 18 (1849)

Norden, John, *A pathway to patience in all manner of crosses* (1626)

North, Roger, *Notes of Me: the Autobiography of Roger North*, ed. P. Millard (Toronto, 2000)

Norwood, Richard, *The Journal of Richard Norwood, Surveyor of Bermuda*, ed. Wesley Frank Craven and Walter Hayward (New York, 1945)

Nourse, Timothy, *A discourse upon the nature and faculties of man* (1686)

Pagit, Eusabius, *A verie fruitful sermon... conserning Gods everlasting predestination* (1583)

Paré, Ambroise, *The workes of that famous chirurgion Ambrose Parey*, trans. Thomas Johnson (1634)

Paston, Robert, *The Whirlpool of Misadventures: Letters of Robert Paston, First Earl of Yarmouth 1663–1679*, ed. Jean Agnew, Norfolk Record Society, vol. 76 (2012)

Pechey, John, *A plain introduction to the art of physic* (1697)

Pechey, John, *The store-house of physical practice* (1695)

Pemell, Robert, *De morbis puerorum, or, a treatise of the diseases of children* (1653)

Penington, Mary, *Experiences in the Life of Mary Penington Written by Herself*, ed. Norman Penney (1992, first publ. 1911)

Perkins, William, *A golden chaine, or the description of theologie* (1600)

Perkins, William, *A treatise of the vocations, or callings of men* (1603)

Phillips, Edward, *The new world of English words* (1658)

Platter, Felix, *Platerus golden practice of physick* (1664)

Puttenham, George, *The arte of English poesie* (1589)

R. N., *Proverbs English, French, Dutch, Italian, and Spanish* (1659)

Read, Alexander, *Most excellent and approved medicines* (1651)

Reynolds, Edward, *A treatise of the passions and faculties of the soule of man* (1640)

Rich, Mary, *Autobiography of Mary Countess of Warwick*, ed. T. Crofton Croker (1848)

Robinson, Nicholas, *A new theory of physic* (1725)

Rogers, Benjamin, *The Diary of Benjamin Rogers Rector of Carlton, 1720–71*, ed. C. D. Linnell Symcotts, Bedfordshire Historical Record Society, vol. 31 (Streatley, 1951)

Rogers, Timothy, *Practical discourses on sickness & recovery* (1691)

Ross, Alexander, *Arcana microcosmi, or, the hid secrets of man's body* (1652, first publ. 1651)

Russell, Rachel, *Letters of Rachel, Lady Russell*, ed. Thomas Selwood, 2 vols. (1853, first publ. 1773)

Ryder, Dudley, *The Diary of Dudley Ryder*, ed. William Matthews (1939)

S. J., *Paidon nosemata; or childrens diseases* (1664)

S. W., *A family jewel, or the womans councellor* (1704)

Sackville, Charles, *The new academy of complements* (1669)

Savage, Sarah, *Memoirs of the Life and Character of Mrs Sarah Savage*, ed. J. B. Williams (1821)

Searle, Arthur (ed.), *Barrington Family Letters, 1628–1632* (1983)

Senault, Jean-François, *The use of passions*, trans. Henry Earl of Monmouth (1671, first publ. 1649)

Seymour, Frances, *The Gentle Hertford: Her Life and Letters*, ed. Helen Hughes (New York, 1940)

Sharp, Jane, *The midwives book* (1671)

Sheafe, Thomas, *Vindiciae senectutis, or, a plea for old-age* (1639)

Shepard, Thomas, *God's Plot: The Paradoxes of Puritan Piety, Being the Autobiography and Journal of Thomas Shepard*, ed. Michael McCiffert (Amherst MA, 1972)

Shirley, John, *The illustrious history of women* (1686)

Shower, John, *Some account of the holy life and death of Mr. Henry Gearing* (1699)

Sibbs, Richard, *A consolatory letter to the afflicted conscience* (1641)

Sidney, Robert, *Domestic Politics and Family Absence: The Correspondence (1588–1621) of Robert Sidney, First Earl of Leicester, and Barbara Gamage Sidney*, ed. Margaret Hannay, Noel Kinnamon, and Michael Brennan (Aldershot, 2005)

Sprengell, Conrade Joachim, 'Natura Morborum Medicatrix: Or, Nature Cures Diseases', in Matthaeus Purmann (ed.), *Chirurgia Curiosa* (1706), 319–43

Starkey, George, *Natures explication and Helmont's vindication* (1658)

Stevens, [Minister], *The great assize; or, Christ's certain and sudden appearance to judgment* (1672–96)

Steward, Thomas, *Sacrificium laudis, or a thank-offering* (1699)

Stout, William, *The Autobiography of William Stout of Lancaster, 1665–1752*, ed. J. D. Marshall (Manchester, 1976)

Symcotts, John, *A Seventeenth Century Doctor and his Patients: John Symcotts, 1592?–1662*, ed. F. N. L. Poynter and W. J. Bishop, Bedfordshire Historical Record Society, vol. 31 (Streatley, 1951)

T. A., *A rich store-house, or treasury for the diseased* (1596)

Taylor, Jeremy, *The rule and exercises of holy dying* (1651)

The aphorismes of Hippocrates, trans. S.H. [possibly Stephen Hobbes] (1655)

The fathers legacy: or counsels to his children (1677)

The happy damsel: or, a miracle of God's mercy (1693)

The lamented lovers: or the young men and maiden's grief (1675–96?)

The nob[l]e[-]mans generous kindness (1672–96)

The shutting up infected houses as it is practised in England (1665)

The woman to the plow and the man to the hen-roost (1675)

Thomas, Keith (ed.), *The Oxford Book of Work* (Oxford, 1999)

Thomson, George, *Galeno-Pale: or, a chymical trial of the galenists* (1665)

Thomson, George, *Ortho-methodoz itro-chymike: or the direct method of curing chymically* (1675)

Thoresby, Ralph, *Letters Addressed to Ralph Thoresby, FRS*, ed. W. T. Lancaster (1912)

Thoresby, Ralph, *The Diary of Ralph Thoresby*, 2 vols., ed. Joseph Hunter (1830)

Thornton, Alice, *The Autobiography of Mrs Alice Thornton*, ed. Charles Jackson, Surtees Society, vol. 62 (1875)

Tuke, Thomas, *The high-way to heauen: or, the doctrine of election* (1609)

Turner, Daniel, *A remarkable case in surgery* (1709)

Twyne, Thomas, *The schoolmaster, or teacher of table phylosophie* (1583, first publ. 1576)

V. J., *Golgotha; or, a looking glass for London…With an humble witness against the cruel… shutting-up* (1665)

Verney, Frances (ed.), *The Verney Memoirs, 1600–1659*, 2 vols. (1925, first publ. 1892)

Vernon, John, *The compleat scholler; or, A relation of the life…of Caleb Vernon* (1666)

Vickers, William, *An easie and safe method for curing the King's evil* (1711)

Walker, Elizabeth, *The vertuous wife*, ed. Anthony Walker (1694)

Walkington, Thomas, *Optick glasse of humors* (1639, first publ. 1607)

Wall, Alison (ed.), *Two Elizabethan Women: Correspondence of Joan and Maria Thynne 1575–1611*, Wiltshire Record Society, vol. 38 (Devizes, 1983)

Waller, Edmund, *The workes of Edmond Waller* (1645)

Waller, William, *Divine meditations upon several occasions* (1680)

Wallington, Nehemiah, *The Notebooks of Nehemiah Wallington, 1618–1654: A Selection*, ed. David Booy (Aldershot, 2007)

Walton, Izaak, *The lives of Dr. John Donne, Sir Henry Wotton, Mr. Richard Hooker, Mr. George Herbert written by Isaak Walton* (1670)

Walwyn, William, *Physick for families* (1669)

Watson, Thomas, *The doctrine of repentance* (1668)

Welwood, James, *A true relation of the wonderful cure of Mary Maillard* (1694)

Wentworth, William, *Wentworth Papers 1597–1628*, ed. J. P. Cooper, Camden Society, vol. 12 (1973)

Whitaker, Tobias, *An elenchus of opinions concerning the cure of the small pox* (1661)

Whitelocke, Bulstrode, *The Diary of Bulstrode Whitelocke, 1605–1675*, ed. Ruth Spalding (Oxford, 1990)

Whythorne, Thomas, *The Autobiography of Thomas Whythorne*, ed. James M. Osborn (Oxford, 1961)

Wilkinson, Robert, *A jewell for the eare* (1602)

Willis, Thomas, *Willis's Oxford Casebook (1650–52)*, ed. Kenneth Dewhurst (Oxford, 1981)

Woodall, John, *The surgions mate... [and] the cures of... diseases at sea* (1617)

Woodford, Robert, *The Diary of Robert Woodford, 1637–1641*, ed. John Fielding, Camden Society, vol. 42 (2012)

Woodman, Philip, *Medicus novissimus; or, the modern physician* (1712)

Woolley, Hannah, *The gentlewomans companion* (1670)

Wotton, Henry, 'A hymn to my God in a night of my late sickness', in Izaak Walton (ed.), *Reliquiae Wottonianae, or, a collection of lives, letters, poems with characters of sundry personages* (1651), 361–2

Wright, Thomas, *The passions of the minde* (1630, first publ. 1601)

ELECTRONIC RESOURCES

Bible Gateway (<https://www.biblegateway.com>); all quoted verses are from the 1611 King James Version of the Bible

Bridgeman Images (<https://www.bridgemanimages.com/en-GB/>)

Early English Books Online (<http://eebo.chadwyck.com/home>)

Eighteenth Century Collections Online (<http://quod.lib.umich.edu/e/ecco/>)

Oxford Dictionary of National Biography (<http://www.oxforddnb.com/>)

Oxford English Dictionary (<http://www.oed.com>)

Proceedings of the Old Bailey (<https://www.oldbaileyonline.org/>); reference numbers:
OA16841217
OA16950712
OA16980126
T16800707-8
T16831010a-16
T16841210-41
T17170911-41

UCSB English Broadside Ballad Archive (<https://ebba.english.ucsb.edu/>)

Wellcome Images (<https://wellcomeimages.org>)

Foxe, John, *The Unabridged Acts and Monuments Online* or *TAMO* (1583 edition), HRI Online Publications, Sheffield, 2011 (<http//www.johnfoxe.org>)

Isham, Elizabeth, *Diary and Confessions: Constructing Elizabeth Isham, 1609–1654*, Warwick University Online Editions, ed. Elizabeth Clarke, Nigel Smith, Jill Millman, and Alice Eardley (<http://web.warwick.ac.uk/english/perdita/Isham/index_bor.htm>)

Pepys, Samuel, *The Diary of Samuel Pepys*, ed. Henry B. Wheatley (1893), Project Gutenberg, managed by Phil Gyford (<http://www.pepysdiary.com/>)

Index

NOTE: Specific diseases can be found under 'diseases', particular emotions and emotional gestures, under 'emotions', and individual bodily organs, fluids, and sensations, under 'bodies'. To aid clarity and understanding, the physiological stages, signs, and mechanisms of recovery are listed sequentially under 'recovery', with cross-references to other places in the Index where these subjects are dealt with in more detail. Matters relating to the five senses appear in the 'senses/sensory' section, types of occupations under 'work', and relationships between different family members, friends, and acquaintances, under 'relationships, personal'. The footnotes are not included in the Bibliography, with the exception of frequently cited authors. All persons are ordered by surname.